Handbook of

Regional Cerebral Blood Flow

Handbook of

Regional Cerebral Blood Flow

edited by

Stevo Knezevic
V. A. Maximilian
Zdenko Mubrin
Isak Prohovnik
John Wade

LAWRENCE ERLBAUM ASSOCIATES, PUBLISHERS
1988 Hillsdale, New Jersey Hove and London

Lawrence Erlbaum Associates, Inc., Publishers
365 Broadway
Hillsdale, New Jersey 07642

Library of Congress Cataloging-in-Publication Data

Handbook of regional cerebral blood flow.

Bibliography: p.
1. Cerebral circulation. 2. Regional blood flow—Measurement. 3. Xenon—isotopes—Measurement. 4. Radioisotopes in medical diagnosis. I. Knezevic, Stevo.
QP108.5.C4H36 1987 612′.824 87-6806
ISBN 0-89859-558-4

Printed in the United States of America
10 9 8 7 6 5 4 3 2 1

Contents

Preface

At a time when our library shelves already bulge under the weight of so many volumes, the introduction of another medical textbook demands justification. Ultimately this will be reflected by the response to the book, but some discussion of its origin and purpose is appropriate in the introduction.

This volume attempts to present a comprehensive, detailed overview of the most common modern technique for quantitative measurement of regional Cerebral Blood Flow (rCBF). This technique involves administration of tracer amounts of ^{133}Xenon for a short period, by inhalation or intravenous injection, and external monitoring of its concentration by stationary detectors. A short monitoring period (10 to 15 minutes) and a noninvasive procedure, as well as relatively simple instrumentation, are among the advantages of such techniques. The proliferation and standardization of the instruments over the last decade, and their growing impact in diverse medical disciplines, are among the reasons for this volume.

Although theoretical insights by Roy and Sherrington predicted our field as early as a century ago, the empirical story began with Kety and Schmidt in the late nineteen forties. Within a decade, much of what we now take for granted about the cerebral circulation had been elucidated. In the early sixties, Lassen and Ingvar introduced the radioactive inert gas method. This allowed examination of separate regions within the brain, and subsequently led to extraordinary pictures of regional CBF in health and disease, and the promise of more rational treatment for patients with cerebrovascular disorders. The utility of the method was limited by the need for arterial puncture, but within a few years the noninvasive era was ushered in by Veall and Mallett, who demonstrated that the isotope could be administered by inhalation. The field came of age in 1975 when Obrist and his colleagues provided the standard compartmental model.

With Obrist's seminal contribution, noninvasive rCBF became practical and standardized, and the period of development was summarized by Deshmukh and Meyer, nearly a decade ago. That volume described what was then known about the methodology and applications of rCBF measurement, and provided an excellent overview.

We feel that the time is now right for a reflective volume describing the progress which has occurred since then, both methodologically and clinically. Technical developments over the last decade have dramatically changed the instruments and their capabilities. Greater availability has meant that cerebral blood flow has been studied in many conditions pertaining to practically all medical disciplines. The growing importance of cerebral circulation to many disciplines is reflected in the diversity of patients studied in rCBF laboratories, and is one of the central reasons for publishing the present volume. The major part of the book is, therefore, devoted to reviews of the significance of cerebral circulatory phenomena and their clinical relevance to diverse medical disciplines. It is our hope that practitioners will benefit not only from the chapters specifically related to their specialty, but also from the exposure to rCBF practices in other disciplines. The affiliations of the editors reflect such a diversity: we work in neurology, psychiatry, neurosurgery and pharmacology. Our common interest in cerebral circulation has led us to realize that we can contribute to each other's particular interests, and that phenomena taken for granted by one specialist may constitute a novel observation to another. We have benefitted from this interdisciplinary view, and we hope to share it with the readers.

Defining the appropriateness of clinical questions for rCBF presupposes a comprehensive knowledge of cerebral physiology, as well as an intimate familiarity with mathematical and physical issues. This is in common with many other techniques in nuclear medicine. The first part of this volume deals with those topics in a way that we hope will be useful for those now venturing into rCBF, as well as for veterans.

A central aim of the present volume is to address the clinical status of rCBF. Each chapter will illuminate this issue from a particular viewpoint, and we would encourage the reader to be influenced by the authors' judgments rather than present our editorial views here. We would suggest, however, that noninvasive rCBF methods, when properly employed, can extend our knowledge of pathophysiological mechanisms. They cannot compete with CT scanning for localization of tissue pathology, nor should they be expected to replace angiography in visualizing vessel disease. But when tissue perfusion is relevant to the clinical presentation or treatment plan, or when an indirect measure of local metabolism is informative, then rCBF results may be extremely helpful. But our methods are prone to misuse because they are relatively inexpensive, free of risk, and deceptively simple. We would urge practitioners to use them only when a specific question can be postulated and answered by such methods. However, we leave the detailed discussions to the specific chapters. Each chapter was written by an experienced researcher and an acknowledged authority; the editors excercised much restraint and intervened only minimally in the content of the chapters. We do not necessarily agree with the positions taken by every author, but feel that all deserve careful consideration.

The book stems from an International Workshop on rCBF which was held on the island of Brac, Yugoslavia in May 1984, an event for which the present editors must also claim responsibility. It was extremely pleasant, great fun, and most instructive. It was there that we realized that a multidisciplinary rCBF community existed, and it is for that community that we present this book. We thank our distinguished colleagues who served as faculty there and subsequently contributed chapters to the present volume, and we thank the participants for making it a pleasant and stimulating event. We are glad to take part in the exciting developments currently occurring and we hope to share our enthusiasm.

Finally, the editors would like to thank each other. We met fortuitously several years ago in London, England and Lund, Sweden, and have become friends through common suffering and aspirations. The order of names is alphabetical; we contributed equally, both to events in Yugoslavia and our editorial duties, and we all owe much to each other.

Stevo Knezevic, M.D.
V.A. Maximilian, Ph.D.
Zdenko Mubrin, M.D.
Isak Prohovnik, Ph.D.
John Wade, M.D.

1 The Physiology and Regulation of Cerebral Blood Flow

James McCulloch
Wellcome Surgical Institute, University of Glasgow

INTRODUCTION

It is axiomatic that the basic principles concerning the mechanisms by which cerebral blood flow is regulated should be thoroughly understood by all those interested in the cerebral circulation. However, from even the most cursory inspection of the scientific literature pertaining to the cerebral circulation, it is clear that there is widespread inability to appreciate well-established features of cerebrovascular regulation. Sophisticated instrumentation for rigorous assessment of cerebral blood flow in humans in two or three dimensions is becoming even more widely available; but no technology, however sophisticated, can compensate for the failure of the clinical investigator to appreciate the basic physiology and pathophysiology. In this chapter, I will review the basic physiology of the cerebral circulation with emphasis on areas directly relevant to the clinical investigator. Initially, I will describe the fundamental responses of the cerebral circulation (i.e., the responses to alterations of arterial carbon dioxide and oxygen tensions, the responses to alterations in perfusion pressure, and the relationship between cerebral metabolic activity and blood flow). Thereafter I will consider in detail how cerebrovascular reactivity can be drastically modified in pathological states. Finally, I will consider the impact made by quantitative autoradiographic techniques for measuring cerebral blood flow and glucose use in all anatomical components of the brains of experimental animals.

Influence of Arterial Blood Gas Tensions on Cerebral Blood Flow

The level of cerebral blood flow is extremely sensitive to changes in arterial carbon dioxide tension, displaying marked increases during moderate hypercap-

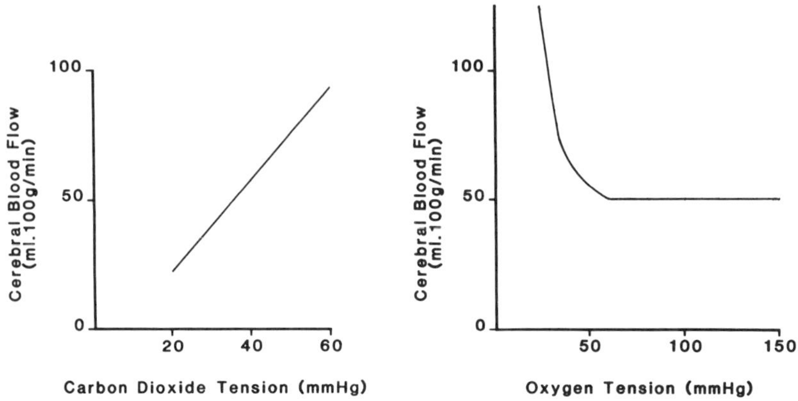

FIGURE 1.1. Diagrammatic representation of the alterations in cerebral blood flow which are associated with changes in (a) arterial carbon dioxide tension and (b) arterial oxygen tension.

nia and reductions during hypocapnia. The magnitude of cerebral circulatory responses is approximately 5% change in cerebral blood flow for each 1 mm Hg change in arterial carbon dioxide (Harper & Glass, 1965) (Fig. 1.1). In contrast, metabolic acidosis and alkalosis (during which arterial carbon dioxide tension remains constant), with pH values ranging from 6.7 to 7.6, have little effect upon the level of cerebral blood flow (Harper & Bell, 1963).

The level of cerebral blood flow is relatively insensitive to changes in arterial oxygen tension over the normal physiological range. If the arterial oxygen tension falls below 50 mm Hg, pronounced increases in cerebral blood flow occur (Fig. 1.1) such that at 30 mm Hg, cerebral blood flow is almost double that observed at 100 mm Hg. Ventilation with 100% oxygen has minimal effects upon cerebral blood flow, with the best available evidence indicating only 10% reductions in cerebral blood flow at this level of hyperoxygenation compared with normoxia (McDowall, 1966).

Modification of the Cerebrovascular Responses to Alterations of Arterial Blood Gas Tensions

The cerebrovascular dilation induced by hypercapnia is markedly attenuated by moderate hypotension (Fig. 1.2) (Harper & Glass, 1965), and dilatation elicited by hypoxia and seizures similarly reduced by hypotension (Plum et al., 1968). Hypotension is itself associated with the dilatation of cerebral arteries and arterioles, i.e., the autoregulatory mechanism via which cerebral blood flow is maintained constant (*vide infra*). Pre-existing dilatation in response to the hypotension diminishes the capacity of the resistance vessels to respond to a further dilatory stimulus simply because there are finite limits to each vessel's capacity

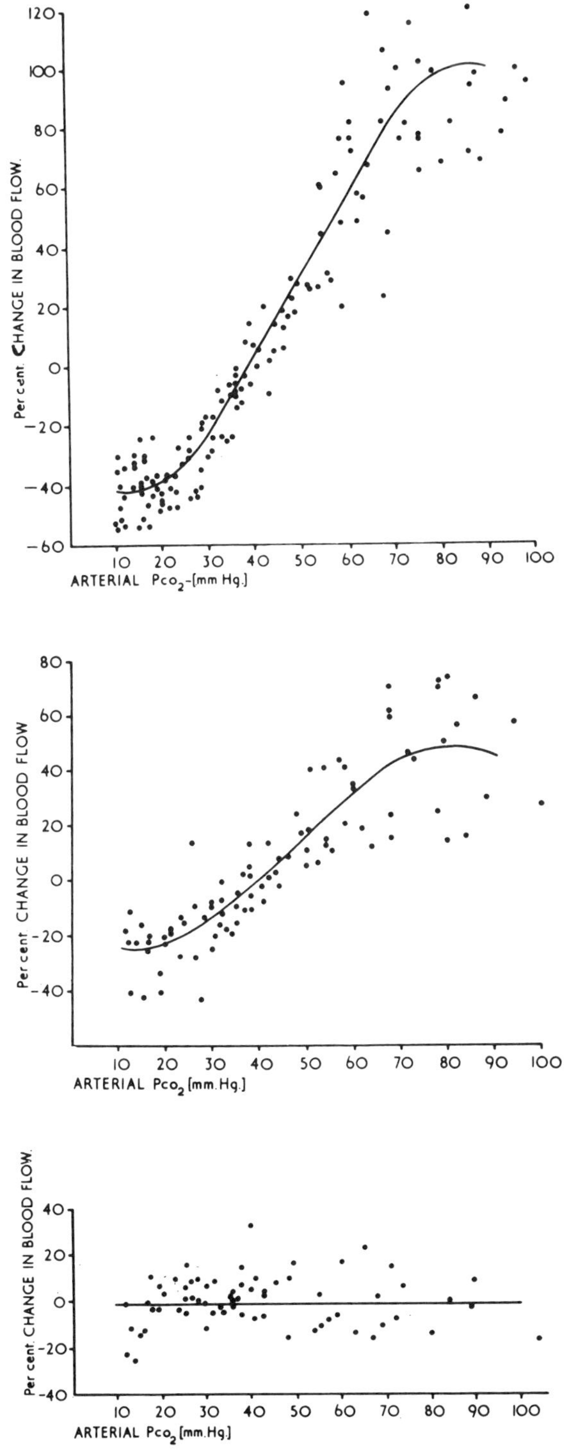

FIGURE 1.2. The effects of alterations in arterial carbon dioxide tension upon cortical blood flow in dogs in normotension (mean arterial pressure: 150 mm Hg) (upper), moderate hypotension (100 mm Hg) (middle), and severe hypotension (50 mm Hg) (lower). (from Harper, 1966; with permission).

to dilate. This simple observation has important implications both clinically (e.g., fruitless attempts to increase cerebral blood flow in the face of iodopathic or drug-induced hypotension) and experimentally (e.g., factors which modify the cerebrovascular response to hypercapnia have been wrongly implicated in the mechanisms of action of this basic response through the failure of the investigator to recognize the effects of the factors upon mean arterial pressure).

The magnitude of the increases in cerebral blood flow elicited by hypercapnia is directly proportional to the level of cerebral metabolic activity, and factors which reduce cerebral oxygen and glucose consumption (such as increasing the depth of anesthesia) reduce the response of the cerebral circulation to hypercapnia (Fujishima et al., 1971; Grubb et al., 1974) (Fig. 1.3). Furthermore, as the local levels of blood flow and glucose utilization are regionally heterogeneous throughout the CNS, so also are the magnitudes (in units of ml $100g^{-1}min^{-1}$, mm HG^{-1}) of the local responses to induced hypercapnia (Fig. 1.4), ranging from a blood flow change of 1.5 ml $100g^{-1}min^{-1}$ per mm Hg of change in arterial carbon dioxide tension in the cerebellar hemisphere where basal blood flow is low, to 4.4 ml $100g^{-1}min^{-1}$ mm Hg^{-1} in anterior cingulate cortex where basal blood flow is high. There is an almost irresistible temptation to express the response to induced hypercapnia in units of *percentage* change from

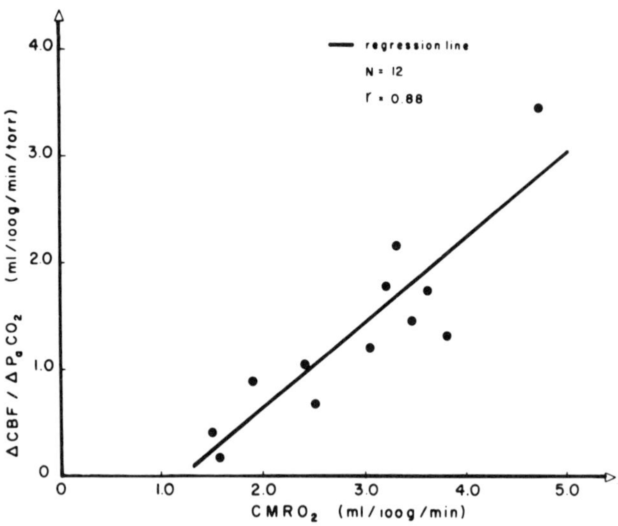

FIGURE 1.3. The relationship between cerebral blood flow and cerebral oxygen consumption in the dog brain both at normocapnia and hypercapnia. Cerebral oxygen consumption was decreased by barbiturate administration. The cerebral circulatory response to hypercapnia is related directly to the level of cerebral oxygen consumption. (from Edvinsson & MacKenzie, 1977; with permission).

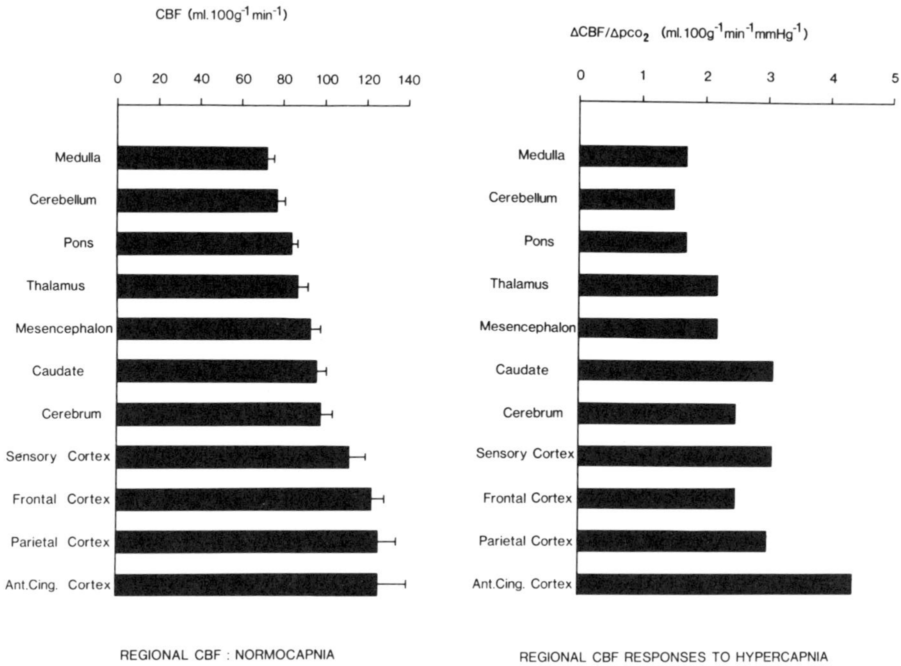

FIGURE 1.4. Local cerebral blood flow and local circulatory responses to induced hypercapnia in conscious rats. The hypercapnic response is related to the level of blood flow in normocapnic conditions. In these experiments, cerebral blood flow was measured by ^{14}C-iodoantipyrine uptake with tissue dissection.

basal level per mm Hg of alteration. Data on hypercapnic responses presented in this manner must be viewed cautiously, as numerical value describing the response is markedly influenced by the basal level of blood flow as well as by the magnitude of the blood-flow changes induced by hypercapnia.

The occlusion of one carotid artery or spasm of major cerebral arteries (induced mechanically or as a consequence of subarachnoid hemorrhage) (Boisvert et al., 1979; Harper et al., 1972; Sengupta et al., 1973, 1974) has profound effects on the magnitude of increases of cerebral blood flow which occur in hypercapnia or hypoxia (Fig. 1.5), while having little effect on the level of cerebral blood flow observed under normocapnic, normoxic conditions. The attenuation of the cerebrovascular reactivity with carotid occlusion must be borne in mind in patients with carotid artery disease whose capacity to compensate during a hypoxic or hypotensive insult may be severely impaired. Moreover, this is a feature in most cerebrovascular pathologies, e.g., in cerebral ischemia the capacity of cerebral vessels to dilate during induced hypercapnia may be almost completely lost (Fig. 1.6) (Hossmann, 1982; Waltz, 1970).

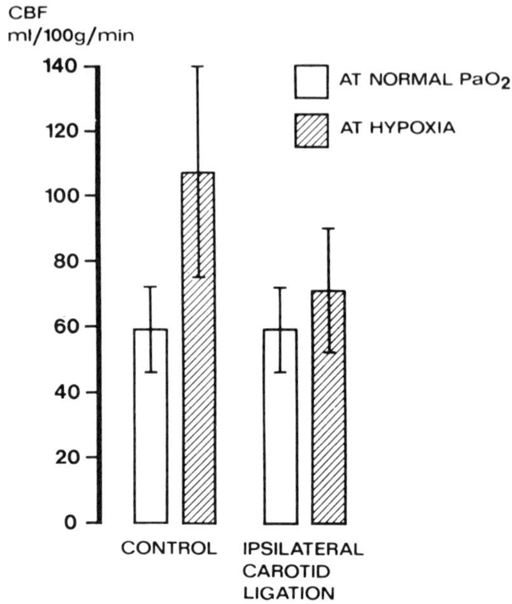

FIGURE 1.5. The effect of hypoxia (arterial oxygen tension approximately 36 mm Hg) upon cerebral blood flow in baboons prior to and after ipsilateral carotid artery ligation. (from Sengupta et al. 1974; with permission).

The most persistent controversy in cerebrovascular physiology has been concerned with the functional role played by the vast array of aminergic and peptidergic nerve fibers which are known to innervate cerebral blood vessels (see McCulloch, 1984). It is now almost universally accepted that the basic physiological responses of the cerebral circulation to hypercapnia, hypoxia, and changes in perfusion pressure (Fig. 1.2) are *not* the direct consequence of neurogenically mediated alterations in arterial and arteriolar caliber. Neurogenic mechanisms, though not responsible per se for the alterations in cerebral blood flow which occur during alterations in arterial blood gas tensions, may influence the magnitude of the responses which are observed. In normoxic, normocapnic, normotensive animals, cervical sympathectomy and sympathetic stimulation result in only minimal alterations in cerebral blood flow (Harper et al., 1972). The marked alterations which are noted in some species with sympathetic stimulation. e.g., in the dog (D'Alecy & Feigl, 1972), can be attributed to the most common methodological artifact of animal studies, namely the failure to measure cerebral blood flow uncontaminated by extracerebral blood flow (Edvinsson & MacKenzie, 1977). However, in hypercapnic animals, when cerebral blood flow is elevated, stimulation of the cervical sympathetic nerves leads to pronounced reductions in cerebral blood flow (Harper et al., 1972).

This differential effect of sympathetic stimulation in normocapnia and hypercapnia has been attributed to an effect upon the caliber of larger pial arteries. Sympathetically induced constriction of these vessels results in a fall, distally, in

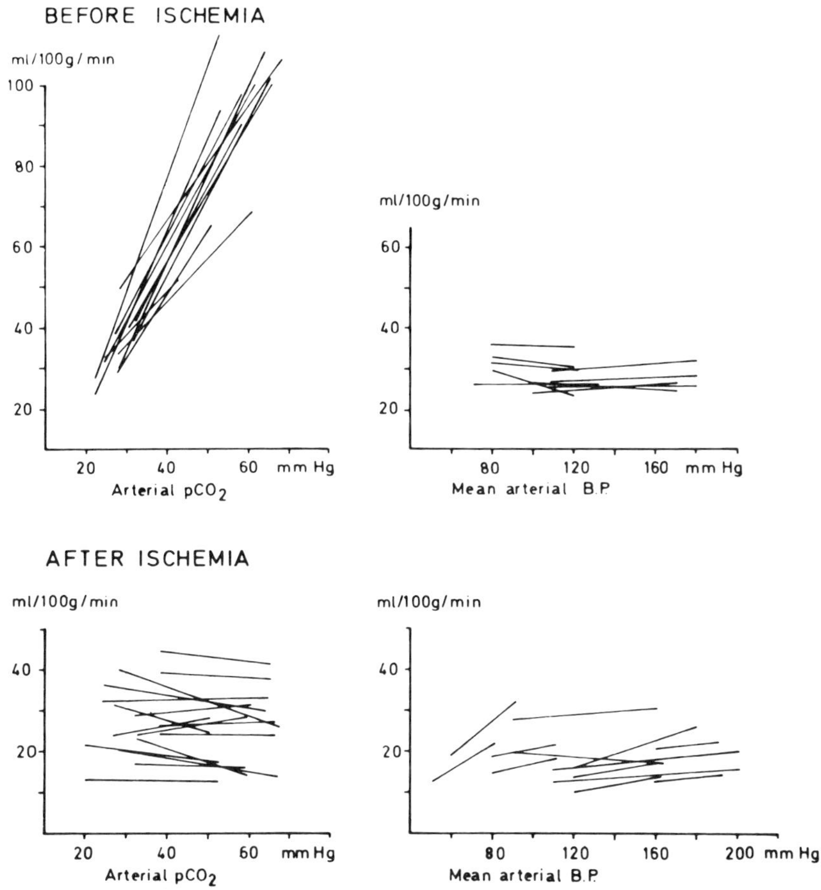

FIGURE 1.6. The cerebral circulatory response to induced hypercapnia and blood pressure alteration before and a few hours after 1 hour of complete ischemia in the cat brain. Note abolition of CO_2 reactivity and preservation of autoregulation in this model of global ischemia. (from Hossman, 1982; with permission).

intravascular pressure which would, in normocapnic conditions, elicit an autoregulatory dilatation of intracerebral vessels to maintain an unchanged level of cerebral tissue perfusion. In hypercapnia, when the intracerebral vessels are already dilated they are unable to dilate further to compensate for the sympathetically induced constriction of the proximal pial arteries. The hypothesis of differential control of pial arteries (where there may be greater sympathetic influence) and of intracerebral vessels (intimately linked to local metabolic demand (see subsequent section) remains the most widely accepted view of neurogenic regulatory mechanisms in the cerebral circulation (see Harper et al.,

1972). It should be emphasized that of all the neurotransmitters/neuromodulators which are present in cerebrovascular nerve fibers (i.e., noradrenaline, acetylcholine, substance P, neuropeptide Y, somatostatin, 5-hydroxytryptamine, vasoactive intestinal polypeptide and cholecytokinin), only for noradrenergic sympathetic fibers has a tentative physiological role been proposed. The available evidence suggests that the sympathetic adrenal discharge which is responsible for physiological elevations in mean arterial pressure provides also protection for the cerebral circulation by constricting major cerebral arteries, and extending the range of autoregulation of cerebral blood flow to much higher levels of arterial pressure (Bill & Linder, 1976; MacKenzie et al., 1979).

Mechanisms Underlying the Cerebrovascular Responses to Alterations in Arterial Gas Tensions

The caliber of cerebral arteries and arterioles is extremely sensitive to alterations in perivascular pH, with acidosis provoking vasodilation and alkalosis vasoconstriction, with arteriolar diameter changing by about 7% for each 0.1 alteration in perivascular pH (see Kuschinsky et al., 1972). The hydrogen ion concentration of the extracellular fluid is determined by the equilibrium of a bicarbonate/carbon dioxide buffer, and the available evidence suggests that effects of arterial carbon dioxide tension upon cerebral blood vessels are a consequence of changes in perivascular pH and not a direct effect of carbon dioxide per se upon cerebrovascular smooth muscle.

The basic mechanisms which underlie the hypoxic vasodilatation have been widely considered to involve perivascular pH alterations, with the decrease in oxygen delivery to cerebral tissue producing a shift from aerobic to anaerobic glycolysis with increased lactate production. However, despite considerable efforts, no definitive evidence of an acidotic shift in perivascular pH has yet appeared, and doubts persist as to the precise nature of the cerebral circulatory response to hypoxia. In contrast to the view expressed by some workers (Ponte & Purves, 1974), there is no reliable evidence that dilatation of cerebral blood vessels induced by activation of perivascular nerve fibers is a major factor in the response to hypoxia, as prior denervation of peripheral chemoreceptors, or surgical division of the principal sympathetic and parasympathetic nerves which innervate cerebral vessels, has minimal effects on the hypoxic vasodilatation (Edvinsson & MacKenzie, 1977; Hoff et al., 1977; Kuschinsky & Wahl, 1978).

In recent years, a number of factors other than perivascular pH have been suggested to play a role in the basic physiological responses of the cerebral circulation. The two most favored conditions have been potassium ions and adenosine (Berne et al., 1974; Kuschinsky & Wahl, 1978; Winn et al., 1981a), each of which is a potent dilator of cerebral vessels, and, certainly in the case of adenosine, displays marked increases in the cerebral concentrations in hypoxia and hypercapnia (Winn et al., 1981b). The cerebral circulatory responses to hypercapnia can be abolished by inhibitions of prostaglandin synthesis, such as indomethacin, without any alteration in the responses to hypoxia or to changes in perfusion pressure being noted, and the data have been used to implicate prostaglandins (prostacyclin being the most favored candidate) in the hypercapnic cerebrovascular dilatation (Pickard et al., 1979). It would seem prudent to view alterations in cerebral blood flow which are provoked by alterations in arterial blood gas tensions as being achieved by a multifactorial mechanism, and not solely via alterations in perivascular pH.

Influence of Cerebral Perfusion Pressure

The level of perfusion pressure (defined as the mean blood pressure minus the cerebral venous pressure) is of vital importance to the maintenance of an adequate supply of blood to the brain. The classical response of the cerebral circulation to alterations is mean arterial pressure is shown in Fig. 1.7. Over a fairly wide range of arterial pressures (50–144 mm Hg) the level of cerebral blood flow remains relatively constant, and this response is effected by dilatation of the cerebral resistance vessels during hypotension and by their constriction during hypertension (MacKenzie et al., 1976). Cerebrovascular resistance is thus either reduced or increased to maintain a constant blood flow to the brain. This phenomenon is customarily referred to as autoregulation, and can be demonstrated similarly when changes in cerebral perfusion pressure are produced by increases in cerebral venous or intracranial pressure (Johnson et al., 1973). There are, however, upper and lower limits to the autoregulatory capacity beyond which cerebral blood flow varies in direct relation to cerebral perfusion pressure. Se-

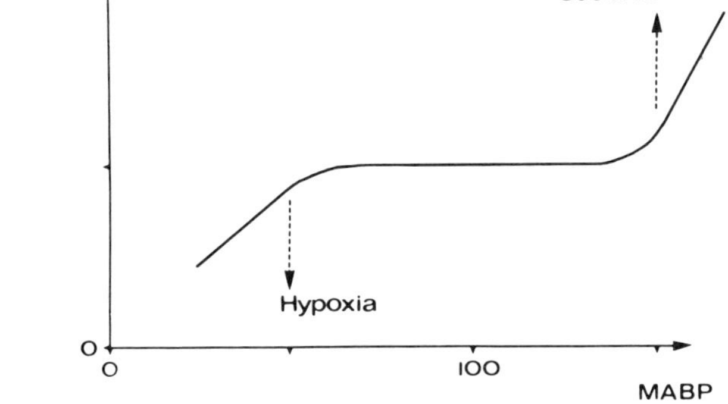

FIGURE 1.7. Diagrammatic representation of the alterations in cerebral blood flow associated with changes in mean arterial pressure. The constancy of blood flow with moderate alterations of perfusion pressure is often termed cerebrovascular autoregulation.

vere hypotension carries the risk of cerebral ischemia as a consequence of reduced cerebral blood flow, whereas in severe hypertension there is a risk of cerebral edema (Fig. 1.7).

Modifying the Cerebrovascular Autoregulatory Response

Modifications of the cerebrovascular autoregulatory response fall into two broad categories. In the first group, which may often be extreme forms of the second group, the ability of the cerebral vasculature to maintain a constancy of cerebral blood flow during changes in perfusion pressure is completely lost, and this type of response is commonly encountered in cerebrovascular disease. In the second group, cerebrovascular autoregulation can be demonstrated, but the upper and lower limits of cerebrovascular autoregulatory response are shifted. Furthermore, the classic cerebrovascular autoregulatory curve (Fig. 1.7) conveys a false sense of security. The upper and lower limits of autoregulation are not fixed or absolute, but rather, the levels of perfusion pressure at which cerebral blood flow fails are crucially dependent on how perfusion pressure is altered and upon the conditions (e.g., anesthesia, etc.) in which they are being investigated. For example, in the baboon anesthetized with phencyclidine, cerebral blood flow is reduced by more than 20% where arterial pressure is reduced by 45% from base line when hypotension is induced by hemorrhage, whereas if hypotension is produced by halothane and trimetaphan, no alteration in blood flow occurs with the same degree of hypotension (Fitch et al., 1975). In chronic hypotension, in

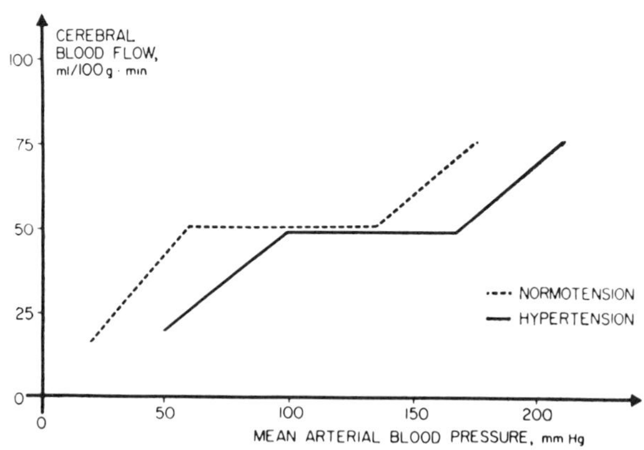

FIGURE 1.8. Diagrammatic representation of autoregulatory curves from normotensive and hypertensive subjects. The entire curve is shifted to higher mean arterial pressures in hypertension.

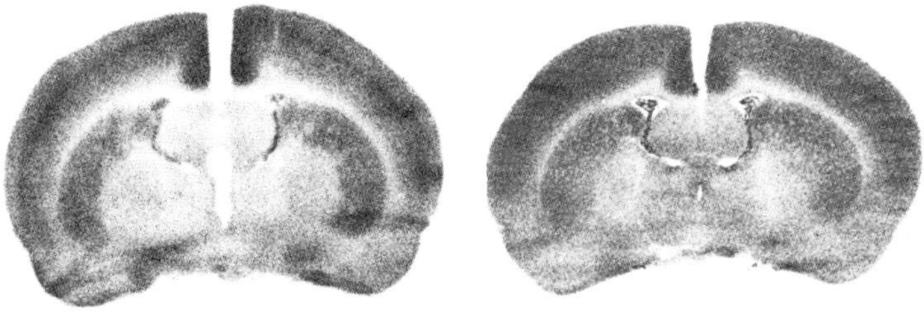

FIGURE 1.9. Regional heterogeneity of cerebral glucose utilization (left) and cerebral blood flow (right) in coronal autoradiograms prepared from the conscious rat. The local levels of cerebral glucose utilization and blood flow are each proportional to local optical density. The values of both variables are greatest in cerebral cortex and caudate nucleus (CN), intermediate in the choroid plexus (CP), and globus pallidus (GP), and least in subcortical white matter (WM). Autoradiograms were prepared using ^{14}C-deoxyglucose (Sokoloff et al., 1977) and ^{14}C-iodoantipyrine (Sakurada et al., 1978) as tracer molecules.

man and in experimental animals, the upper and lower limits of cerebrovascular autoregulation occur at higher levels of mean arterial pressure such that the entire autoregulatory curve is shifted to the right (Fig. 1.8) (Jones et al., 1976; Strandgaard et al., 1975). The adaptation of autoregulation to high blood pressures can result in the symptoms of cerebral ischemia being observed in hypertensive patients during antihypertensive treatment at blood pressure levels which are within the autoregulatory limits in normotensive individuals.

One of the earliest demonstrations of disturbed cerebrovascular autoregulation was the impairment which occurs during hypercapnia. With marked hypercapnia (arterial carbon dioxide tensions about 75 mm Hg), where the cerebral blood vessels are already dilated, the capacity to maintain a constant level of cerebral blood flow during induced hypotension is lost, and cerebral blood flow will decline as perfusion pressure declines (Harper, 1966). (See previously for the counterpart of this response in which the hypercapnic vasodilatation is attenuated by moderate hypotension: Harper & Glass, 1965.) Similarly, autoregulation is severely impaired where there is occlusion of a carotid artery (Sengupta et al., 1974). Under these circumstances, a fall in intravascular pressure occurs in the circle of Willis distal to the occlusion with a subsequent compensatorv autoregulatory dilatation and, therefore, an inability to compensate in full for any reduction in systemic arterial pressure. The autoregulatory capacity of the cerebral circulation is markedly disturbed in a number of cerebrovascular pathologies; for example, following periods of hypoxia, following subarachnoid hemorrhage (Fig. 1.9) in cerebral ischemia, during hypoglycemic coma (see

Boisvert et al. 1979; Siesjö et al., 1983; Waltz, 1970, as some of the many examples).

Mechanism of Autoregulation

Three major mechanistic hypotheses (metabolic, myogenic, and neurogenic) have been advanced to account for cerebrovascular autoregulation and, although each has a body of evidence in its support, no single theory holds sway at the present time. Of the three hypotheses, the view that activity in perivascular nerve fibers is *responsible* for the maintenance of constant blood flow presently has few adherents. The ablation of either the afferent or efferent components of the reflex loop which would be putatively involved (i.e., baroreceptors → CNS → cerebrovascular nerve fibers) does not result in a loss of cerebrovascular autoregulation, provided the surgical procedures are carefully performed (see Edvinsson & MacKenzie, 1977). However, it should be emphasized yet again that the level of activity in sympathetic nerve fibers does determine the perfusion pressure at which the lower and upper limits of autoregulation are observed (Bill & Linder, 1976; Fitch et al., 1975). The basis of the metabolic hypothesis for cerebrovascular autoregulation is that the principal determinant of local levels of cerebral blood flow appears to be local metabolic activity of cerebral tissue (e.g., glucose utilization, oxygen consumption), and it is believed that this is achieved by the local generation of vasoactive chemical factors (hydrogen and potassium ions, adenosine, etc.) as products of metabolic activity. (See section on flow metabolism coupling for detailed discussion.) The metabolic hypothesis of cerebrovascular autoregulation postulates that a reduction in perfusion pressure results in a transient fall in cerebral blood flow, effecting elevation in the perivascular concentrations of vasoactive metabolites with subsequent arteriolar dilatation, with consequent restoration of a normal level of cerebral blood flow. This sequence of events would be consistent with the slow time constant (10–30 seconds) of cerebrovascular autoregulation, and with the importance of local metabolic activity as a determinant of local cerebral blood flow. However, it has proven extremely difficult to identify which chemical agents are involved in cerebrovascular autoregulation. The perivascular concentrations of the two most favored candidates—hydrogen and potassium ions—do not appear to change during induced hypotension, and much interest is now focused on adenosine, which does display rapid suitable alterations in its cerebral tissue levels during changes in perfusion pressure (Winn et al., 1981a, 1981b). In the myogenic hypothesis, cerebrovascular autoregulation is considered to result from an intrinsic property of vascular smooth muscle, first noted by Bayliss in 1902, that increases of intraluminal pressure in vessels in vitro provoke the contraction of vascular smooth muscle (for evidence in favor, see Symon et al., 1973). The mygenic hypothesis is perhaps the most widely accepted at present, principally as a consequence of the negative evidence which has emerged concerning its two principal rivals.

Relationship Between CBF and Cerebral Metabolism

As the brain contains only small amounts of energy generating substrates, the maintenance of cerebral function is dependent on the continuity of its blood supply. Under normal circumstances, the level of cerebral blood flow is adjusted to the level of cerebral oxygen and glucose consumption, i.e., the two substrates whose catabolism is responsible for almost all energy generation in cerebral tissue. When cerebral function is depressed and the total energy requirements are reduced, as in coma, for example, total cerebral blood flow, oxygen consumption, and glucose utilization are reduced from the level observed in the conscious state. In contrast, during seizures, which represent the most severe form of CNS functional activation, total oxygen and glucose utilization are markedly elevated, and these are met from a parallel increase in cerebral blood flow (see Edvinsson & MacKenzie, 1977).

With the advent of autoradiographically based techniques for determining local levels of cerebral glucose utilization and blood flow in conscious animals (Sakurada et al., 1978; Sokoloff et al., 1977) and of positron emission tomography for assessing cerebral blood-flow oxygen and glucose use (Phelps et al., 1982), the coupling which exists between blood flow and the energy-generating metabolic processes can now be demonstrated to exist in all anatomical and functional subunits of the CNS. Thus, the level of blood flow is greatest in areas of greatest glucose utilization (such as primary auditory nuclei and the neocortex), intermediary in regions where glucose use is intermediary (such as caudate nucleus and thalamus), and lowest in regions where glucose use rates are least (such as globus pallidus and white matter) (Fig. 1.9) (Baron et al., 1984; McCulloch, Kelly, & Ford, 1982). With these techniques it has been possible to examine the relationship between cerebral glucose utilization (or oxygen consumption) and tissue blood flow in a manner which circumvents many of the problems that were inherent in most of the earlier investigations and, most crucially, any regional heterogeneity in the cerebral circulatory and metabolic responses can be fully assessed. A further advantage in animal investigations is that studies can be carried out in conscious animals, and thus the complicating effects of general anesthesia can be avoided. Modification of the relationship between blood flow and metabolism by physiological, pharmacological, or pathological factors falls into one of three broad categories. Finally, a number of agents whose primary actions are upon cerebral tissue, such as barbiturates, effect quantitatively similar alterations in cerebral blood flow and glucose utilization in any given region such that the normal relationship and ratio between cerebral blood flow and glucose use is kept constant (Fig. 1.10) (Sokoloff, 1981).

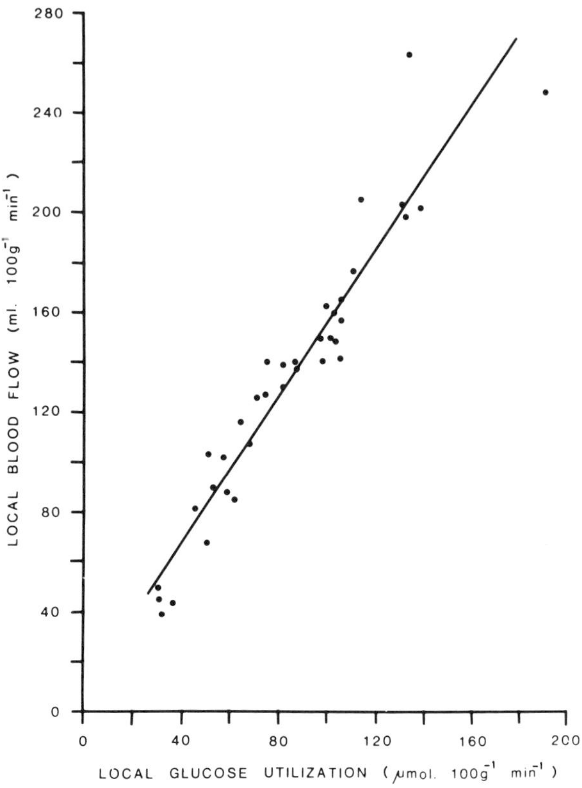

FIGURE 1.10. The relationship between mean local cerebral blood flow and glucose utilization in normal, conscious rats. Each point represents mean blood flow and glucose use in a single, anatomically discrete brain region. Data were obtained from autoradiographic investigations using ^{14}C–2–deoxyglucose and ^{14}C–iodoantipyrine as tracers for glucose use and blood flow, respectively. An excellent correlation exists between these two variables in every region of the CNS.

Secondly, in a number of conditions, such as long-standing metabolic acidosis or following prostaglandin synthesis inhibition (Kuschinsky et al., 1981; McCulloch, Kelly, Grome, & Pickard, 1982), the normal hierarchy of blood flow and glucose use is preserved, but the ratio between these two parameters has been altered to a similar extent in every region of the CNS. It is from these global, uniform alterations of the flow-metabolism couple that an appreciation of the mechanisms regulating cerebral tissue perfusion is beginning to emerge. The third type of response is one in which coupling between cerebral blood flow and glucose use has been selectively disturbed in a small number of regions, and occurs in many pathological conditions such as following subarachnoid hemorrhage (Fig. 1.11), in the vicinity of brain tumors, during and after seizures, and in spreading cortical depression (Baron et al., 1984; Lear et al., 1981; Mies et al., 1981; Raichle et al., 1976). A common feature of cerebrovascular disorders is the inability of the cerebral tissue in the region ultimately damaged to maintain the normal relationship between flow and metabolic activity.

The hypothesis that cerebral metabolic activity plays the dominant role in determining cerebral blood flow is generally credited to Roy and Sherrington (1890), and it is their view of the mechanism by which this is achieved that presently holds sway. Roy and Sherrington proposed that "the chemical products of cerebral metabolism contained in the lymph which bathes the walls of the arterioles of the brain can cause variations of the calibre of the cerebral vessels . . . in this reaction the brain possesses an intrinsic mechanism by which its vascular supply can be varied locally in correspondence with local variations of functional activity." Although this view is generally accepted, it has proved extremely difficult to identify which chemical products of cerebral metabolism mediated the vascular reactions. The principal candidates are perivascular pH (which is determined by carbon dioxide and lactate generated from glucose catabolism), potassium and calcium ions, adenosine, and osmolarity. Each of these factors is extremely vasoactive upon cerebral arterioles and often display alterations in perivascular concentrations during changes in cerebral metabolic activity, although these changes are often of insufficient rapidity or magnitude to account for the observed changes in cerebral blood flow. Thus, doubts persist as

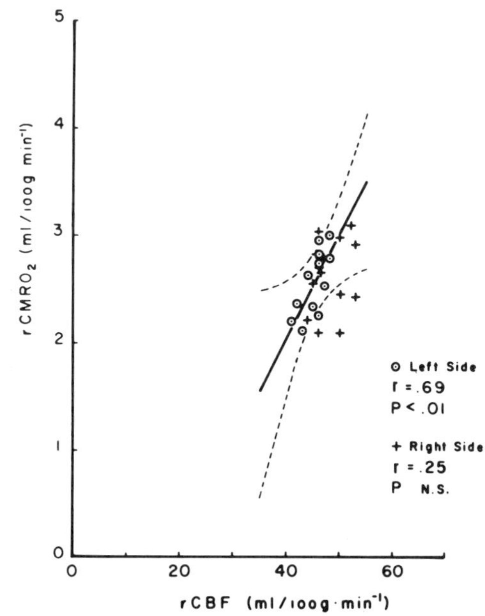

FIGURE 1.11. In vivo correlation between regional cerebral blood flow (rCBF) and regional cerebral metabolic rate for oxygen ($rCMRO_2$) in one patient who bled from a right middle cerebral artery aneurysm 24 hours before study. Linear regression line (solid) and 95% confidence limits (broken lines) calculated from left hemisphere data (open dot) only. Four right hemisphere data points significantly to right of 95% confidence limits represent data obtained from regions in vicinity of ruptured aneurysm. (From Raichle et al., 1976; with permission.)

to the precise mediators of flow-metabolism coupling. (For references, see the discussion of metabolic theory of cerebrovascular autoregulation.)

Cerebrovascular Pharmacology

There has been, and will continue to be, extensive investigation of drug effects within the cerebral circulation in attempts to define, in man and in animals, the mechanisms by which cerebral blood flow is controlled and to identify compounds which can be used to treat cerebrovascular disorders. In experimental animals a major portion has been directed toward elucidating the physiological role of the putative neurotransmitters, noradrenaline, acetylcholine, 5-hydroxytryptamine, histamine, substance P, and vasoactive intestinal polypeptide (VIP), which have all been found in nerve fibers innervating cerebral blood vessels or in perivascularly located mast cells (McCulloch, 1984). Over the last decade, a number of broad principles which have emerged from investigation of the cerebral circulatory effects of neurotransmitters in experimental animals form the basis of all cerebrovascular pharmacology.

The first concept is that the cerebral circulation is generally unresponsive to systemically administered neurotransmitters (monoamines, prostaglandins, neuropeptides) or drugs which possess a limited ability to penetrate the blood-brain barrier, because the cerebrovascular smooth muscle of cerebral resistance vessels is located on the contraluminal side of the endothelial cells which are the key element in the blood-brain barrier. The influence of blood-brain barrier mechanisms on cerebrovascular responses was first definitely demonstrated by MacKenzie et al. (1976), investigating the effects of noradrenaline. Intracarotid noradrenaline has minimal effects upon cerebral blood flow under normal circumstances, although in extreme vasodilatation small reductions in CBF can be demonstrated because the major in-flow arteries are unprotected by blood-brain barrier mechanisms. However, when noradrenaline is administered in a manner which circumvents the blood-brain barrier (e.g., intraventricularly or by local perivascular microapplication around pial arterioles, or systemically after opening of the blood-brain barrier, the amine has marked cerebrovascular effects; MacKenzie et al., 1976). Thus, the measurement of CBF with the intravascular administration of monoamines whose blood-brain barrier passage is very low (or negligible) is almost futile if the blood-brain barrier is intact. The second concept (which was really the rediscovery of the ideas underlying Kety's work in the 1940s) was the importance of the effects of the neurotransmitter or drug upon metabolic activity (cerebral oxygen and glucose utilization) in determining the level of blood flow. For example, noradrenaline constricts cerebral arteries in vitro, or when administered perivascularly. If the blood-brain barrier is disrupted or circumvented, noradrenaline increases CBF (opposite to what would be anticipated from direct vascular effects) accompanied by, and probably secondary to, increases in oxygen and glucose use (MacKenzie et al., 1976) (Fig. 1.12).

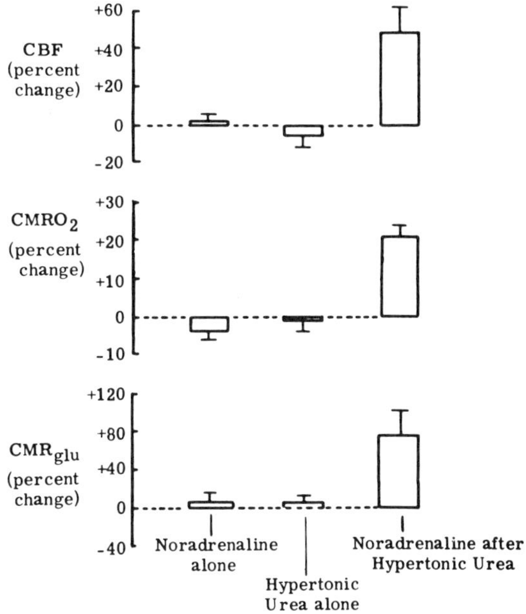

FIGURE 1.12. Alterations from base line in cerebral blood flow (CBF), cerebral oxygen consumption ($CMRO_2$) and cerebral glucose utilization (CMR_{glu}) after intracarotid noradrenaline, intracarotid urea (to increase the permeability of the blood-brain barrier), and noradrenaline after intracarotid urea. (From MacKenzie et al., 1976; with permission).

The third important principle for cerebrovascular pharmacology concerns the topography of blood-flow and metabolism alterations. As the regional distribution of alterations in local cerebral tissue matabolism following administration of a particular drug does not correspond either with the topography of the receptor mechanisms for the drug or with its regional deposition in the CNS (McCulloch, 1982), it is difficult to predict interregional differences in the cerebral circulatory and metabolic responses to drugs. Fortunately, the increasing use of the 2-deoxyglucose autoradiographic technique (Sokoloff et al., 1977), as an investigative technique in its own right for mapping local functional events within the central nervous system as they are reflected in local rates of glucose utilization, provides extensive data on the topography of cerebral metabolic activity.

A comprehensive review of the pharmacology of the cerebral circulation is beyond the scope of the present chapter, but the importance of the general principles outlined herein can be clearly seen when the cerebrovascular actions of neurotransmitters and of anesthetic agents are considered in the response to drugs of local cerebral blood flow and metabolism.

The cerebrovascular effects and the global and local changes in cerebral metabolism which are associated with pharmacological manipulation of various neurotransmitter systems are summarized in Table 1.1. From this table it is apparent that, for most neurotransmitters, it is the direction of the alterations in cerebral metabolic activity which is of primary importance in determining the overall cerebral circulatory response. Thus, stimulation of noradrenergic (Mac-

TABLE 1.1
Neurotransmitters in the Cerebral Circulation

Putative Neurotransmitter	*Direct Cerebrovascular Effects*	*Effects on Cerebral Metabolic Activity*		*Net Alteration in Cerebral Blood Flow*
		Global	*Local*	
Noradrenaline	Contraction (Alpha)	Increase	——	Increase
Dopamine	Dilatation	Increase	Increase (Predominantly)	Increase
Serotonin	Dilatation (Normal tone) Contraction (Low tone)	Reduction	Reduction	Reduction
Acetylcholine	Dilatation (muscarinic)	No change	Increase (Predominantly)	Increase
Histamine	Dilatation	No effect	——	Increase
γ-aminobutyric Acid (GABA)	Dilatation	Reduction	Reduction	Reduction
Vasoactive Intestinal Polypeptide	Dilatation	Increase	Increase	Increase
Substance P	Dilatation	——	——	Increase

The direct cerebrovascular effects denote patterns of response which have been described with both in vitro and in situ techniques. The effects on cerebral metabolic activity and net alterations in cerebral blood flow are based on investigations where problems of blood-brain barrier permeability have been circumvented. Global alterations in cerebral metabolic activity are generally based on $CMRO_2$measurements, and local alterations have been obtained with the 2-deoxyglucose technique. (For reference, see text.)

Kenzie et al., 1976), dopaminergic (McCulloch & Harper, 1977; McCulloch et al. 1982) and VIP (McCulloch & Edvinsson, 1980) receptors results in concomitant increases in cerebral oxygen and glucose consumption and cerebral blood flow; activation of serotonin (Harper & MacKenzie, 1977) or GABAergic (Kelly & McCulloch, 1983) receptors leads to parallel reductions in indexes of cerebral metabolism and cerebral blood flow. In contrast, there is some evidence that acetylcholine (Heistad et al., 1980) and histamine (Gross et al., 1981) activation of cerebrovascular receptors can lead to increased cerebral blood flow without any disturbance of cerebral metabolism (Table 1.1), although this is far from definitive at present.

Similarly, the effects of general anesthesia upon cerebral blood flow and the cerebral oxidative catabolism of glucose have been the subject of considerable investigation, with coherent data emerging. It has long been known that a direct relationship exists between the level of consciousness and global oxygen and glucose consumption by the CNS (for reviews, see Siesjö, 1978; Smith & Wollman, 1972). The administration of intravenous anesthetics (most notably barbiturates and althesin), or inhalational anesthetics (such as halothane, ether, and cyclopropane) in anesthetic concentrations, results in reductions of global cerebral oxygen and glucose consumption by 20–50%, depending on the anesthetic employed and the depth of anesthesia achieved (Siesjö, 1978; Smith & Wollman, 1972). Marked regional heterogenicity of the alterations of glucose utilization following the administration of general anesthetics can be readily demonstrated with 2-deoxyglucose autoradiography, and these fall broadly into two general patterns of response.

Firstly, a group of anesthetic agents, including barbiturates (Sokoloff et al., 1977), chloral derivatives (Grome & McCulloch, 1982) and halothane (Shapiro et al., 1978), produce widespread reductions in glucose utilization throughout the CNS and, although the magnitude of these responses may display considerable interregional differences (see Table 1.2), no region displays a significant increase in its rate of glucose utilization. In contrast, anesthetics which produce "dissociative anesthesia" (such as ketamine and phencyclidine) have been reported to produce local increases in glucose utilization in some limbic areas, although the more widespread response remains a reduction in glucose utilization (Table 1.2) (Crosby et al., 1982; Meibach et al., 1979). However, it should be

TABLE 1.2
Effects of General Anaesthetics upon the Cerebral Vasculature and Cerebral Metabolic Activity

Anesthetic	*Direct cerebrovascular effects*	*Effects upon local cerebral metabolism*
Barbiturates	Dilatation	Reductions throughout all CNS regions.
Althesin	—	Reductions, particularly in cortex, thalamus, and extrapyramidal systems.
Ketamine	Little effect	Increases, particularly in limbic system. Reductions in sensory thalamo-cortical circuits.
Phencyclidine	Little effect	Increases, particularly in limbic system. Reductions in sensory thalamo-cortical circuits.
Chloral derivatives	Little effect	Reductions, particularly in cortex, thalamus, and extrapyramidal systems.
Halothane	Dilatation	Reductions throughout most CNS regions.
Cyclopropane	Dilatation (particularly at higher concentrations).	Reduced.
Ether	Dilatation (particularly at higher concentrations).	Reductions throughout all CNS regions.

For reference, see text.

emphasized that the most pronounced reductions in glucose utilization with *all* anesthetic agents so far examined are observed in thalamo-cortical systems and sensory relay nuclei in the brain stem. In addition to the marked alterations of cerebral metabolism produced by general anesthetics (which are presumably linked to the disturbances of CNS function), many anesthetics, particularly the inhalational anesthetics, can elicit the dilatation of cerebral blood vessels. With halothane, cyclopropane, and ether, increases in cerebral blood flow are often observed in spite of marked depression of cerebral oxygen and glucose consumption. These observations, with are indicative of a disturbance in the coupling of blood flow to metabolic demand by general anesthetics, must be considered carefully in relation to the majority of cerebral circulatory investigations in animals which, of necessity, are conducted under conditions of general anesthesia.

A vast number of compounds, barbiturates, steroids, vasodilators, free radical scavengers, calcium antagonists, ergot derivatives, monoamine receptor blockers, etc., have been advanced as possessing properties for the amelioration of the consequences of cerebrovascular disease. No compound has yet achieved wide acceptance as being of value in the clinical treatment of cerebrovascular disorders (Hossmann, 1982). Major advances have been made toward understanding the pathophysiology of cerebral ischemia, edema, and vasospasm. There is general agreement that vasodilatation, per se, in conditions of cerebral ischemia, is of little therapeutic relevance because the vessels in the ischemic area are likely to be already maximally dilated as a consequence of tissue acidosis. Indeed, in cerebral ischemia, dilatation of the vessels in nonischemic regions may even be deleterious, as this provokes the diversion of flow away from the ischemic region (''steal''). Similarly, many agents which increase cerebral blood flow in normal animals together with concomitant increases in metabolic demand, are of little practical value in cerebrovascular disease as they are only likely to exacerbate the imbalance between substrate supply and substrate demand (Hossmann, 1982).

CONCLUDING COMMENTS

With the vast array of approaches which are now available for CBF measurement in patients (including positron emission tomography, inhalational ^{133}Xenon clearance, stable Xenon enhanced CT mapping, etc.), clinicians are now better equipped, technically, to map reliable CBF determinations with spatial resolutions hitherto impossible. What advice, derived from investigations in animals, can be offered to clinical cerebrovascular investigators? Firstly, the measurement of the basal cerebral blood flow under ''resting'' conditions may not fully reflect cerebrovascular dysfunction, and may provide a false sense of normality. The question to be addressed, particularly where cerebrovascular abnormality is suspected, is not just what is the basal level of CBF, but whether the cerebral circulation can respond normally to a physiological stimulus such as hypercapnia. Secondly, too much attention is often directed to cerebral blood flow per se at the expense, particularly, of alterations in oxidative metabolism. In many clinical investigations of CBF the key to accurate interpretation is often consideration of what changes are occurring in cerebral metabolic activity. Thirdly, particularly in psychiatry and clinical pharmacology of the cerebral circulation (remember the importance of the blood-brain barrier), one should not interpret a blood-flow change within a region as being indicative of a primary functional change in that area; distant changes in blood flow mediated via polysynaptic neuronal circuits (and consequent changes in energy generation) must be fully considered.

REFERENCES

Baron, J. C., Rougemont, D., Soussaline, F., Bustany, P., Crouzel, C., Bousser, M. G. and Comar, D. (1984). Local interrelationships of cerebral oxygen consumption and glucose utilization in normal subjects and in ischemic stroke patients: A position tomography study. *J. Cereb. Blood Flow Metabol. 4,* 140–149.

Bayliss, W. M. (1902). On the local reactions of the arterial wall to changes of internal pressure. *J. Physiol. 37,* 264–277.

Berne, R. M., Rubio, R., & Curnish, R. R. (1974) Release of adenosine from the ischemic brain. Effect on cerebral vascular resistance and incorporation into cerebral adenine nucleotides. *Circulation Res., 35,* 262–271.

Bill, A., & Linder, J. (1976). Sympathetic control of cerebral blood flow in acute arterial hypertension. *Acta Physiol. Scand., 96,* 114–121.

Boisvert, D., Pickard, J. D., Graham, D. I., & Fitch, W. (1979). Delayed effects of subarachnoid haemorrhage on cerebral metabolism and the cerebrovascular response to hypercapnia in the primate. *J. Neurol. Neurosurg. Psychiat., 42:* 892–898 (1979).

Crosby, G., Crane, A. M., & Sokoloff, L. (1982). Local changes in cerebral glucose utilization during ketamine anesthesia. *Anesthesiol., 56,* 437–443.

D'Alecy, L. G., Feigl, E. O. (1972). Sympathetic control of cerebral blood flow in dogs. *Circulation Res., 31,* 267–283.

Edvinsson, L., & MacKenzie, E. T. (1977). Amine mechanisms in the cerebral circulation. *Pharmacol. Rev. 28,* 275–348.

Fitch, W., MacKenzie, E. T., & Harper, A. M. (1975). Effects of decreasing arterial pressure on cerebral blood flow in the baboon: Influence of the sympathetic nervous system. *Circulation Res., 37,* 550–557.

Fujishima, M., Scheinberg, P., Busto, R., & Reinmuth, O. M. (1971). The relation between cerebral oxygen consumption and cerebral vascular reactivity to carbon dioxide. *Stroke 2,* 251–257.

Grome, J. J., & McCulloch, J. (1983). The effects of apomorphine upon local cerebral glucose utilization in conscious rats, and rats anaesthetized with chloral hydrate. *J. Neurochem. 40,* 569–576.

Gross, P. M., Harper, A. M., & Teasdale, G. M. (1981). Cerebral circulation and histamine. I. Participation of vascular H_1 and H_2 receptors in vasodilatatory responses to carotid arterial infusion. *J. Cereb. Blood Flow Metab., 1,* 97–108.

Grubb, R. L., Jr., Raichle, M. E., Eichling, J. O., & Ter–Pogossian, M. M. (1974). The effect of changes in P_aCO_2 on cerebral blood volume, blood flow and vascular mean transit time. *Stroke 5*, 630–639.

Harper, A. M. (1966). Autoregulation of cerebral blood flow: Influence of arterial pressure on blood flow through the cerebral cortex. *J. Neurol. Neurosurg, Psychiat, 29*, 398–403.

Harper, A. M., & Bell, R. A. (1963). The effect of metabolic acidosis and alkalosis on the blood flow through the cerebral cortex. *J. Neurol. Neurosurg. Psychiat., 26*, 341–344.

Harper, A. M., Deshmukh, V. D., Rowan, J. O., & Jennett, W. B. (1972). The influence of sympathetic nervous activity on cerebral blood flow. *Arch. Neurol., 27*, 1–6.

Harper, A. M., Deshmukh, V. D., Sengupta, J., Rowan, J. O., & Jennett, W. B., (1972). The effect of experimental spasm on the CO_2 responses of cerebral blood flow in primates. *Neuroradiology, 3*, 134–136.

Harper, A. M., & Glass, H. I. (1965). Effect of alterations in the arterial carbon dioxide tension on the blood flow through the cerebral cortex at normal and low arterial blood pressures. *J. Neurol. Neurosurg. Psychiat., (28*, 449–452.

Harper, A. M., & MacKenzie, E. T. (1977). Cerebral circulatory and metabolic effects of 5-hydroxytryptamine in anaesthetized baboons. *J. Physiol., 271*, 721–733.

Heistad, D. D., Marcus, M. L., Said, S. I., & Gross, P. M. (1980). Effect of acetylcholine and vasoactive intestinal polypeptide on cerebral blood flow. *Am. J. Physiol., 239*, H73–H80.

Hoff, J. T., MacKenzie, E. T., & Harper, A. M. (1977). Responses of the cerebral circulation to hypercapnia and hypoxia after VIIth cranial nerve transection in baboons. *Circulation Res., 40*, 258–262.

Hossmann, K.–A. (1982). Treatment of cerebral ischaemia. *J. Cereb. Blood Flow. Metabol., 2*, 275–298.

Johnston, I. H., Rowan, J. O., Harper, A. M., & Jennett, W. B. (1973). Raised intracranial pressure and cerebral blood flow. 2. Supratentorial and infratentorial mass lesions in primates. *J. Neurol. Neurosurg. Psychiat., 36*, 161–170.

Jones, J. V., Fitch, W., MacKenzie, E. T., Strandgaard, S., & Harper, A. M. (1976). Lower limit of cerebral blood flow autoregulation in experimental renovascular hypertension in the baboon. *Circulation Res., 39*, 555–557.

Kelly, P. A. T., & McCulloch, J. (1983). The effects of the GABAergic agonist muscimol upon the relationship between local cerebral blood flow and glucose utilization. *Brain Res., 258*, 338–342.

Kuschinsky, W., Suda, S., & Sokoloff, L. (1981). Local cerebral glucose utilization and blood flow during metabolic acidosis. *Am. J. Physiol., 241*, H772–H777.

Kuschinsky, W., & Wahl, M. (1978). Local chemical and neurogenic regulation of cerebral vascular resistance. *Physiol. Rev., 58*, 656–689.

Kuschinsky, W., Wahl, M., Bosse, O., & Thurau, K. (1972). Perivascular potassium and pH as determinants of local pial arterial diameter in cats. *Circulation Res., 31*, 240–247.

Lear, J. L., Jones, S. C., Greenberg, J. H., Fedora, T. J., & Reivich, M. (1981). Use of ^{123}I and ^{14}C in a double radionuclide autoradiographic technique for simultaneous measurement of LCBF and $LCMR_{glu}$. *Stroke, 12*, 589–597.

MacKenzie, E. T., McCulloch, J., O'Keane, M., Pickard, J. D., & Harper, A. M. (1976). Cerebral circulation and norepinephrine: Relevance of the blood-brain barrier. *Am. J. Physiol., 231*, 438–488.

MacKenzie, E. T., McGeorge, A. P., Graham, D. I., Fitch, W., Edvinsson, L., & Harper, A. M. (1979). Effects of increasing arterial pressure on cerebral blood flow in the baboon: Influence of the sympathetic nervous system. *Pflügers Arch., 378*, 189–195.

MacKenzie, E. T., Strandgaard, S., Graham, D. I., Jones, J. V., Harper, A. M., & Farrar, J. K. (1976). Effects of acutely induced hypertension in the cat on pial arteriolar caliber, local cerebral blood flow and the blood-brain barrier. *Circulation Res., 39*, 33–41.

McDowall, D. G. (1966). Interrelationships between blood oxygen tensions and cerebral blood flow. In J. P. Payne & D. W. Hill (Eds.). *Oxygen measurements in blood and tissues* (pp. 205–219). London: Churchill.

McCulloch, J. (1982). Mapping functional alterations in the CNS with [^{14}C] deoxyglucose. In L. L. Iversen, S. D. Iversen, & S. H. Snyder (Eds.). Handbook of Psychopharmacology Plenum Press, 15, 321–410.

McCulloch, J. (1984). Perivascular nerve fibres and the cerebral circulation. *Trends in Neurosci, 7,* 135–138.

McCulloch, J., & Edvinsson, L. (1980). Cerebral circulatory and metabolic effects of vasoactive intestinal polypeptide. *Am. J. Physiol., 238,* H449–H456.

McCulloch, J., & Harper, A. M. (1977). Cerebral circulation: Effect of stimulation and blockade of dopamine receptors. *Am. J. Physiol., 233,* H222–H227.

McCulloch, J., Kelly, P. A. T., & Ford, I. (1982). Effect of apomorphine on the relationship between local cerebral glucose utilization and local cerebral blood flow (with an appendix on its statistical analysis).*J. Cereb. Blood Flow Metabol., 2,* 487–499.

McCulloch, J., Kelly, P. A. T., Grome, J. J., & Pickard, J. D. (1982). Local cerebral circulatory and metabolic effects of indomethacin. *Am. J. Physiol., 243,* H416–H423.

Meibach, R. C., Glick, S. D., Cox, R., & Maayani, S. (1979). Localization of phencyclidine induced changes in brain energy metabolism. *Nature, 282,* 625–626.

Mies, G., Niebuhr, I., & Hossmann, K.–A. (1981). Simultaneous measurement of blood flow and glucose metabolism by autoradiographic techniques. *Stroke, 12,* 581–588.

Phelps, M. E., Mazziotta, J. C., & Huang, S.–C. (1982). Study of cerebral function with positron computed tomography. *J. Cereb. Blood Flow Metabol., 2,* 113–162.

Pickard, J. D., Boisvert, D. P. J., Graham, D. I., & Fitch, W. (1979). Late effects of subarachnoid haemorrhage on the response of the primate cerebral circulation to drug induced changes in arterial blood pressure. *J. Neurol. Neurosurg. Psychiat., 42,* 899–903.

Plum, F., Posner, J. B., & Troy, B. (1968). Cerebral metabolic and circulatory responses to induced convulsions in animals. *Arch. Neurol., 18,* 1–13.

Ponte, J., & Purves, M. J. (1974). The role of the carotid body chemoreceptors and carotid sinus baroreceptors in the control of cerebral blood vessels. *J. Physiol.* (London), *237,* 315–340.

Raichle, M. E., Grubb, R. L., Gado, M. H., Eichling, J. O. and Ter–Pogossian, M. (1976). Correlation between regional cerebral blood flow and oxidative metabolism. *Arch. Neurol., 33,* 523–526.

Roy, C. S., & Sherrington, C. S. (1890). On the regulation of blood supply of the brain. *J. Physiol., 11,* 85–108.

Sakurada, O., Kennedy, C., Jehle, J., Brown, J. D., Carbin, G. L., & Sokoloff, L. (1978). Measurement of local cerebral blood flow with iodo[^{14}C]antipyrine. *Am. J. Physiol., 234,* H59–H66.

Sengupta, D., Harper, M., & Jennett, B. (1973). Effect of carotid ligation on cerebral blood flow in baboons. 1. Response to altered arterial PCO_2. *J. Neurol. Neurosurg. Psychiat., 36,* 736–741.

———. (1974). Effect of carotid ligation on cerebral blood flow in baboons. 2. Response to hypoxia and haemorrhagic hypotension. *J. Neurol. Neurosurg. Psychiat., 37,* 578–584.

Shapiro, H. M., Greenberg, J. H., Reivich, M., Ashmead, G., & Sokoloff, L. (1978). Local cerebral glucose uptake in awake and halothane anesthetized primates. *Anesthesiol., 48,* 97–103.

Siesjö, B. K. (1978). *Brain energy metabolism.* New York: Wiley.

Siesjö, B. K., Ingvar, M., & Pelligrino, D. (1983). Regional differences in vascular autoregulation in the rat brain in severe insulin-induced hypoglycaemia. *J. Cereb. Blood Flow Metabol., 3,* 478–485.

Smith, A. L., & Wollman, H. (1972). Cerebral blood flow and metabolism. *Anesthesiol., 36,* 378–400.

Sokoloff, L. (1981). Localization of functional activity in the central nervous system by measurement of glucose utilization with radioactive deoxyglucose. *J. Cereb. Blood Flow Metabol., 1,* 7–36.

Sokoloff, L., Reivich, M., Kennedy, C., Des Rosiers, M. H., Patlak, C. S., Pettigrew, K. D., Sakurada, O., & Shinohara, M. (1977). The [^{14}C]-deoxyglucose method for the measurement of local cerebral glucose utilization: Theory, procedure, and normal values in the conscious and anesthetized albino rat. *J. Neurochem., 28,* 897–916.

Strandgaard, M., Jones, J. V., MacKenzie, E. T., & Harper, A. M. (1975). Upper limit of cerebral blood flow autoregulation in experimental renovascular hypertension in the baboon. *Circulation Res., 37,* 164–167.

Symon, L., Held, K., & Dorsch, W. C. (1973). A study of regional autoregulation in the cerebral circulation to increased perfusion pressure in normocapnia and hypercapnia. *Stroke, 4,* 139–147.

Waltz, A. G. (1970). Effect of P_aCO_2 on blood flow and microvasculature of the ischemic and non-ischemic cerebral cortex. Stroke 1: 27–37.

Winn, H. R., Rubio, G. K., & Berne, R. M. (1981a). The role of adenosine in the regulation of cerebral blood flow. *J. Cereb. Blood Flow Metabol., 1,* 239–244.

———. (1981b). Brain adenosine concentration during hypoxia in rat. *Am. J. Physiol., 241,* H235–H242.

2 Basic Principles of CBF Measurement by Xenon-133 and External Recording by Multiple Stationary Detectors

Niels A. Lassen
Department of Clinical Physiology,
Bispebjerg Hospital,
Copenhagen

The masterful article by Kety from 1951 outlines the conceptual basis for the use of inert gases as tracers of blood flow (Kety, 1951). He dates the principles back to Zuntz (1897), who already in 1897 expressed that the washout curve from a single compartment would be monoexponential. Kety also refers to the early history of the use of radioactive inert gases and external counting for flow measurements. Jones (1950) appears to have been the first to study cerebral blood flow by this approach. Using radioactive Krypton he found a biexponential curve. In 1955 Conn proposed to use ^{133}Xenon inhalation, a procedure subsequently developed into a practical method by others (Mallett & Veall, 1965; Obrist, Thompson, Wang, & Wilkinson, 1975; Risberg, Ali, Wilson, Wills, & Halsey, 1975; Veall & Mallett, 1966).

This is not the place for outlining the subsequent and still ongoing efforts for computer-based curve analysis and for modifying collimator design and probe placement. Instead this chapter will summarize the method's theoretical background, i.e. considerations of diffusion equilibrium in a single tissue, multicompartmental analysis, and devoncolution thus reformulating some of the ideas of Kety with specific reference to ^{133}Xenon CBF. It is elementary to state, that if flow is zero in a tissue, then no ^{133}Xenon will enter that tissue, and, consequently no clearance curve from that area is obtained. In other words, the clearance *principle* is "blind" to total ischemia. But total ischemia, nevertheless, does influence the curve as it reduces the counting rate. This can theoretically be taken into account by using the bolus distribution principle.

This chapter will focus on this dilemma, that in particular due to superposition of tissue layers, cannot be resolved in practice. Hence it follows, that cases of grossly inhomogeneous CBF in particular with areas of very low flow, as in many stroke cases, cannot be adequately studied by this technique. This is indeed generally accepted and underlies current efforts to develop a tomographic CBF technique based on SPECT (Lassen et al., 1981; Stokely, Sveinsdottir, Lassen, & Rommer, 1980), an approach that eliminates the superposition problem. Thus, to formulate the basic limitations of the conventional ^{133}Xenon inhalation CBF technique is essential to understand the proper use of this technique.

INERTNESS

^{133}Xenon is a radioactive species of Xenon, an inert gas that exists in low concentration in atmospheric air. Xenon does not, under normal conditions, form any chemical compounds.

The air can be considered a carrier substance that rapidly dilutes any ^{133}Xenon escaping via exhalation or from the containers in which it is kept. This means that contamination of counting equipment by ^{133}Xenon is very unlikely to occur in the laboratory, provided adequate ventilation is assured. It may in this context be mentioned that due to the high solubility of ^{133}Xenon in oil, we have occasionally seen greasy, oiled hair retaining some ^{133}Xenon. In such cases extra precautions to reduce leaks and to assure ventilation are appropriate. ^{133}Xenon may be trapped by adsorption to the surface of coal particles (''active charcoal''). This is in some systems used to reduce atmospheric pollution by exhaled waste (this constitutes, however, only a very small problem due to the dilution effect mentioned). Some systems even have recycling traps in which the adsorbed ^{133}Xenon may be set free by heating the charcoal and used again.

^{133}Xe SOLUBILITY

^{133}Xenon is in the steady state distributed solely according to solubility. A fundamental property is here, as for most other inert gases, the *lipophilicity,* i.e. the higher solubility in lipids than in water. If one equilibrates a biphasic system with water in one phase and lipid in the other, then the oil:water concentration ratio can be measured. This so-called oil:water partition coefficient exceeds 10 for Xenon.

Equilibrating water with ^{133}Xenon with air as the second phase shows that Xenon is not very water-soluble, its water:gas partition coefficient is below 0.1. The same holds for all water-dominated body tissues, such as blood and parenchymatous tissues as muscle, myocardium, and liver (if not fat-infiltrated). Even brain tissue has a fairly low Xenon solubility. Body fat has as the only tissue a fairly high solubility with a tissue/air partition coefficient of almost 1.0.

Due to its low solubility in body fluids ^{133}Xenon administered by inhalation will have a more than tenfold higher concentration in the air in the lungs and in the airways than in the arterial blood that equilibrates with the alveolar air. The same holds when ^{133}Xenon is administered by intravenous injection as it diffuses over into the lung's air spaces. Thus i.v. injection is almost equivalent to a brief inhalation. In both cases the radiation exposure to the lung much exceeds that to all other organs. The lung is thus the critical organ for radiation exposure. In this context it must be emphasized that the lung is not very sensitive to ionizing radiation. For the same absorbed dose organs with rapidly dividing cell populations, the gonads, bone marrow, and intestinal epithelium are much more affected.

^{133}Xe—THE TISSUE-BLOOD PARTITION COEFFICIENT, λ.

In the steady state as after prolonged inhalation ^{133}Xenon is distributed in the body as the pre-existing "cold" (nonradioactive) Xenon; i.e., it has the same gas tension ("partial pressure") everywhere. This is also expressed by stating that steady state means that diffusion equilibrium is reached throughout, so that this state represents a true thermodynamic equilibrium. Thus ^{133}Xenon in the steady state is distributed strictly according to *the relative solubility of the various tissues*. The absolute amount of ^{133}Xenon present, its partial pressure, does not matter as, in all tissues, the concentration is proportional to partial pressure (Henry's Law).

For reasons that will become clear in deriving the equation for blood flow, Kety introduced the concept of the *Tissue/Blood Partition Coefficient,* λ. This coefficient is defined as the equilibrium ratio of the concentration in tissue and in blood, i.e.

$$\left[\frac{C_{\text{tissue}}}{C_{\text{blood}}}\right]_{\text{equil.}} = \lambda_{\text{tissue}} \tag{1}$$

The tissue concentration is customarily measured as the amount of Xenon per *gram* of tissue and that of the blood as amount of substance per *milliliter* of blood. Hence λ has the dimension of ml/g, i.e. it is not a unit-free ratio as might have been expected, had the usual physical definitions been followed.

C_{tissue} and C_{blood}—and therefore also λ—are at any given gas tension a function solely of the physicochemical composition of the two phases. This has been studied in some detail by Yeh and Peterson (1965). For the tissue the important parameters are the water concentration, the protein concentration, and above all the concentration of triglyceride fat:

$$C_{\text{tissue}} = \Sigma\, W_i C_i \tag{2}$$

where W_i is the fraction of a gram each tissue element contributes ($\Sigma\, W_i = 1.0$). For blood the solubility in red blood cells and in normal plasma is so constant that one with good appromation can write

$$C_{\text{blood}} = Hct{\cdot}C_{rbc} + (1-Hct){\cdot}C_{\text{pl}} \tag{3}$$

where Hct is the fractional cell volume, $(1 - Hct)$ the fractional plasma volume, and where the red blood cell and plasma concentration of ^{133}Xenon can be considered a constant from one individual to the next at any given tension. The solubility in red blood cells is somewhat greater than in normal plasma. It may be mentioned that in gross hyperlipidemia C_{pl} will increase with the fractional lipid concentration (according to equation (2). This is, however, a rare condition. *In practice, both the gross composition of most tissues (water, protein, fat) and of blood (hemacotrit) is sufficiently constant to render both* C_{tissue} *and* C_{blood} *constant at a given tension.* Hence also their ratio, λ, can be considered to be constant, a constant that once measured in normal man can be applied to the subject we want to study!

This fair degree of constancy of λ was recognized by Kety (1951) and it underlies all the uses of inert gases as tracers of tissue blood flow. In particular it should be stressed that the blood volume in the tissues does not materially alter λ. This is seen by inserting equation (2) into equation (1) to obtain

$$\lambda_{\text{tissue}} = W_b\,\lambda_b + (1 - W_b)\lambda_{bft} \tag{4}$$

where λ_b and W_b are the partition coefficient respectively the fractional volume of the blood in the tissue and λ_{bft} and $1 - W_b$ the same parameters for the blood free tissue. Because λ_b is almost the same as λ_{bft} and because W_b only is anyhow only a very small fraction, it follows that C_{tissue} (tissue + its contained blood) is almost constant.

To give a numerical example, consider the brain cortex having at normal hematocrit a λ of about 0.85 for the blood free tissue, λ_{bft}. The hematocrit of the cortex blood is slightly lower than that of the blood in the large vessels, the hematocrit ratio being about 0.95. Using equation (3) and inserting that $C_{rbc}/C_p \sim 2.0$, a large vessel hematocrit of 0.40 and a small vessel hematocrit of 0.38 gives

$$\lambda_{\text{b}} = \frac{C_b}{C_{\text{blood}}} = \frac{0.38 \cdot 2 \cdot C_p + 0.62 \cdot 1 \cdot C_p}{0.40 \cdot 2 \cdot C_p + 0.60 \cdot 1 \cdot C_p} = 0.98$$

Calculating λ_{tissue} according to equation (4) for two different values of the fractional blood volume 2% and 4%, one gets a λ for 2% of 0.8526 and for 4% of 0.8552; i.e., a 100% increase in tissue blood content only increases λ by 0.3%. This constancy of λ despite alterations of tissue blood content is clearly of basic importance.

In relation to studies of the brain it is also of importance to note, that the white matter of the brain, even though it has a high concentration of lipids, does not contain triglycerides as adipose tissue; myelin has not nearly as high a Xenon solubility as adipose tissue lipid-triglycerides. A typical value for λ_w is 1.50 and not 10.0 as adipose tissue (Veall & Mallett, 1965). Table 2.1 lists values of λ for ^{133}Xenon (from Høedt-Rasmussen, Sveinsdottir, & Lassen, 1966).

TABLE 2.1

Hct	λ_g	λ_w	λ_{brain}*
0.26	0.92	1.71	1.24
0.32	0.88	1.64	1.18
0.38	0.84	1.57	1.13
0.41	0.82	1.53	1.10
0.44	0.80	1.50	1.08
0.50	0.77	1.44	1.04

λbrain is calculated assuming 60% gray and 40% white matter.

In diseases the only gross alteration in physiochemical composition of brain tissue affecting λ to be expected is demyelinization. This would tend to alter λ_w from 1.50 toward the value for gray matter of 0.85. This is, however, not of great significance for CBF measurements as the contribution of white matter to mean flow is fairly small:

$$\bar{f} = W_g f_g + W_w f_w$$

or, expressed in words, the mean flow, $\bar{f}$, is a weighted average of the flow in the gray f_g and white f_w matter with the tissues fractional weights W_g and W_w as weighing factors (i.e., $W_g + W_w = 1.0$) Now with normal values inserted $W_g = W_w = 0.5$ and $f_g = 0.80$ ml/g/min and $f_w = 0.20$ ml/g/min it follows, that a 76% overestimation of f_w due to using 1.50 instead of 0.85 will lead to $f_w = 0.20 \cdot (0.85/1.50) = 0.11$ and hence $\bar{f} = 0.455$ ml/g/min instead of 0.50, i.e. it leads only to a 10% overestimation of mean flow in this extreme case of complete demyelinization, a case that one cannot ever expect to encounter in actual practice.

Xe^{133} Exponential Washout Curve of ^{133}Xenon from Single, Homogeneous Tissue

As discussed by Kety (1951), it has long been recognized, that all inert gases diffuse completely freely across cell membranes. In fact, since these membranes contain lipids, the diffusional transport is considerably faster than across a water layer of the same minute thickness.

Calculations also show that the dimensions of the tissue mass subserved by a single capillary are so small that *diffufusion equilibrium is reached between tissue and effluent venous blood in a single passage of the blood through the tissue.* In other words, the steady state relation (equation 1) also holds in the dynamic nonsteady state, i.e., for any given tissue *i*.

$$\left[\frac{C_{\text{tissue}}(t)}{C_{\text{vein}}(t)}\right] = \left[\frac{C_{\text{tissue}}(\infty)}{C_{\text{blood}}(\infty)}\right] = \lambda \qquad (5)$$

This relation can be applied to derive the washout function of ^{133}Xenon from a tissue by unlabeled arterial blood. In this case the rate of *increase* in tissue concentration $d\,C_{\text{tiss.}}/dt$ is negative; i.e., mass balance gives

$$d\,C_{\text{tiss.}}/dt = -f\cdot C_{\text{vein}}(t) \tag{6}$$

where f is the blood flow per gram of tissue and per unit time (usually dt is measured in minutes). From equation (3) we substitute $C_{\text{vein}}(t) = C_{\text{tiss.}}(t)/\lambda$, to get, with C denoting $C_{\text{tiss.}}$, that

$$dC/dt = -f/\lambda\ C \tag{7}$$

This simple first-order differential equation has the solution of the exponential function with the constant $(-f/\lambda)$ being the exponential coefficient:

$$C(t) = C(O)\exp(-f/\lambda\cdot t) \tag{8}$$

Thus it follows, that for a single, homogeneous tissue i washed out by unlabeled arterial blood $C(t)$ will decrease monoexponentially with time with exponential coefficient $K = f/\lambda$, i.e., with a half-time $t½ = \ln 2/K \simeq 0.693/K = 0.693\cdot\lambda/f$.

BIEXPONENTIAL WASHOUT

A brief bolus of ^{133}Xenon injected via the arterial input to the brain will distribute to the two main tissues as does the blood. The fractional amount reaching the gray matter is therefore $I_g = f_g W_g/(f_g W_g + f_w W_w)$ and that reaching the white matter $I_w = f_w W_w/(f_g W_g + f_w W_w)$ with $I_g + I_w = 1.0$. This partitioning represents the bolus distribution principle. Reaching the two tissues the ^{133}Xenon diffuses into the tissue and will be washed out by the unlabeled arterial blood arriving after the bolus. For both tissues a monoexponential curve is followed. For the total system, the brain, the washout curve is the sum of the two exponential curves, i.e., *a biexponential curve,* with the relative weight of each tissue being given by the bolus distribution principle:

$$C(t) = \mathrm{I}_g \exp(-f_g \lambda_g \cdot t) + I_w \exp(-f_w/\lambda_w \cdot t)$$

with

$$I_g = f_g W_g/(f_g W_g + f_w W_w)$$

and

$$I_w = f_w W_w/(f_g W_g + f_w W_w) \tag{9}$$

THE CONVOLUTION INTEGRAL

A prolonged input function to the brain as achieved by inhalation or i.v. injection can be considered as a *series* of i.a. bolus injections. For a single tissue i this means, that the washout function (the residue of ^{133}Xenon as a function of time) has the form of a sum of the response to this series of brief inputs:

$$\begin{aligned} C_i(t_n) = &+ f_iC_a(t_1)\ \Delta t \exp(-f_i/\lambda_i(t-t_1)) \\ &+ f_iC_a(t_2)\ \Delta t \exp(-f_i/\lambda_i(t-t_2)) \\ &+ \\ &\cdot \\ &\cdot \\ &\cdot \\ &+ f_iC_a(t_n)\ \Delta t \exp(-f_i/\lambda_i(t-t_n)) \end{aligned}$$

or, in integral notation

$$C_i(t) = f_i \int_0^t C_a(\tau) \cdot \exp(-f_i/\lambda_i(t-\tau))d\tau$$

or

$$C_i(t) = f_i \exp(-f_i/\lambda_i \cdot t) \int_0^t C_a(\tau)\exp(f_i/\lambda_i(t-\tau))d\tau$$

or

$$C_i(t) = f_i\, C_a(t) * \exp(-f_i/\lambda_i \cdot t) \tag{10}$$

This is the well-known convolution integral. When written as a sum of n multiplications the principle is best understood. $f_iC_a(t_1)\Delta t$ is the input in the first brief time interval of length Δt time units(from 0 to t_1) during which $C_a(t)$ can be considered constant at the value $C_a(t_1)$; this input occurs at time t_1 and hence the response is calculated by multiplying the *unit-input response* $\exp(-f_i/\lambda_i{\cdot}t)$ by the input $(f_iC_a(t_1))$ and then calculating the contribution of this input at time t, i.e., $(t - t_1)$ time units after the onset of the unit response; this time shift is crucial; for the input at time t_2 the response is obtained by inserting $(t-t_2)$ etc. The convolution integral is thus a rather complex way of multiplying the two functions "in the reverse," so to say. This operation is in a shorthand manner denoted by the symbol $*$.

The convolution integral was derived by Kety (1951) for use in his so-called autoradiographic method for measurement of local tissue blood flow. In this method the tissue concentration C_i is measured at time t, say after 30 seconds, by the density (grayness) on the photographic film exposed by the tissue section for many days at low temperature (e.g., using liquid nitrogen). It is important to note that for very short times the exponential terms are practically unity (as $f_i/\lambda{\cdot}t \simeq 0$) and that equation (10) therefore reduces to

$$C_i(t) = f_i \int_0^t C_a(\tau)d\tau = \text{flow} \times \text{area} \tag{11}$$

Thus, in the autoradiogram taken at short time the local tissue concentration C_i is practically *directly proportional* to the local blood flow f_i. Measuring the entire arterial blood curve $C_a(t)$ in the same units as $C_i(t)$ and integrating allows to solve for f_i. This is the bolus distribution principle as currently used for radioactive microspheres or for chemical tracers that are efficiently retained in the tissue such as Iodine-123-isopropyl-iodo-amphetamine (IMP).

CBF by stationary detectors recording ^{133}Xenon administered by inhalation or by intravenous injection.

In this case the impulse-response of each detector is considered to be a biexponential curve as has been shown to be the case with good approximation in normal humans. The end-expiratory ^{133}Xenon concentration $C_A(t)$ is considered to indicate the shape of the arterial input curve to the brain with a time delay being included of approximately 5 seconds, i.e.,

$$C_a(t) = A \cdot C_A(t - td) \tag{12}$$

where A is the unknown proportionality constant that depends on the efficiency of the detector and on the air/blood partition coefficient. In some laboratories the end-expiratory curve is substituted by a lung curve as suggested recently by Obrist and Jaggi (1981).

The equation for the counting rate $N(t)$ as a function of time is

$$N(t) = \alpha \sum_{i=1}^{i=2} W_i \, C_i(t) \tag{13}$$

where α is a proportionality constant relating units of counts over the head to concentration in the brain: this counting efficiency constant is complicated by the fact, that only part of the truncated cone of tissue is seen fully by the detector (there is a half-shadow effect toward the periphery), by tissue absorption and by Compton scatter. Because α is not strictly the same for the superficially located cortex and for the deeper located gray matter, one cannot *a priori* assume that W_i, the fractional weight of the two tissues, are equal to the true anatomical ratio. The gray/white ratio is about 0.6/0.4 in man.[15]

Using the convolution integral with a biexponential pulse response yields Obrist's equation (Obrist et al., 1975):

$$N(t) = \sum_{i=1}^{i=2} P_i \, C_A(t - td) \exp(-f_i/\lambda_i \cdot t) \tag{14}$$

where $P_i = A \cdot \alpha \cdot W_i \cdot f_i$ ($i = 1$ and 2).

Note, that if A and α were accurately known then for a short time for which the exponential term remains close to 1.0 (equation 14) could be solved directly as it the reduces to

$$N(t) = A \cdot \alpha \int_{o}^{t} C_A(t - td)dt \cdot \sum_{i=1}^{i=2} W_i f_i \qquad (15)$$

$$= (A \text{ known constant}) \cdot (\text{Mean blood flow of area, } \bar{f})$$

Obrist et al. (1975), as Mallet and Veall (1965) instead used the integral equation on a prolonged washout curve using 1 minute of ^{133}Xenon inhalation followed by a 10 minutes lasting washout period. Fitting the experimental curve to a family of biexponential functions (with different P_1, P_2, K_1 $(= f_i/\lambda_i)$ and K_2 (f_2/λ_2)) the best fit is estimated using the classical least-square criterion, i.e. minimizing the sum of the square of the difference between the presumed response and the actually observed response.

This well-known approach in which A and α cancel out when calculating W_1 and W_2 from P_1 and P_2 suffers the limitation that it renders the method "blind" to areas of zero flow or just of very low flow; in this case the curve recorded is dominated by the curve shape arising from other tissues and the curves low *absolute amplitude* is ignored, cf. that equation (15) predicts that $\bar{f}$ = (a constant)$\cdot N(t)$.

This point is emphasized in order to show that just as the intracarotid bolus ^{133}Xenon injection method, the ^{133}Xenon inhalation method is based on a clearance principle in which it is the curve's shape, and not the absolute amount of indicator, as in the bolus distribution principle, that is taken into account. This renders both methods "blind" to very low flow components if coexisting with higher flows. In this context it may be mentioned that rotating detector systems yielding a tomographic reconstruction do allow to use bolus distribution principle. Thus, despite the complications due to Compton scatter and tissue absorption, this approach is basically better suited to detect grave ischemia.

Here is not the place to discuss the limitations inherent in assuming that the biexponential model is strictly correct. The important contributions (cf. Risberg et al. (1975)) in proposing an "initial slope index" that is insensitive to precise value of the four parameters (as long as they give a good fit) should be emphasized. Among the significant recent contributions one may mention the attempts at using the entire head curve after correction for artifacts. This is clearly of importance for getting a better representation of high blood-flow components that, however, still would tend to become hidden in the high-frequency components comprised by the artifacts mentioned.

The conclusion reached is that the classical ^{133}Xenon inhalation method is insensitive to smaller high-flow components (that are well seen by the i.a. method) and insensitive to smaller very low-flow components (that are better seen tomographically); with this limitation it yields a measure of mean blood flow, a measure that perhaps is best derived by using an initial slope approach as Risberg et al. (1975) or a modification thereof.

CONCLUDING COMMENTS

This chapter sought to present the basic principles behind the classical ^{133}Xenon inhalation method for CBF measurement. They were expressed in some detail, among other things, in order to show that variations in the brain:blood partition coefficient λ cannot cause any substantial error.

Many important aspects of the method have not been touched upon. In particular the massive cross-talk between hemispheres and the effect of Compton scatter. For this topic the recent study by Bolmsjö (1984) should be consulted. These factors imply, that even if using many, say 32 detectors, over each side of the head, the actual resolution is quite gross, perhaps limited to six or eight areas. In particular, in relation to focal cerebral diseases as cerebrovascular disease or epilepsy, this constitutes a limitation. As repeatedly emphasized by Risberg, this all means, that the conventional ^{133}Xenon inhalation method is best suited for the study of fairly diffuse cerebral disorder as dementia. A tomographic approach is necessary in particular for accurate assessment of focal reductions of CBF.

We currently use the conventional ^{133}Xenon inhalation method for studying CBF autoregulation in long-term diabetics with arteriolar disease in order to extend previous studies showing deficient regulation in some patients. In this study intravenous injection is used combined with end-expiratory sampling and four detectors are placed over each side of the head. Four studies are made over approximately 3 hours. This series shows an intraindividual coefficient of variation of only approximately 4% and in normal humans the expected horizontal flow/pressure curve with moderate BP variations proving the method's overall reliability. This very preliminary personal experience and the massive experience of other groups, in particular that of Risberg and coworkers in dementia and of Obrist and coworkers in head trauma makes me conclude, that for certain problems involving more or less the whole brain, it is the method of choice.

The subsequent papers in this volume will further illustrate the ^{133}Xenon inhalation method. Both limitations and advantages relative to alternative approaches will be discussed. In particular the practical aspects, the actual performance of the ^{133}Xenon inhalation CBF study will be mentioned. It is fairly inexpensive, very easy to carry out and to repeat and completely atraumatic. The main point is, however, what is it good for? I have outlined my own opinion, implying, as stated, a rather limited role for clinical routine studies, but a wider use for clinical research where the limitations mentioned can better be tolerated as in this case groups of patients are dealt with.

REFERENCES

Bolmsjö, M. (1984). Hemisphere cross talk and signal overlapping in bilateral regional cerebral blood flow measurements using Xenon-133. *Eur. J. Nucl. Med. 9:*1–5.

Conn, H. L. (1955). Measurement of organ blood flow without blood sampling. *J. Clin. Invest. 34*:916 (abstr.).

Høedt-Rasmussen, K., Sveinsdottir, E. & Lassen, N. A. (1966). Regional cerebral blood flow in man determined by intraarterial injection of radioactive inert gas. *Circulat. Res. 18*:237–247.

Jones, H. B. (1950). Respiratory system: Nitrogen elimination in Medical Physics (O. Glasser Ed.). Year Book Publishers, Chicago. *2*:855–871.

Kety, S. S. (1951). The theory and applications of the exchange of inert gas at the lungs and tissues. *Pharmacol. Rev. 3*:1–41.

Lassen, N. A., Henriksen, L. & Paulson. O. (1981). Regional cerebral blood flow in stroke by ^{133}Xenon inhalation and emission tomography. *Stroke 12*:284–288.

Mallett, B. L. & Veall, N. (1965). The measurement of regional cerebral clearance rates in man using Xenon-133 inhalation and extracranial recording. *Clin. Sci. 29*:179–191.

Obrist, W. D. & Jaggi, J. L. (1981). External monitoring of the lung as a substitute for end-tidal ^{133}Xe sampling in noninvasive CBF studies: preliminary findings. *rCBF Bull. 2*:25–27.

Obrist, W. D., Thompson, H. K., jr., King, C. H. & Wang, H. S. (1967). Determination of regional cerebral blood flow by inhalation of 133-Xe. *Circulat. Res. 20*:124–135.

Obrist, W. D., Thompson, H. K., jr., Wang, H. S. & Wilkinson, W. E. (1975). Regional cerebral blood flow estimated by 133-Xenon inhalation. *Stroke 6*:245–256.

Risberg, J., Ali, Z., Wilson, E. M., Wills, E. L. & Halsey, J. H., jr. (1975). Regional cerebral blood flow by 133-Xenon inhalation. *Stroke 6*:142–148.

Risberg, J., Halsey, J. H., Wills, E. L. & Wilson, E. M. (1975). Hemispheric specialization in normal man studied by bilateral measurement of the regional cerebral blood flow. *Brain 98*:511–524.

Stokely, E. M., Sveinsdottir, E., Lassen, N. A., & Rommer, P. (1980). A single photon dynamic computer-assisted tomograph (DCAT) for imaging brain function in multiple cross-sections. *J. Comput. Assist. Tomogr. 4*:230–240.

Veall, N. & Mallett, B. L. (1966). Regional cerebral blood flow determination by 133-Xe inhalation and external recording: The effect of arterial recirculation. *Clin. Sci. 30*:353–369.

Veall, N. & Mallett, B. L. (1965). The partition of trace amounts of Xenon between human blood and brain tissue at 37°C. *Phys. Med. Biol. 10*:375–382.

Yeh, S. Y. & Peterson, R. E. (1965). Solubility of krypton and xenon in blood, protein solutions, and tissue homogenates. *J. Appl. Physiol. 20*:1041–1047.

Zuntz, N. (1897). Zur Pathogenese und therapie der durch rasche Luftdruckänderungen erzeugten Krankheiten. *Fortsch. d. Med. 15*:632–639.

3 The Noninvasive ^{133}Xe Method: Influence of the Input Function on Computed rCBF Values

Walter D. Obrist
University of Pennsylvania Philadelphia

Hsioh Shan Wang
Duke University, Durham, N.C.,

William E. Wilkinson
Duke University, Durham, N.C.

Dan Harel
Haifa University, Israel

The ^{133}Xe inhalation and IV injection methods have become widely used for determination of regional cerebral blood flow (rCBF) in humans. Both of these methods are dependent on estimates of the arterial input function, derived noninvasively from measurements of end-tidal (expired) air ^{133}Xe concentration. Although generally assumed to be valid, little attention has been paid to the influence of such estimates on computed blood-flow values. This chapter examines the effect on rCBF of three common variations in the end-tidal air curve: (1) differences in shape of the curve due to the route of ^{133}Xe administration, ie., inhalation vs. IV injection, (2) distortions of the curve in elderly subjects and patients with pulmonary disease, and (3) temporal displacement of the air and head curves attributable to lung-brain circulation time.

COMPARISON OF ^{133}Xe INHALATION AND IV INJECTION

Following the systematic studies of Austin and coworkers (Austin, Horn, Rouhe, & Hayward, 1972), intravenous injection has gained wide acceptance as a convenient alternate to ^{133}Xe inhalation. Except for the route of isotope administration and consequent difference in shape of the end-tidal air curves, the two methods are essentially identical, including the technique of clearance curve analysis. The question arises whether comparable rCBF values are obtainable by these two methods, and to what extent their respective findings are interchangeable. A systematic comparison between inhalation and IV injection was therefore undertaken (Obrist & Wang, 1981), and forms the basis of the present report.

Methods

Two cerebral blood flow studies, separated by an interval of 30 minutes, were performed on eight healthy males, age 21–25. In four subjects, inhalation preceded IV injection, while in the remaining four the order of testing was reversed. ^{133}Xe inhalation consisted of breathing 3 mCi/liter in air for 1 minute. IV injection consisted of a rapidly infused 12 mCi bolus of ^{133}Xe in saline. An indwelling catheter was inserted into the antecubital vein well in advance of both studies. Residual radioactivity from the first test was subtracted from the second.

Extracranial monitoring was carried out by eight NaI detectors (15 mm diameter), four being placed over each hemisphere. As previously described (Obrist, Thompson, Wang, & Wilkinson, 1975), a two-compartment analysis of the clearance curves was performed that employed a correction for recirculation, based on isotope concentration in the end-tidal air. Curve fitting began when the end-tidal ^{133}Xe concentration fell to 20% of its peak value, and ended 11 minutes after the start of isotope administration. In two subjects, simultaneous arterial sampling was performed, which served to check the shape of the end-tidal ^{133}Xe curve. Continuous capnographic recordings provided an estimate of arterial pCO_2.

An analysis was performed of five CBF variables. Two of them, f_1 and IS, are indexes of fast compartment flow, while two others, CBF_{15} and ISI, represent average blood flow of the fast- and slow-clearing compartments. The relative weight of the fast compartment, w_1, served to indicate any shifts in compartmental size. Definitions of f_1, IS, CBF_{15} and w_1 may be found in Obrist and Wilkinson (1980). ISI was determined according to Risberg and coworkers (Risberg, Ali, Wilson, Wills, & Halsey, 1975). For purposes of statistical analysis, single blood-flow values were computed for each subject by averaging across the eight brain regions.

Although $PaCO_2$ differences between ^{133}Xe inhalation and IV injection were small, varying from −2 to +3 mm (mean difference = 0.2 mm Hg), CBF was nevertheless corrected for CO_2 in order to obtain more accurate comparisons. Blood flows associated with the lower CO_2 were corrected upward to the higher value in individual subjects. CBF correction factors were 4.0% per mm $PaCO_2$ for f_1 and IS, and 3.0% for CBF_{15} and ISI. The mean $PaCO_2$ of the group after correction was 37.8 mm Hg.

Results

Fig. 3.1 illustrates the essential difference in shape of the input function for the two routes of isotope administration, plotted separately for one of the subjects. Relative to a 1-minute inhalation, the curve for a bolus IV injection rises more abruptly and peaks approximately 30 seconds earlier. Values for both the arterial and end-tidal ^{133}Xe concentrations are shown superimposed in each graph. The

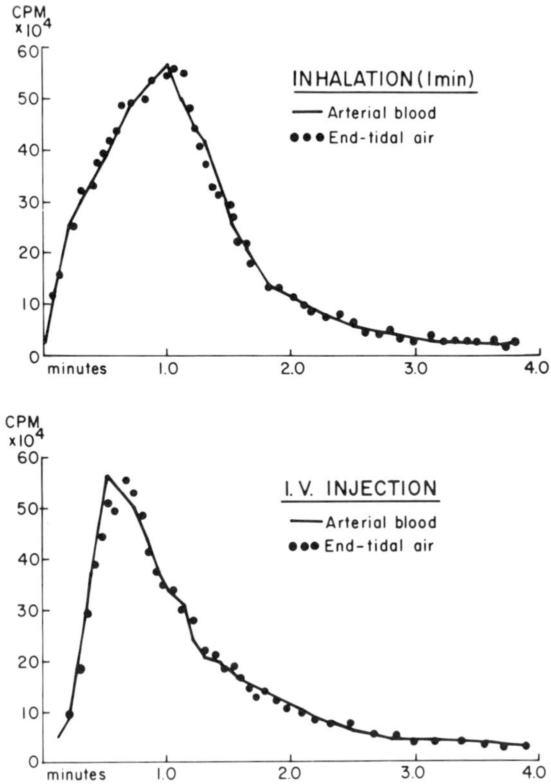

FIGURE 3.1. Comparison of arterial and end-tidal ^{133}Xe concentrations for a 1-min inhalation (above) and a bolus IV injection (below) in a healthy young adult. Peak count rates have been equalized.

close agreement between arterial and end-tidal curves confirms previous observations on healthy young adults (Obrist, Thompson, King, & Wang, 1967).

Table 3.1 compares the blood flow values obtained by the two CBF methods. For three of the variables (f_1, IS, and CBF_{15}) there was a tendency for IV injection to yield slightly higher values (4% to 5%), two of which were statistically significant. Rank-order correlations between injection and inhalation exceeded 0.90 for all three of these variables ($p < 0.02$). In contrast, neither ISI nor w_1 revealed systematic differences or significant correlations between the two CBF methods.

The slightly higher blood-flow values for IV injection are difficult to interpret, since the effect of procedural differences between the methods cannot be separated from differences in the time course of the input function. In order to clarify this issue, a computer simulation was performed in which CBF was held

TABLE 3.1
Comparison of 133-Xenon Inhalation and IV Injection in 8 Healthy Young Adults

CBF Variable[1]	Mean and Standard Deviation		
	IV Injection	Inhalation	Difference (Inj.-Inhal.)
f_1	74.1 ± 7.2	70.9 ± 7.0	+3.2 ± 2.7 (4.5%)[2]
IS	73.6 ± 8.7	70.3 ± 7.8	+3.3 ± 1.9 (4.7%)[2]
CBF_{15}	47.2 ± 6.1	45.4 ± 4.6	+1.8 ± 2.8 (4.0%)
ISI	50.7 ± 6.8	51.4 ± 5.2	−0.7 ± 4.6 (1.4%)
w_1	43.5 ± 3.8	43.6 ± 2.1	−0.1 ± 3.8 (0.2%)

[1] f_1 and CBF_{15} are expressed in ml/100 g/min; IS and ISI are × 100; w_1 is in percent. All blood-flow values have been corrected for $PaCO_2$ (mean = 37.8 mm Hg).
[2] Significant difference ($p < 0.02$), t-test).

constant while the input function varied, comparable to that in Fig. 3.1. Two multicompartmental clearance curves were synthesized, one based on a brief arterial input which simulated IV injection (rapid rise with peak at 30 seconds), and the other based on a longer input which simulated a 1-minute inhalation (slower rise with peak at 60 seconds). The curves were synthesized by a method perviously described (Obrist et al., 1975), involving the convolution of arterial input with three exponentials, representing two cerebral and one extracerebral (scalp) compartment.

Table 3.2 presents the results from the computer simulation. Negligible differences (<0.3%) were found between the two types of input for all CBF variables except ISI, which was approximately 10% lower for injection than for inhalation. The latter is consistent with the findings in Table 3.1, where ISI differed from the other CBF variables (f_1, IS and CBF_{15}) in the direction of lower, as opposed to higher, values for IV injection.

TABLE 3.2
Computer Simulation of 133-Xenon Inhalation and IV Injection

CBF Variable	Synthetic Head Curves[1]		Difference (Inj.-Inhal.)
	IV Injection	Inhalation	
f_1	72.4	72.2	+0.2 (0.3%)
IS	71.7	71.5	+0.2 (0.3%)
CBF_{15}	44.8	44.7	+0.1 (0.2%)
ISI	43.3	48.0	−4.7 (9.8%)
w_1	42.0	42.0	0.0 (0.0%)

[1] The two clearance curves were synthesized with identical CBF parameters, but different input functions (end-tidal air curves).

Discussion

Given the results from the computer simulation (Table 3.2), it seems unlikely that the small differences observed between injection and inhalation (Table 3.1) can be due to the shape of the input function. A possible explanation for the slightly higher CBF values following IV injection are differences in the procedure for ^{133}Xe administration. Whereas inhalation involved turning a valve some distance from the subject, injection required the presence of the investigator at bedside. In this particular setting, the subjects were unaware of the onset of inhalation but, because of mild physical discomfort, were cognizant of the IV injection. An increased blood flow of 4% to 5% in the latter condition is entirely consistent with psychological activation (Risberg, Maximilian, & Prohovnik, 1977).

The finding of a lower ISI for the simulated IV injection (Table 3.2) can be explained by the mathematical properties of this variable. By definition, ISI is a composite slope of the fast- and slow-clearing compartments between 2 and 3 minutes on the recirculation-corrected head curve. At 2 minutes following a rapid IV injection, the fast compartment will contribute less to the slope of the curve than it does after a 1-minute inhalation, the isotope having undergone greater clearance by this time. Thus, caution should be exercised in the interpretation of ISI differences when the time course of the input function varies, even with the same route of ^{133}Xe administration. Other CBF variables, including IS (initial slope of the impulse-equivalent curve), will be less sensitive to the shape of the input function, as demonstrated by the simulation.

Conclusion

The results indicate that there is little or no systematic difference in computed rCBF values between the inhalation and intravenous routes of ^{133}Xe administration. The choice of method therefore depends on other facfors, such as technical, economic, or psychological considerations.

DISTORTION OF THE END-TIDAL ^{133}Xe CURVE

rCBF measurements by either ^{133}Xe inhalation or IV injection require knowledge of the arterial input function. Because of the risk and complexity of arterial sampling, noninvasive measurements of end-tidal air have been routinely used to estimate arterial ^{133}Xe concentration. A question arises concerning the validity of such estimates, particularly in elderly subjects and patients with pulmonary disease, where the end-tidal ^{133}Xe concentration may no longer accurately reflect arterial levels.

Although there is good agreement between end-tidal and arterial ^{133}Xe curves in healthy young adults (Obrist et al., 1967), there is reason to believe that end-tidal measurements consistently underestimate arterial concentration in elderly subjects and patients with pulmonary disease. In the case of pCO_2, it is well established that end-expiratory values are lower than arterial values in such individuals, a phenomenon attributed to increased alveolar dead space (Nunn, 1977). A comparable situation can be expected in the case of ^{133}Xe, such that expired gas from the enlarged dead space will dilute gas from well-perfused and ventilated regions of the lung. Futhermore, inequalities of ventilation perfusion ratio in different parts of the lung, including shunts, can contribute to discrepancies between end-tidal and arterial ^{133}Xe concentration (Rochester, Brown, Wichern, & Fritts, 1967).

This chapter illustrates a patient with emphysema in whom the end-tidal ^{133}Xe curve is markedly distorted, relative to the arterial curve, with the result that there is a significant reduction in computed rCBF values. Additional data are presented on discrepancies between end-tidal and arterial pCO_2 measurements.

Methods

Simultaneous arterial and end-tidal CO_2 determinations were made in eight healthy young adults (age 21–25) and nine elderly subjects (age 65–75) during routine rCBF studies. Three of the elderly subjects were normal and six had mild-to-moderate degrees of obstructive lung disease, verified by pulmonary function tests. Arterial pCO_2 was measured on a Laboratory Instruments Blood Gas Analyzer, and end-tidal CO_2 on a Beckman Capnograph. Four determinations of each were averaged for a given subject.

In one of the elderly subjects with pulmonary disease, simultaneous arterial and end-tidal ^{133}Xe measurements were made during a 1-minute inhalation rCBF study. The subject was a 65-year-old male with X-ray evidence of emphysema, severe hypoxemia, and dyspnea. Rapid sequential arterial samples were drawn anaerobically through a manifold of syringes and stopcocks, care being taken to flush the dead space between samples. Arterial ^{133}Xe concentration was measured off-line on a Packard Auto-gamma Spectrometer, a technique that provided excellent counting statistics. Continuous on-line monitoring of end-tidal ^{133}Xe was carried out in the usual manner.

Results

Fig. 3.2 presents a comparison between end-tidal and arterial estimates of pCO_2. Whereas all eight of the healthy young subjects lie close to the line of agreement, only three of the elderly subjects did. Deviations from this line were in the direction of an underestimation of pCO_2 by end-tidal measurements. Five of the six subjects with large deviations had evidence of mild-to-moderate pulmonary disease.

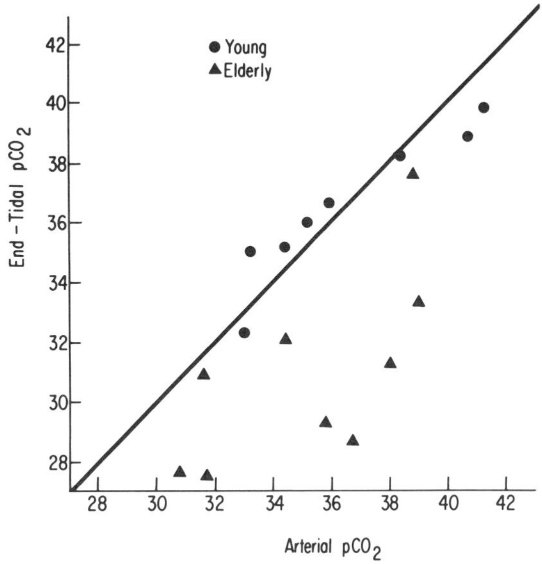

FIGURE 3.2. Capnographic estimates of pCO_2 (expressed in mm Hg) plotted against arterial pCO_2 in eight healthy young adults and nine elderly volunteers. Three of the elderly subjects were normal and six had chronic pulmonary disease. The line of perfect agreement is shown.

Fig. 3.3 plots the end-tidal and arterial ^{133}Xe concentrations for the patient with emphysema. It should be noted that the end-tidal peaks are oriented downwards during ^{133}Xe inhalation, and upwards when breathing room air. Because absolute concentrations of ^{133}Xe were not measured, the magnitude of the curves was arbitrarily adjusted by equalizing the areas under them. Although other normalization factors could have been used, it is clear that superimposition of the curves is not attainable, due to a marked difference in their shape. Relative to the arterial curve, the end-tidal values both rise and fall more steeply, indicating an underestimation of the end-tidal peaks. This graph is in striking contrast to the curves plotted for the healthy young subject shown in Fig. 3.1. In the latter case, the arterial and end-tidal curves were easily superimposed, their shape being essentially identical.

When the two input functions plotted in Fig. 3.3 were used to compute rCBF, discrepant values were obtained. As shown in the graph, the mean value for CBF_{15} (average of eight regions) was 38.8 ml/100 g/min when based on the arterial curve, but only 29.2 when based on the end-tidal curve. Assuming that the arterial concentration represents true input to the brain, use of the end-tidal curve resulted in an underestimation of rCBF by 25%. In contrast, the two input

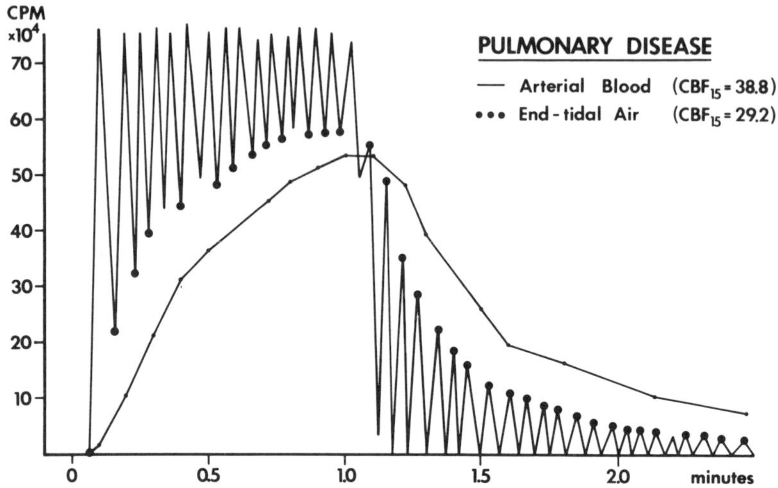

FIGURE 3.3. Comparison of arterial and end-tidal ^{133}Xe concentrations during a 1-min inhalation study in a 65-year-old man with obstructive lung disease. Areas under the curves have been equalized. CBF_{15} was 25% lower when end-tidal, as opposed to arterial, values were used in the computation.

functions plotted for the healthy young subject in Fig. 3.1 (upper graph) yielded mean CBF_{15} values of 48.3 and 48.8 ml/100 g/min for the arterial and end-tidal curves, respectively, which is a difference of less than 1%.

Discussion

The observed discrepancies between end-tidal and arterial pCO_2 in elderly subjects (Fig. 3.2) serves to emphasize a well-established finding (Nunn, 1977) that has relevance for the interpretation of rCBF data. Although interpretation of regional patterns and test–retest variations within a subject are less dependent on accurate CO_2 determinations, any assessment of blood-flow level requires unbiased estimates of arterial pCO_2. Caution should therefore be exercised in accepting capnographic CO_2 measurements in elderly subjects suspected of having even mild pulmonary disease. In such cases, a suitable substitute might be arterialized venous blood, obtained with minimal trauma from the dorsum of a warmed hand (Brooks & Wynn, 1959).

Consistent with the pCO_2 findings, is the observation that end-tidal ^{133}Xe peaks are attenuated relative to arterial values in the presence of pulmonary disease. As shown in Fig. 3.3, this attenuation causes a distortion of the end-tidal curve, such that during ^{133}Xe inhalation the arterial input is overestimated, while during clearance it is underestimated. The effect of such distortion on computed rCBF values can be predicted from the operational blood-flow equation, modified and rearranged to emphasize the effect of arterial input. For a simplified one-compartment model:

$$C_{(t)} = C_{(x)}e^{-K(t-x)} + C_{(x)}e^{-K(t-x)} \frac{\int_{x}^{t} C_{A(u)}e^{Ku}du \downarrow}{\int_{0}^{x} C_{A(u)}e^{Ku}du \uparrow},$$

in which $C_{(t)}$ = tissue concentration of ^{133}Xe at any time, t,
$C_{(x)}$ = tissue concentration at the end of inhalation, time x,
$C_{A(t)}$ = arterial concentration estimated from the end-tidal air curve, and
K = f/λ, where f is blood flow per unit weight of tissue and λ is the tissue-blood partition coefficient.

In the above equation, the head curve, $C_{(t)}$, is seen as the sum of two components: tissue concentration at the end of inhalation exponentially decayed (first term), plus a correction for subsequent recirculation (second term). The arrows indicate the direction of under- or overestimation of the integrals due to distortion of the end-tidal curve, C_A. The net effect of such distortion is to reduce the correction for recirculation, which in turn attenuates estimates of the rate constant, K, obtained by curve fitting. Simply stated, K is forced to decline in order to describe the slow clearance of isotope from the tissue when it is not sufficiently accounted for by the recirculation term of the equation. This interpretation was verified by computer simulations in which the input function was overestimated during ^{133}Xe inhalation and underestimated during clearance. Solutions for K, and therefore rCBF, were reduced in direct proportion to the degree of air curve distortion.

Since pulmonary disease has the effect of prolonging both the uptake and clearance of ^{133}Xe from the lung (Matthews & Dollery, 1965), distortions of the end-tidal curve in the direction of a steeper rise and fall might deceptively cause it to appear normal. Thus, it may be difficult to assess the extent of air curve distortion without knowledge of arterial ^{133}Xe concentration. A clue to the occurrence of distortion, however, is a discrepancy between end-tidal and arterial pCO_2.

The possibility arises that air curve distortions may be less for IV injection than for ^{133}Xe inhalation. With IV injection, the end-tidal peaks are consistently oriented in the upward direction, as opposed to their inversion during ^{133}Xe inhalation (see Fig. 3.3). If attenuation of the end-tidal peaks is proportional throughout, then the shape of the curve following IV injection should not be affected by pulmonary disease, and computed rCBF values would remain unchanged. This may not be true, however, since marked distortion of the end-tidal curve has also been observed following IV injection in a patient with black lung disease, which led to an underestimation of CBF_{15} by 23% (Jaggi & Obrist, 1983). Interestingly, external monitoring of the lung in this case gave a good approximation of the arterial curve, but considering the heterogeneity of ^{133}Xe clearance from different regions of the abnormal lung (Matthews & Dollery, 1965), this may have been fortuitous.

The implication of the present findings for research and clinical evaluation of elderly subjects and patients with pulmonary disease is not entirely clear. Certainly, the occurrence of pulmonary disease sufficient to distort the end-tidal ^{133}Xe curve must be taken into account. The question is at what point are the computed rCBF values significantly affected? Although studies in normal aging may be minimally influenced, subjects with various "risk factors" (Shaw, Mortel, Meyer, Rogers, Hardenberg, & Cutaia, 1984) are likely to have greater pulmonary pathology, and these results should be interpreted cautiously. The extent to which pulmonary function affects rCBF computation is clearly an important subject for future investigation.

Conclusion

There is a potential for persons of advanced age and/or patients with pulmonary disease to show reduced concentrations of both end-expiratory CO_2 and ^{133}Xe. Since end-tidal measurements are used to estimate arterial concentrations of these gases in rCBF studies, such an underestimation can affect both the computed values of blood flow and their interpretation. In particular, the end-tidal ^{133}Xe curve may become distorted relative to the true arterial input, and this will result in attenuation of rCBF values. It remains for future research to define the dimensions of this problem.

TIME DISPLACEMENT OF THE HEAD, AND AIR CURVES

In most rCBF studies with ^{133}Xe, the head curve can be expected to lag behind the expired air curve by variable amounts due to lung-brain circulation time. Depending on specific recording techniques, this time displacement, referred to as "delta" (Δ), may range from 3 to 12 seconds (Obrist et al., 1967). A question arises concerning the effect of Δ on computed blood-flow values, and whether a correction for it is necessary in the clearance curve analysis. Obrist et al. (1975) found that K_1 (fast compartment rate constant) was relatively insensitive to Δ when a delayed start-fit time was used, but could be influenced markedly by starting the curve fit early. Meric and coworkers (Meric, Seylaz, Correze, Luft, & Mamo, 1979) confirmed this dependence on start-fit time, and recommended delaying the fit as a solution to the problem. Recently, Hazelrig and coworkers (Hazelrig, Katholi, Blauenstein, Halsey, Wilson, & Wills, 1981) proposed an analysis with early start-fit times that explicitly solved for △.

The present report examines the effect of time displacement of the head and expired air curves on computed rCBF values. Two different types of analysis were performed, one that assumed a constant △ and the other that provided a solution for △. Parallel analyses were carried out on computer simulations and on data from normal control subjects. Only those results relating specifically to △ are presented here; other aspects of the study, including the effects of random noise, will be reported elsewhere.

Methods

A noise-free, multicompartmental clearance curve was synthesized by a method previously described (Obrist et al., 1975) that involved the convolution of a typical 1-minute inhalation air curve with three exponentials, representing two cerebral and one extracerebral (scalp) compartment. Air passage artifact was added to the head curve, and normal values were assumed for the rate constants, compartmental weights and partition coefficients.

Two different analytical approaches were used in the clearance curve analysis: *Model I,* the standard four-parameter, two-compartment model with a delayed start-fit time, i.e., 20% point on the air curve (Obrist et al., 1975), and *Model II,* a new six-parameter model which started curve fitting at time zero (start of ^{133}Xe inhalation). In addition to the standard four parameters, the latter model included a correction for air passage artifact that involved the solution of a linear unknown (Prohovnik, Knudsen, & Risberg, 1983), plus variable time displacement between head and air curves that involved a solution for △, a nonlinear unknown (Hazelrig et al., 1981).

The synthetic curve was analyzed by each model under three different conditions: (1) no time displacement between head and air curves, (2) a 6-sec shift of the head curve (0.1 min), and (3) a 12-sec shift of the head curve (0.2 min), the shifts being to later times. Because the four-parameter model did not include a solution for △, a fixed value of 0.1 min was assumed in all analyses, representing a typical lag of the head curve. The computed CBF variables were: f_1, an index of fast compartment flow, and CBF_{15}, an index of average flow for the fast and slow compartments (Obrist & Wilkinson, 1980).

The two analytical models were also applied to rCBF data from 14 normal volunteers, age 21–35, who were studied by the IV injection method. Values for both f_1 and CBF_{15} were averaged across 16 brain regions.

Results

Figure 3.4 presents the results from the computer simulation. For Model II (six parameters), both f_1 and CBF_{15} remained constant as the time displacement

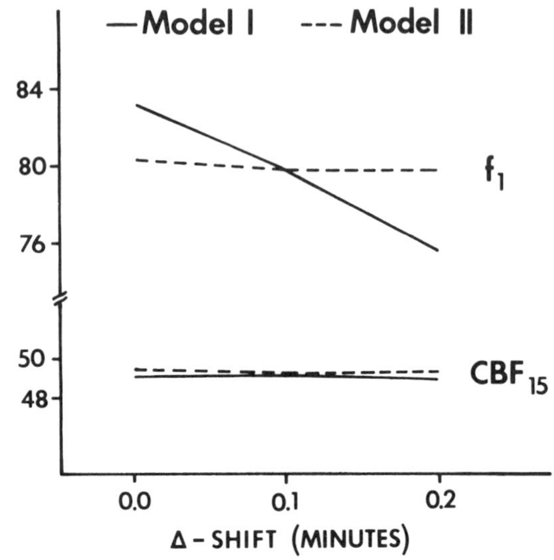

FIGURE 3.4. Effect of time displacement between head and air curves (△-shift) on the computed values of f_1 and CBF_{15} determined by two different methods: Model I = standard start-fit time (4 parameters); Model II = start-fit at time zero (six parameters). Three different time displacements were analyzed with each model (0.0, 0.1, and 0.2 min). A fixed △ of 0.1 min was assumed in Model I; solutions for △ were provided by Model II. Based on synthetic data in which the "true" value for f_1 = 80.0 and for CBF_{15} = 50.5 ml/100 g/min.

between head and air curves (△-shift) varied from 0.0 to 0.2 min. This can be attributed to the solution for △ in this analysis, which automatically shifted the curves so that they were properly aligned. Of special interest is the finding that Model II consistently gave an f_1 of 80 ml/100 g/min, which is the true value in the simulation. CBF_{15}, on the other hand, was underestimated by approximately 3% by both models, presumably due to the inclusion of extracerebral components in the synthetic curve.

In contrast to these findings, Model I (four parameters) yielded constant values only for CBF_{15}, the values for f_1 showing a clear dependence on △ (Fig. 3.4). It should be noted that in Model I, a fixed △ of 0.1 min was assumed, ie., the air curve was shifted by this amount in each analysis. Thus, it is not surprising that when the true time displacement was 0.1 min, the two models were in complete agreement. On the other hand, when the assumed △ deviated from the true value, Model I yielded over- or underestimates of f_1, depending on the direction of the deviation.

Table 3.3 compares the Model I and II analyses in 14 normal volunteers. For Model II, a mean △ of approximately 0.1 min was obtained, while air passage artifact (APA) at the end of inhalation averaged approximately 7%. In parallel with the simulation results, CBF_{15} did not differ appreciably between Models I and II. The findings for f_1 also paralleled the simulation, in that there was agreement between the two models when the correct △ was assumed in the Model I analysis (Table 3.3). In contrast, when no △-shift was assumed, f_1 was lower for Model I, similar to the simulation results when an incorrect △ was assumed (0.2 min condition).

TABLE 3.3
Comparison of Model I and Model II Analyses
in Normal Adult Subjects

Method of Analysis	*Mean and S.D. (14 Cases)*[1]			
	Δ (min)	*% APA*	f_1	CBF_{15}
Model II	.097 ± .028	6.8 ± 1.8	74.8 ± 8.8	45.5 ± 6.3
Model I				
With Δ-shift[2]	—	—	75.0 ± 7.2	46.5 ± 5.5
No Δ-shift	—	—	71.4 ± 7.1	45.9 ± 5.5

[1]Sixteen brain regions were averaged for each subject; mean $PaCO_2$ for the group = 35.5 mm Hg. APA = Air Passage Artifact.

[2]In this analysis, the air curves were shifted .097 min (mean Δ estimated by Model II).

Discussion

The primary difference between the two analytical models is their start-fit time, and the necessity of including two additional unknown parameters in Model II in order to accommodate earlier curve fitting. As revealed in Fig. 3.4 and Table 3.3, rCBF values computed by the two models are in essential agreement, except for differences in f_1 that arise when the wrong $\triangle$ is assumed in Model I. Specifically, an f_1 error of approximately 5% can be expected if the assumed $\triangle$ in Model I deviates from the true value by 0.1 min. Since deviations of this magnitude could occur in patients with prolonged lung-brain circulation times, caution should be exercised in the interpretation of f_1 when the standard Model I is used. Because CBF_{15} does not show comparable sensitivity to $\triangle$, it is the preferred variable in Model I analyses of such patients, a choice that is reinforced by its greater statistical stability in pathological conditions (Obrist & Wilkinson, 1980).

Conclusion

Variations in the time displacement of the head and air curves ($\triangle$) have little or no effect on computed rCBF values, provided that an appropriate allowance is made for such displacement, either by explicitly solving for $\triangle$, or by correctly assuming its value. In contrast to f_1, CBF_{15} is relatively unaffected by $\triangle$ in the standard four-parameter, two-compartment analysis.

ACKNOWLEDGMENT

The authors are indebted to Jurg L. Jaggi for his assistance in the computer analysis and preparation of graphs.

REFERENCES

Austin, G., Horn, N., Rouhe, S., & Hayward, W. (1972). Description and early results of an intravenous radioisotope technique for measuring regional cerebral blood flow in man. *European Neurology, 8,* 43–51.

Brooks, D., & Wynn, V. (1959). Use of venous blood for pH and carbon-dioxide studies. *Lancet 1,* 227–230.

Hazelrig, J. B., Katholi, C. R., Blauenstein, U. W., Halsey, J. H., Jr., Wilson, E. M., & Wills, E. L. (1981). Total curve analysis of regional cerebral blood flow with ^{133}Xe inhalation: Description of method and values obtained with normal volunteers. *IEEE Transactions on Biomedical Engineering, 28,* 609–615.

Jaggi, J. L., & Obrist, W. D. (1983). External monitoring of the lung as a substitute for end-tidal Xe-133 sampling in non-invasive CBF studies. *Journal of Cerebral Blood Flow and Metabolism, 3*(Suppl. 1), 123–124.

Matthews, C. M. E., & Dollery, C. T. (1965). Interpretation of ^{133}Xe lung wash-in and wash-out curves using an analogue computer. *Clinical Science, 28,* 573–590.

Meric, P., Seylaz, J., Correze, J.-L., Luft, A., & Mamo, H. (1979). Measurement of regional cerebral blood flow by intravenous injection of Xe^{133}. *Medical Progress through Technology, 6,* 53–63.

Nunn, J. F. (1977). *Applied respiratory physiology* (2d ed.). London: Butterworth.

Obrist, W. D., Thompson, H. K., King, C. H., & Wang, H. S. (1967). Determination of regional cerebral blood flow by inhalation of 133-Xenon. *Circulation Research, 20,* 124–135.

Obrist, W. D., Thompson, H. K., Wang, H. S., & Wilkinson, W. E. (1975). Regional cerebral blood flow estimated by ^{133}Xenon inhalation. *Stroke, 6,* 245–256.

Obrist, W. D., & Wang, H. S. (1981). Comparison of 133-Xenon inhalation and IV-injection in regional CBF studies. In J. S. Meyer, H. Lechner, M. Reivich, E. O. Ott & A. Aranibar (Eds.), *Cerebral vascular disease 3* (pp. 140–144). Amsterdam: Excerpta Medica.

Obrist, W. D., & Wilkinson, W. E. (1980). The non-invasive Xe-133 method: Evaluation of CBF indices: In A. Bes & G. Geraud (Eds.), *Cerebral circulation* (pp. 119–124). Amsterdam: Excerpta Medica.

Prohovnik, I., Knudsen, E., & Risberg, J. (1983). Accuracy of models and algorithms for determination of fast-compartment flow by noninvasive ^{133} Xe clearance. In P. L. Magistretti (Ed.), *Functional radionuclide imaging of the brain* (pp. 87–115). New York: Raven Press.

Risberg, J., Ali, Z., Wilson, E. M., Wills, E. L., & Halsey, J. H., Jr. (1975). Regional cerebral blood flow by ^{133}Xenon inhalation. *Stroke, 6,* 142–148.

Risberg, J., Maximilian, A. V., & Prohovnik, I. (1977). Changes of cortical activity patterns during habituation to a reasoning test: A study with the ^{133}Xe inhalation technique for measurement of regional cerebral blood flow. *Neuropsychologia, 15,* 793–798.

Rochester, D. F., Brown, R. A., Jr., Wichern, W. A., Jr., & Fritts, H. W., Jr. (1967). Comparison of alveolar and arterial concentrations of ^{85}Kr and ^{133}Xe infused intravenously in man. *Journal of Applied Physiology, 22,* 423–430.

Shaw, T. G., Mortel, K. F., Meyer, J. S., Rogers, R. L., Hardenberg, J., & Cutaia, M. M. (1984). Cerebral blood flow changes in benign aging and cerebrovascular disease. *Neurology, 34,* 855–862.

4 Data Quality, Integrity, and Interpretation

I. Prohovnik
Department of Biological Psychiatry, New York State Psychiatric Institute, and Department of Psychiatry, College of Physicians and Surgeons, Columbia University

INTRODUCTION

The intra-arterial administration of diffusible tracers, introduced by Kety and Schmidt (1945) and transformed into regional capabilities by Lassen et al. (1963), was an extremely elegant procedure from a theoretical point of view. An intracarotid bolus injection of ^{133}Xe is a clean physiological procedure, and can be described by simple mathematical equations. It is straightforward, robust, sensitive, and easy to interpret. It is, however, invasive and rather unpleasant from the patient's viewpoint, and involves some risk. Largely through the pioneering efforts of Mallett and Veall (1965) and Obrist et al. (1967, 1975), it has been replaced by the noninvasive inhalation or IV injection methods. These current methods are safe and convenient for the patient, but present formidable complexity of physiological modeling, mathematical algorithms, and technological options for the user.

The complexity of current noninvasive methods is a reasonable price to pay for their safety, efficacy, and convenience from the patient's viewpoint. Another recent trend has made the situation somewhat more difficult, however. Perhaps more than any other method of in vivo organ imaging, rCBF instruments are operated by clinical (e.g., neurology) rather than technical (e.g., nuclear medicine) departments. The advantage of greater immediate access is sometimes compromised by the absence of specialized technical knowledge. This may result in errors and frustration on the part of the clinical practitioner; this chapter is intended for such practitioners, and for others interested in a nontechnical presentation of methodological and procedural guidelines.

The purpose of this chapter is to present the considerations that usually determine data quality, and thus the reliability of clinical interpretation. It is not a rigorous presentation of equations and technology, and it is limited to two-dimensional, nontomographic imaging. Following the reasoning and procedures outlined here, the reader should be able to perform the procedure and evaluate the data with a reasonable degree of confidence in their validity.

CHOICE OF METHODS

Administration Routes

The first decision usually faced is the choice between tracer administration by inhalation or by intravenous injection. According to Obrist (1980, this volume), there appears to be no theoretical basis for choosing one over the other. The choice appears grounded in practical considerations. In the United States, unfortunately, ^{133}Xe dissolved in saline for intravenous administration is not commercially available at present. Investigators wishing to use IV administration must import the tracer from Europe or produce their own. The inhalation method is indicated from this practical viewpoint. ^{133}Xe in gas form is commercially available from several manufacturers, both in single-dose quantities (10 and 20 mCi) and in bulk quantities that are less expensive. The use of bulk quantities is also convient because, if the instrumentation for storage is available, it shortens the time necessary between procedures and allows greater patient throughput.

On the other hand, the IV method may require somewhat lower dosages of ^{133}Xe than inhalation. Precise data are not available, but it appears that adequate statistical reliability can be achieved with administration of about 15–20 mCi IV, compared with about 30 mCi by inhalation. Note that the administered (dispensed) dose is similar to the uptake dose (the amount temporarily retained by the patient) in the IV method, but not in inhalation. Uptake doses are probably in the 10–15 mCi range for both administration routes. The IV method of Xenon administration is more efficient because it avoids the equilibration process between lungs and spirometer, and the associated dead space. The lower dosages with the IV method provide a somewhat more favorable dosimetry. The lungs and tracheal mucosa, which are the target organs for radioXenon and the tissues critical in determining its safety, are exposed to both inhaled and exhaled ^{133}Xe with inhalation, but only to exhaled air when administered intravenously. Thus, the IV method involves less radiation exposure (cf. Atkins et al., 1980, for more quantitative estimates). In addition, due to the lower average tracer concentrations in nasopharyngeal spaces, the IV method may be expected to create fewer artifactual counts in frontotemporal locations (see the subsequent discussion of the Air-Passage Artifact). Finally, patient preferences must be considered. Sampling of exhaled air (and, therefore, a mask or mouthpiece) is necessary with both methods, but the IV method requires venipuncture which may present additional discomfort for the patient.

To conclude, the choice between IV and inhalational administration appears to be a practical issue. The IV method has more favorable dosimetry, is probably less artifact-prone, but involves an additional discomfort for the patient. The current unavailability of commercially produced tracer for IV injection in the United States appears to be the major factor in favor of the inhalation method, in addition to its economic advantage.

Technological Choices

Worldwide, there are currently five or six manufacturers of rCBF equipment, some of whom offer more than one instrument. Those having a good engineering facility can also construct their own instruments because the technology is widely known. Issues involved in such choices include price, portability, number and resolution of detectors, flexibility, and software quality.

Portability may be important in some contexts, irrelevant in others. The possibility of moving the instrument, and of conducting bedside monitoring, is attractive and may be essential when studying severely ill patients. It is associated, however, with limited flexibility. Portable instruments are usually limited to the IV mode only, since gas administration systems are bulky. Portable instruments may also offer a limited number of detectors, and thus limited investigational capability. Portable instruments usually have fewer radiation safety and artifact rejection features. The number of detectors is also variable in stationary instruments, the current maximum being 32. With fewer detectors one is limited to partial cortical coverage. All commercial systems offer resolution of 20–30 mm at the cortical surface; there is currently no high-resolution feature commercially available. One such system is under development (Risberg et al., this volume), and appears to offer substantial advantages for some research purposes. Its potential cost/benefit ratio for clinical applications is yet to be evaluated, as is the general value of increased resolution in rCBF (cf. Hoffer et al., 1984).

The quality of software and its associated hardware features are currently the major distinctive characteristics of available instruments. There are various implementations, differing in physiological models, mathematical algorithms, type of computer and associated peripherals. Perhaps the most visible aspects of such implementations is their differing display features. Displays of final flow results range from basic numerical tables to sophisticated color displays. The most important aspect of software, however, from the present viewpoint, is its technical Quality Control (QC) features. Some systems offer more than others; no commercially available system includes all the features to be recommended.

PROCEDURES AND ON-LINE MONITORING

Dosage Considerations

No information has been published about the doses of ^{133}Xe necessary for sufficient quality of rCBF results. Most experienced investigators would probably recommend administration (for adult patients) of about 20 mCi IV, or 20–50 mCi by inhalation. The large range of administered doses by inhalation refers to initial spirometer amounts and is due to differences among various administration systems. Indeed, one of the problems in setting dosimetry standards for inhalation involves the calibration of tracer amounts in the administration system (this is one problem that does not exist with IV injection, of course). Little can be offered here beyond the advice to experiment, calibrate, and document each laboratory's dosages.

As a general rule, closed breathing systems retain most of the Xenon after the period of rebreathing; less than half of the Xenon is taken up by the patient (in our system, this figure is around one third). Even this figure overestimates the amount actually absorbed by the patient, as most of the tracer is exhaled during the procedure. Most probably, with an administered dose of about 30 mCi by inhalation, no more than around 5 mCi is retained in the patient's body after the 10 min washout period. We have tried to estimate this amount by taking gamma camera pictures of a normal subject after a series of rCBF measurements. A young healthy male participated in three rCBF procedures, each using 30–35 mCi of administered (spirometer) dose, for a total of 100 mCi administered over about 1 hour. One hour following the end of the last procedure, the subject was scanned by a planar Anger camera, set for a window of 77-120 KeV, and precisely calibrated by imaging a known amount of ^{133}Xe. Calculated activities in different organs were all substantially under 1 mCi. About 100–200 μCi were detected in chest, abdomen and pelvis, compared to about 50 μCi in the head and about 10 μCi in the hands. There was, thus, less than 1 mCi remaining in the total body one hour following three rCBF procedures.

Radioactive counts are characterized by the Poisson distribution: Variance is equal to the mean. Thus, reliability is roughly proportional to the square root of the peak counts, all else being equal. In turn, peak counts are positively related to the amount of Xenon that reaches brain tissue. There are other factors that determine peak cerebral count rates, such as cerebral blood flow, pulmonary function, and respiratory patterns, but for purposes of the present discussion better counts are obtained with higher uptake dosage. The units of count rate are counts per second (cps), but all commercial rCBF systems accumulate cerebral counts for longer periods, usually 5 or 6 sec, which we shall call epochs. Longer epochs provide higher counts for a given dosage, and therefore more reliable data. However, one cannot use epochs that are too long to measure dynamic processes such as clearance. In our case, since the half-time for clearance of gray matter is on the order of 1 min, epochs longer than about 30 sec cannot be used. Epochs of 5 or 10 sec can be used without losing much information, but ideally one would use the fastest sampling possible, such as 1 sec. Because this would entail raising the dosage to obtain satisfactory counts, commercial systems all use the accepted compromise of 5 or 6 sec. In our experience (Prohovnik & Knudsen, unpublished data, 1982) epochs varying between 5 and 10 sec all yield comparable results. One-sec epochs or less may provide more information and more accurate solutions, but they are not commonly used due to the requirement for faster electronics, higher dosages, and more computer memory.

Although statistical reliability is related to count rates, the relation is non-linear. The marginal reduction of variance decreases rapidly with increasing counts, so that there is no advantage in raising count rates from 20 Kcps to 40 Kcps, for example: the coefficient of variation would only be reduced from about .75% to .50%. Both numbers are negligible. On the other hand, the effect of count rate on variance at low rates is substantial: raising count rates from 200 cps to 400 cps would reduce the coefficient of variation from about 23% to about 16%. The upper limit of count rates is usually determined by local medicolegal considerations, however, rather than by theoretical calculations. It is generally agreed by most experienced investigators that peak counts below about 200 cps (corresponding to 1000–1200 per sampling epoch in commercial systems) are not acceptable. The desirable range varies between about 400 cps to 1000 cps, yielding epoch counts of 2000–5000.

Determining the required dosage in order to obtain desired peak counts is relatively simple for the IV method. Given an injected dose and volume of ^{133}Xe in saline, variables such as respiratory pattern and cerebral perfusion will determine peak cerebral count rates. The relationship between injected dose and peak counts should be fairly strong, and the injected dose is always precisely known. A similar determination for the inhalation method is more complex. First, most commercial inhalation systems are poorly calibrated, if at all, and investigators employing the inhalation method often have no more than a vague idea of their administered dosage. Secondly, given a known administered dose, the amount reaching the brain will vary more than it would by injection. Pulmonary absorption and diffusion into the arterial blood are influenced by dead-space volume, respiratory patterns, pulmonary disease, spirometer volume, etc.

In an attempt to illustrate these variables, and as part of an ongoing calibration project, we have derived the data presented in Figs. 4.1–4.3. These figures indicate reasonable correlations between administered dose, uptake dose (defined as the amount of ^{133}Xe originally loaded, minus the amount remaining in the spirometer after the study) peak end-tidal count rates (as an index of arterial concentrations) and peak cerebral count rates. Note that, as expected, end-tidal count rates are the best predictor of cerebral count rates; it is, therefore, possible to predict roughly peak cerebral count rates immediately following the 1-min inhalation period (or immediately following IV injection). Surprisingly, uptake

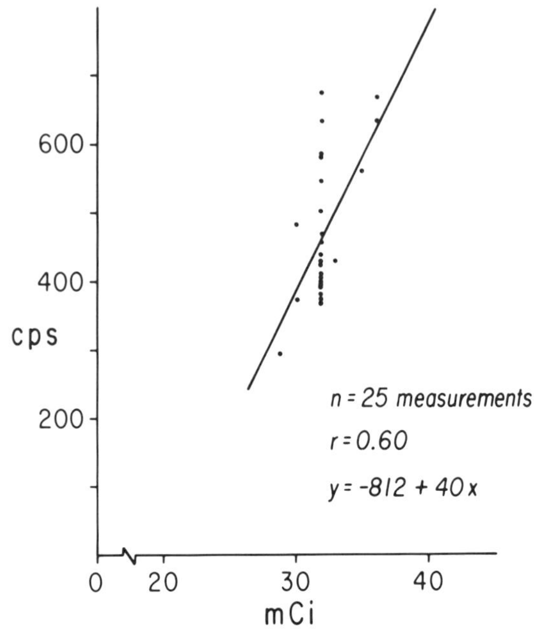

FIGURE 4.1. Cerebral (gray and white, excluding artifact compartments) peak count rates as a function of administered ^{133}Xe dose. This is the amount of ^{133}Xe contained in the spirometer prior to the start of inhalation. Most of the subjects have received our standard dose of 32 mCi; the scatter of cerebral peak counts with this dose indicates the influence of other variables, physiological and anatomical.

dose does not predict cerebral counts as well as administered dose (defined as initial spirometer Xenon amount); we are in the process of further investigating this result. At this point, it appears that prediction of cerebral peak count rates from administered dose is possible in both inhalation and IV methods, but that the specific regression lines may be instrument- and technique-dependent.

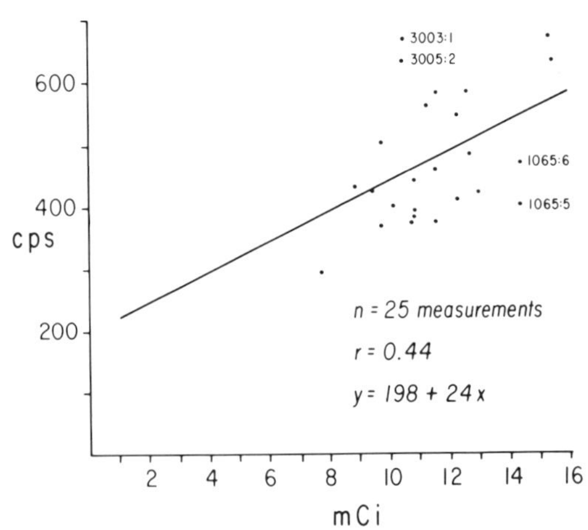

FIGURE 4.2. Cerebral peak count rates (gray and white, excluding artifact compartments) as a function of uptake dose. This is the difference in amount of ^{133}Xe in the spirometer before and after the 1-min inhalation period.

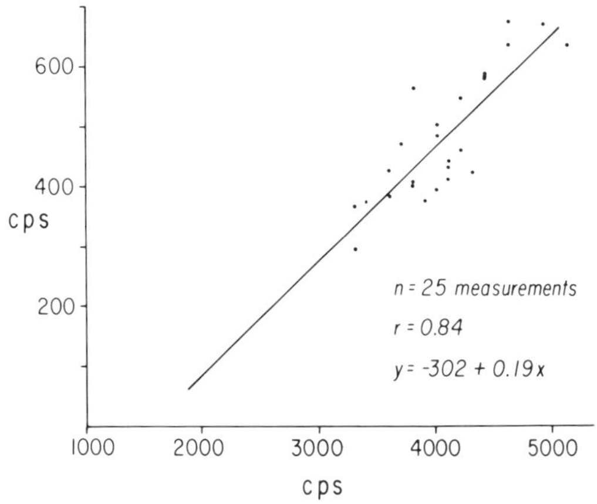

FIGURE 4.3. Cerebral peak count rates (gray and white, excluding artifact compartments), as a function of the end-tidal air-curve count rates, reflecting arterial ^{133}Xe concentrations and therefore the cerebral input function. This is the best predictor of cerebral count rates (r = .84).

Finally, desired peak cerebral counts will also be a function of other variables. Peak counts are proportional to flow; patients with low flows will need greater dosage for satisfactory count rates. Similarly, when a study is performed immediately following another study, a larger dose will be necessary due to the significant amount of activity remaining in cerebral and noncerebral tissue. Young children will require less Xenon than adults for a comparable cerebral count rate. In a recent review of our dosimetry data which are routinely collected, we found in a sample of nine children (age range 6–17, presenting with sickle cell disease and other disorders) that Xenon delivery to the brain, and the ensuing cerebral peak count rates, were 60% higher than in adults when normalized by dose. Thus, whereas we use an uptake dose of about 12 mCi for adults to achieve sufficient peak counts, we need only use 7–8 mCi in children and adolescents.

To summarize this section, although the precise relationship between administered ^{133}Xe dose and data quality has not been demonstrated, general guidelines are known. Administered doses should be about 10–20 mCi intravenously or 30–40 mCi by inhalation. Both result in uptake doses of 10–15 mCi in adults, and the bulk of this amount is cleared out by the end of the 10-min washout period. The end-tidal peak count is an excellent predictor of cerebral peak count rates, but even administered dose can be used for this purpose, after careful calibration of inhalation systems. It is relatively easy to establish a dose–response curve for count rates, and this should probably be done by every laboratory. When this is done, it is possible to identify insufficient counts within a minute or two of administration by noting the peak end-tidal or cerebral counts. If the counts are clearly inadequate, the measurement should be aborted and restarted with sufficient dosage.

Detector Positioning

The importance of precise detector positioning in the current context is impossible to overemphasize; it is a critical determinant of data quality. One obvious reason is the possibility of technically inadequate data arising from such errors. For example, several common commercial systems use 32 detectors in parallel banks. Such banks are known to be prone to errors along the convexity, caused by superior detectors being located so that their fields of view include little cerebral tissue, but much skull and air. Those detectors typically suffer from low count rates, low flow estimates and frequent "slippage." A helmet-like device with detectors perpendicular to the skull helps minimize this problem (cf. Prohovnik et al., 1983a). Secondly, clinical interpretation requires the assumption that the cortical fields measured by the detectors correspond to certain anatomical structures. Thirdly, positioning must be precise and reproducible to allow comparison of results across time and patients. Much of the noise currently contained in rCBF data probably results from imprecise positioning, and the problem will be more critical as resolution increases.

Two general solutions are possible. One is implemented in software, and involves post hoc correction for positioning errors (Farrar, 1981). Another is implemented in hardware, and involves mechanical aids that rely on skull landmarks to position the detectors (Prohovnik et al., 1983a). The ideal solution may be to use mechanical positioners for optimal results, and add a software correction for skull shape. Such a solution is not commercially available.

Study Conditions and Environment

Many laboratories conduct rCBF studies under one condition only; others use various manipulations and provocation conditions. In any case, a standard baseline condition is defined, even if only implicitly. Such a base-line condition should be rigorously and consistently applied; consistency may be more important than the specific nature of the condition. Commonly, base line involves visual, but not auditory, deprivation. Although the utility of this condition has recently been challenged (e.g., Mazziotta et al., 1982), it is still the one probably used by most rCBF laboratories. In this condition, the patient is instructed to keep his eyes closed, and most investigators also cover the eyes or maintain darkness in the room to ensure compliance. The ears are unplugged, but the laboratory is kept as quiet as possible.

In addition to the sensory features, the psychological setting is likely also of consequence. Many patients react emotionally to the appearance of the instrumentation, and to the confinement and immobilization inherent in the procedure. Psychological variables are significant in rCBF due to its sensitivity to such mental states. There is some evidence that rCBF may be affected by motivation (Risberg et al., 1975b) and anxiety (Johanson et al., in preparation). In patients with dementia or lateralized strokes, the setting may interact with clinical features to produce variable affective states. Thus, the measurement condition should be standardized for psychological factors, and any unusual reactions should be documented.

Pharmacological standardization should also be attempted. Many standard medications, as well as alcohol (Berglund & Risberg, 1981), caffeine (Mathew et al., 1983) and nicotine (Hall, 1972; Kubota et al., 1983; Skinhoj et al., 1973) may affect rCBF chronically and acutely. Heavy eating probably also has an effect, and hyperglycemia has been shown to reduce CBF (Duckrow et al., 1985). Although this is sometimes impossible to control, an effort should be made to do so. Compliance is better controlled with inpatients, but even outpatients should be instructed to avoid substances and conditions that may affect rCBF. It is feasible to request abstinence from alcohol for several hours, as well as coffee and nonprescription medication. Heavy smokers present an ambiguous situation; since nicotine withdrawal symptoms may appear rapidly, it is unclear whether a chronic smoker who abstains for several hours is closer to a standard base line than one who has recently smoked. The purpose should be to obtain rCBF results in a state that is typical for the patient, and such a state is not always easy to define. At any rate, such variables should be controlled as much as possible, and deviations should be noted. This also applies to unusual stress conditions, affective complications, sleep deprivation, etc.

Blood gases are known to be relevant to rCBF; $PaCO_2$, in particular, is an important determinant of vascular tone. It should always be monitored and documented. An unusually low value may indicate hyperventilation, which should be corrected prior to the study. An unusually high value may indicate pulmonary disease. CO_2 tension should be monitored throughout the rCBF measurement, or at least several times; significant changes may invalidate the requirement of steady state. Checking blood pressure may be helpful if severe pathology, which may interfere with normal autoregulation, is suspected. In addition, sufficient oxygenation is sometimes at doubt. This may occur when using a closed rebreathing system, and not replenishing it after repeated studies. Although the spirometer volume may be largely unchanged, the closed system replaces inhaled oxygen with exhaled carbon dioxide. After several studies, oxygen concentration in the breathing system may have dropped radically. Although rCBF may not be affected before arterial PO_2 drops to hypoxic levels, and is certainly less sensitive to oxygen than to CO_2 concentrations, attention to oxygenation is warranted.

Finally, other blood constituents may need to be documented for proper interpretation of results. Hemoglobin and hematocrit may significantly affect the blood-brain partition coefficient of Xenon, as well as blood viscosity (for a detailed discussion of the complex issues of viscosity see Kee & Wood, 1984) and oxygen delivery capacity. In hematological disease it may be important to document blood constituents at the time of rCBF measurement; we have found, for instance, a close correlation between Hct, Hb, and CBF in patients with sickle cell disease undergoing hypertransfusion therapy (Prohovnik et al., unpublished data, 1985). According to some authors, other factors should be taken into account (e.g., fibrinogen, Ackerman et al., 1983).

Artifact Rejection

There are several sources of artifacts that may be identified on-line and corrected. First, movement artifacts should be avoided. The patient's head should be moderately restrained, to discourage movement. Because the method is relatively insensitive to small movements (partly due to the limited resolution), severe restraint is probably contraindicated, as it may exacerbate anxiety. If movements are deemed likely, and a good detector-positioning system is available, frequent checks of detector position during the measurement are helpful. Fidgety patients can be discouraged from moving, or the measurement can be aborted and immediately repeated. It is crucial to control head movements online, as their latter correction is usually impossible.

The need for a tight mask or mouthpiece with good nose clamping is obvious with the inhalation method, but perhaps less obvious with IV. It is actually equally important. The sampling of end-tidal Xenon concentrations is equally critical in both methods, and end-tidal CO_2 monitoring has already been mentioned. Poor fit not only leads to poor estimates of these critical variables, but also may degrade the data by allowing Xenon to leak and be visible by the head detectors, distorting the cerebral clearance curves beyond repair. This is, in our experience, the most common cause of excluded detectors, and usually happens at the most anterior and inferior positions. Some investigators attempt to overcome this potential problem by the use of adhesive tapes or substances to ensure mask tightness. Some commercial systems include a "leak detector." This useful feature consists of a system for removal of air from around the patient's face, and fills two functions: in addition to removing the air and thus minimizing the risk of contaminating clearance curves, it also detects the presence of leaked Xenon and warns the operator. Other commercial systems remove the air by means of a fan but do not monitor for Xe concentrations. In our experience, the full implementation of a leak detector is extremely useful.

Investigators whose equipment does not have a leak detector can use other maneuvers to minimize leaks. One method requires the patient to exhale forcefully prior to the procedure; leaky masks can be detected by sensing the escaped air around the mask edges. A more precise and quantified method consists of administering a known concentration of carbon dioxide to the patient, and noting inhaled concentrations. Although end-tidal concentrations vary as a function of respiratory patterns, inhaled concentrations should always be identical to the known administered concentrations. If the end-tidal monitor is placed correctly (in close proximity to the mouth), and demonstrates inhaled concentrations lower than the administered amount, the operator may be fairly certain of a poor mask fit. Similarly, shifts of the end-tidal PCO_2 during the measurement may indicate a developing leak.

Another physiological artifact that may be visible during the measurement is the Air-Passage Artifact (APA). This artifact results when cerebral detectors are contaminated, directly within their fields of view or through scattered radiation, by Xenon in nasopharyngeal air spaces. This artifact was originally suspected by Obrist et al. (1975). Since then, it has been repeatedly verified. The topographic distribution of this artifact corresponds to its anatomical substrate, and it mostly affects frontotemporal locations (Prohovnik et al., 1981). Its magnitude, and the associated distortion of clearance curves, is partly a function of variable anatomy, and it cannot always be avoided. It can be recognized during the measurement, however. Curves in frontotemporal locations that are greatly affected by the APA demonstrate a very rapid rise during the beginning of inhalation, and then a rapid but limited drop immediately at the end of the inhalation period, followed by a moderate clearance or even a short rise. This appearance was utilized by Risberg (1980) for a local correction routine, and it is easily recognized with practice. When this appearance is recognized during the measurement, however, the artifactual influence has already occurred.

It is important to record and monitor the background activity levels during the study. This applies to background activity in exhaled air (reflecting arterial activity) as well as cerebral counts. Relatively high levels should be expected when an rCBF procedure is repeated, due to remaining ^{133}Xe in tissue, or following other nuclear procedures. When high levels are present without such an explanation, the study should be aborted prior to tracer administration, and the cause determined. This should be done not because a high background activity is disruptive per se, but because it often indicates serious equipment malfunctions, such as electronic imbalance or leakage of ^{133}Xe.

Finally, there are numerous other artifacts, of mechanical and electronic origin, that may be detectible on-line. A discussion of all is beyond the scope of this chapter. Generally, any unusual appearance of the air or head curves is a cause for concern, and recognition of such artifacts comes with practice. For more detailed presentations, see Baron et al. (1979) and Dunn et al. (1985).

OFF-LINE TECHNICAL EVALUATION

This section refers to quality control procedures performed after the study is terminated and the patient released. The purpose of this verification is to determine that the data are of adequate technical quality, and if problems are identified, to attempt correction or to eliminate the unreliable detectors from consideration. In extreme cases, the complete measurement may have to be discarded.

Numerical Indexes of Quality

Air Curve and Start-fit Time. When using the Obrist bicompartmental model with Start-Fit Time (SFT), it is important to examine the SFT carefully. It is a central part of the detailed examination of the end-tidal fitting of the air curve, usually performed by the software. Commercially available algorithms for end-tidal fitting are imperfect, and have a nonnegligible rate of failure (i.e., erroneous fitting of a few points). They should not be left entirely unsupervised, especially under certain conditions (such as slow breathing or talking). The examination should include the height and shape of peak, every point during the first 4 or 5 min, the SFT and the background detected in the air detector. The point-by-point examination requires simultaneous presentation of the raw and end-tidal air curves. For those using whole-curve analysis, the averaged air curve should be displayed and examined as well (this is used to estimate the shape of the Air-Passage Artifact). The height, shape and time of the peak can be used for diagnosing tracer administration and arrival problems. The background must be consistently low for all first measurements; high values may indicate Xenon contamination of the air or electronic artifacts. Numerical values are not provided here, as they depend on the particular detector employed and vary across manufacturers. For repeated measurements, a remaining activity correction has been developed (Risberg, 1980) and implemented by some manufacturers. Air background may be slightly higher in repeated measurements, but not substantially so; most of the ^{133}Xe has already been exhaled by this point, and arterial concentrations should be very low.

As part of this air-curve examination, the SFT may reveal inadequate end-tidal or average air-curve fitting, if it is unusually early or delayed. SFT should normally vary between 40–90 sec for IV injection (depending on the type of injection) and between 90 and 150 sec with inhalation. These are only rough ranges, but large deviations from them usually indicate errors in fitting either the end-tidal or the average air curve (whichever was used to derive SFT). A substantial delay of the SFT, indicating slow pulmonary clearance of Xenon, may suggest pulmonary dysfunction. We have so far seen three such patients: delayed SFT, high $PeCO_2$ and other factors suggested pulmonary disease, which was confirmed by pulmonary function testing and changed the interpretation of flow results. Finally, examination of the SFT is crucial because it has a significant influence on the flow results (if calculated by the traditional model, as discussed subsequently). The usual definitions of SFT (e.g., Obrist et al., 1975; Risberg & Prohovnik, 1981) place it at some point determined by the clearance of Xenon from respiratory air. Changes of respiratory patterns may therefore change SFT, without necessarily affecting CBF in the same way. This phenomenon may cause erroneous estimates of flow parameters, and may substantially degrade the reliability of inter- and intrasubject comparisons.

As an illustration, Fig. 4.4 depicts a single clearance curve from a normal subject, analyzed by the Obrist method with three different SFTs. The middle

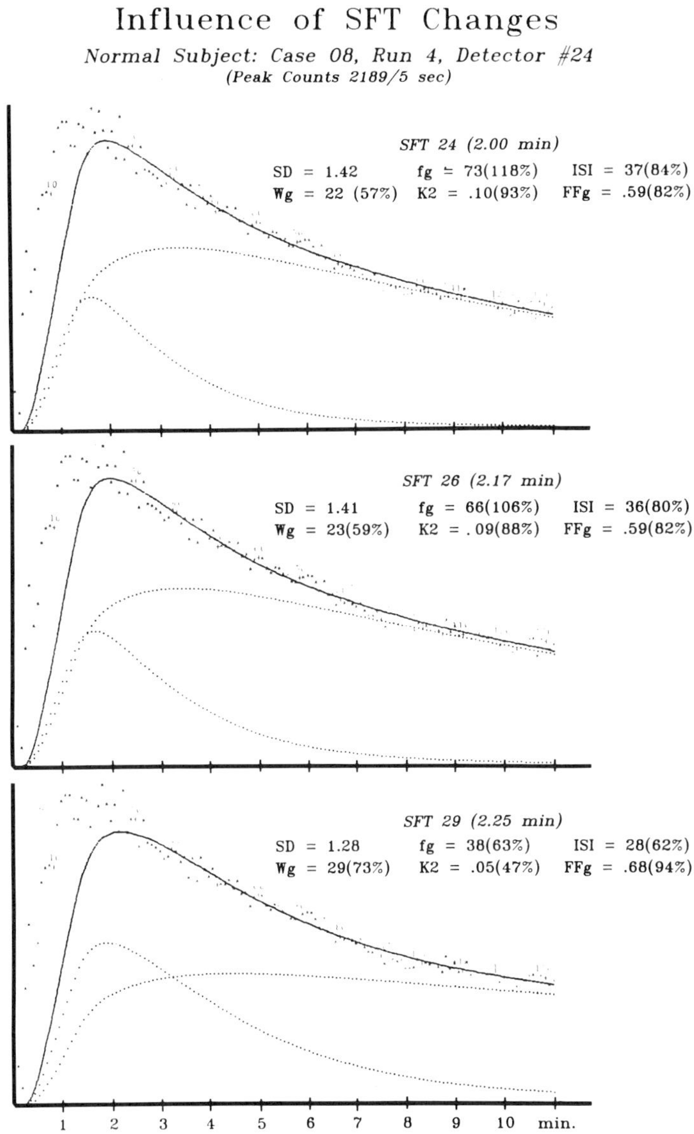

FIGURE 4.4. A single clearance curve from a healthy control subject, analyzed by the Obrist model. The middle panel shows the solution with SFT determined by the Obrist criterion. The upper and lower panels demonstrate substantial changes of flow results when SFT is shifted by −10 seconds and +15 seconds, respectively.

solution was dictated by the usual SFT criterion; the other two solutions were obtained by shifting the SFT only 10 sec earlier or 15 sec later. Obviously, such small shifts of the SFT may well occur solely due to the noise inherent in the air curve, even without physiological changes of respiration. As the figure demonstrates, these small SFT shifts can cause substantial changes of the derived flow parameters, even if the SD (a measure of curve fit) is satisfactory and the visual appearance of the fit is adequate. Generally, later SFTs are associated with lower flow estimates.

Background values for all cerebral detectors must be documented and checked. They should be low and similar in all detectors (again, numerical cutoffs are not provided due to equipment differences). High background values indicate a possible electronics failure, a contamination of air (in which case they are accompanied by high air background) or contamination of the patient, usually because of a recent radionuclide study, rCBF or otherwise. One of the more alarming indicators is high background in the air curve prior to inhalation or injection of the isotope, and its source must be checked. A more complicated situation arises on repeated measurements. As mentioned, a correction for remaining activity has been developed, but has not been implemented by all manufacturers. Some investigators simply wait for the ^{133}Xe to clear from the patient before starting another study. This involves a reduction of throughput, and raises the question of the required waiting interval. Those intervals vary in different laboratories from 15 to 60 min, and our experience (Prohovnik, unpublished data) indicates that 15 min is not enough. The investigators using such short intervals justify them by assuming that by this time the background activity has dropped to some arbitrary level (usually 10–20%) below the expected peak counts of the next measurement. However, this reasoning ignores the fact that it is not the magnitude alone that is of consequence, but the clearance constant as well. A perfectly constant background of high magnitude is less disruptive than a lower background with a clearance rate comparable with that of the phenomena under study. Although the background level may be reasonably low after 15 min, it is still being cleared from the scalp overlying the cerebral tissue, and these clearance rates are confounded in all current models with white-matter cerebral clearance. This may be even more disruptive for those investigators employing longer measurement times (typically, 14 or 15 min). Our experience indicates that a delay interval of about 1 hour is necessary for good results, if a Remaining-Activity Correction (RAC) is not utilized.

When such a correction is employed, its results should be displayed and examined. This correction is essentially a fitting of a monoexponential function (Risberg, 1980), similar in principle to the analysis of the main curve. Its peak, clearance rate, and goodness of fit should be examined just as they are for the main measurement. If the fit is good, the peaks very low (less than 5–10 cps) and the clearance rate uniformly close to zero, the correction was not necessary, and a regular background (linear extrapolation) would have been adequate. If the fit is unsatisfactory, and/or the clearance rates unusual, the procedure should be considered unreliable. In this circumstance, one must access the actual observed data during the background period, and examine them for correctible artifacts. If the data are bad and cannot be corrected, it is usually possible to determine whether the RAC slope was over- or underestimated. From this, the actual flow error can be estimated: the flow results will be distorted in the opposite direction, i.e., underestimation of background slope (such as when using a linear background correction instead of an exponential RAC) will result in overestimation of flow. The magnitude of those errors in flow determination cannot easily be computed, however, and the results cannot be considered numerically adequate. In our experience, normal clearance rates for the RAC are typically .03–.04 sec^{-1}, and peak amplitudes when a measurement is immediately repeated are around 30–60 cps.

Flow Results: Relations Among Parameters and Monoexponential Solutions

The rCBF results themselves may serve as indexes of data quality. When the results are physiologically impossible, or clearly inconsistent with clinical presentation and other evidence, one may suspect technical ambiguities. However, this section is devoted to analysis of data quality that is self-contained, and independent of patient status.

There are several possible indications of technical problems in the results themselves; most of the useful ones necessitate generation and examination of several parameters, and examination of their interrelationships. Normally, the four primary parameters (p_1, p_2, k_1, k_2) are positively correlated. This positive relationship is illustrated for a particular implementation of the simple model in Figs. 4.5–4.7. Thus, higher estimates of fast clearance are usually associated with higher estimates of slow clearance, and clearance is positively associated with compartment size. All else being equal, each p is directly proportional to its respective k, as can easily be seen in the model equations (e.g., Obrist et al., 1975; Prohovnik et al., 1983b). However, with the p value constant, each k will demonstrate a reciprocal relation with its respective w (relative compartment weight), since they are multiplied to obtain p. Normally, thus, one would expect the p to be proportional to k, and a zero correlation between k and w. If p is constrained and cannot covary with k, a negative correlation will emerge between k and w. In addition, under favorable conditions all indexes that reflect level of perfusion (e.g., f_1, k_2, ISI and CBF_{15}, as opposed to w_1) will tend to demonstrate the same phenomena in a given region. If flow is high, it should normally be reflected in all parameters. This is demonstrated most easily by normalizing all parameters to their hemispheric or whole-brain mean, and expressing regional values as percentage of deviation from a mean. It is then expected that all perfusion values will reflect the same tendency (albeit at differ-

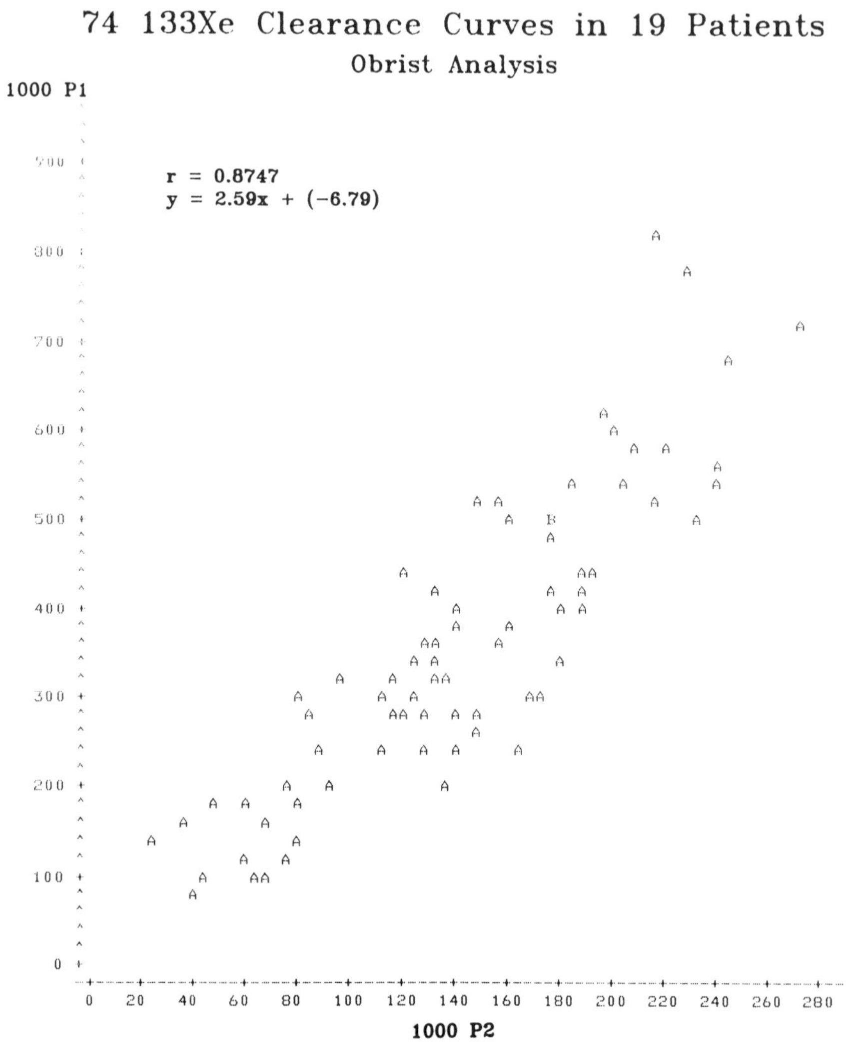

FIGURE 4.5. Compartmental magnitudes of fast and slow clearing matter (p_1 and p_2) are highly correlated. These results were obtained in a sample of 74 curves from 19 patients, using the simple Obrist model. Curves with monoexponential solutions were excluded.

ent sensitivities); i.e., all should be above or all below the mean. A different pattern may indicate degraded solutions.

An extreme breakdown of this relationship is found in the case of monoexponential solutions. Monoexponential solutions of clearance curves can be detected by examining the slow-compartment clearance or the compartmental weights,

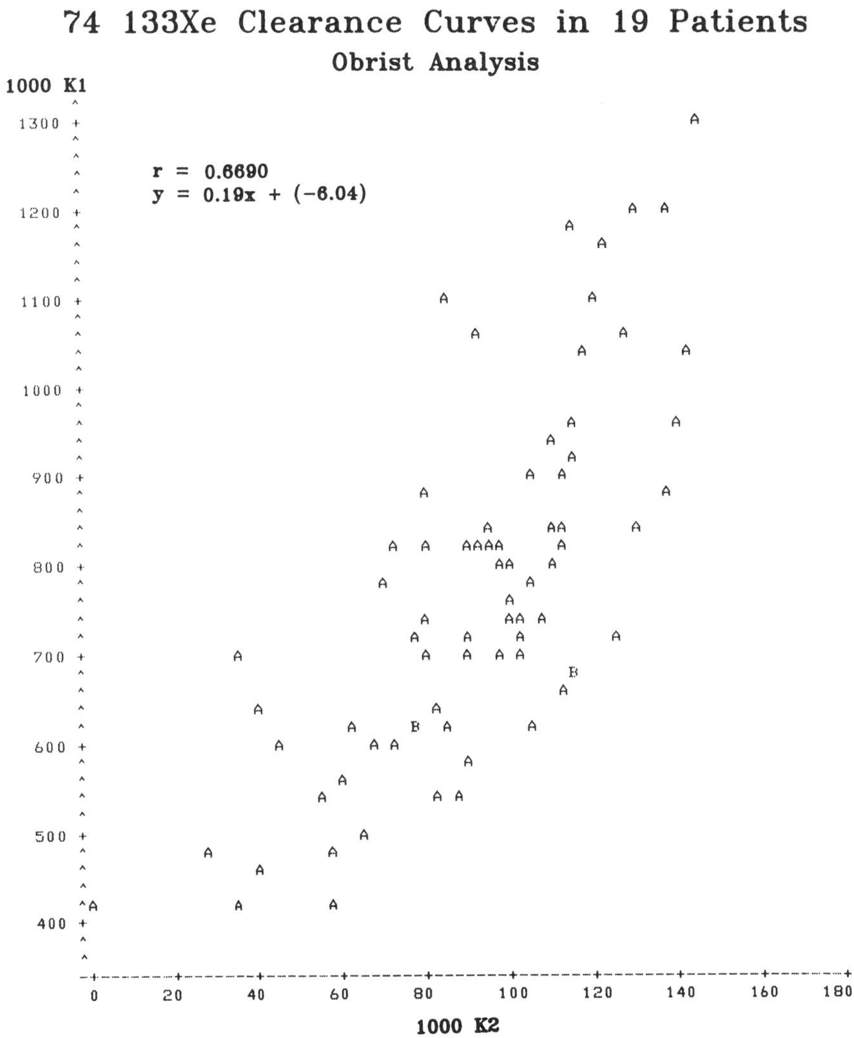

FIGURE 4.6. Clearance rates of the two compartments are also well correlated. Higher white-matter clearance is usually associated with higher gray-matter clearance.

and they represent one of the most extreme forms of degraded data (see Prohovnik, 1984, for a illustrative case). Monoexponential solutions occur when the algorithm cannot distinguish the normally occurring two compartments. The clearance curves are then interpreted as representing a single perfused compartment (actually, the solution will usually indicate a second compartment with slow tracer loading and no clearance). In the absence of technical problems, this

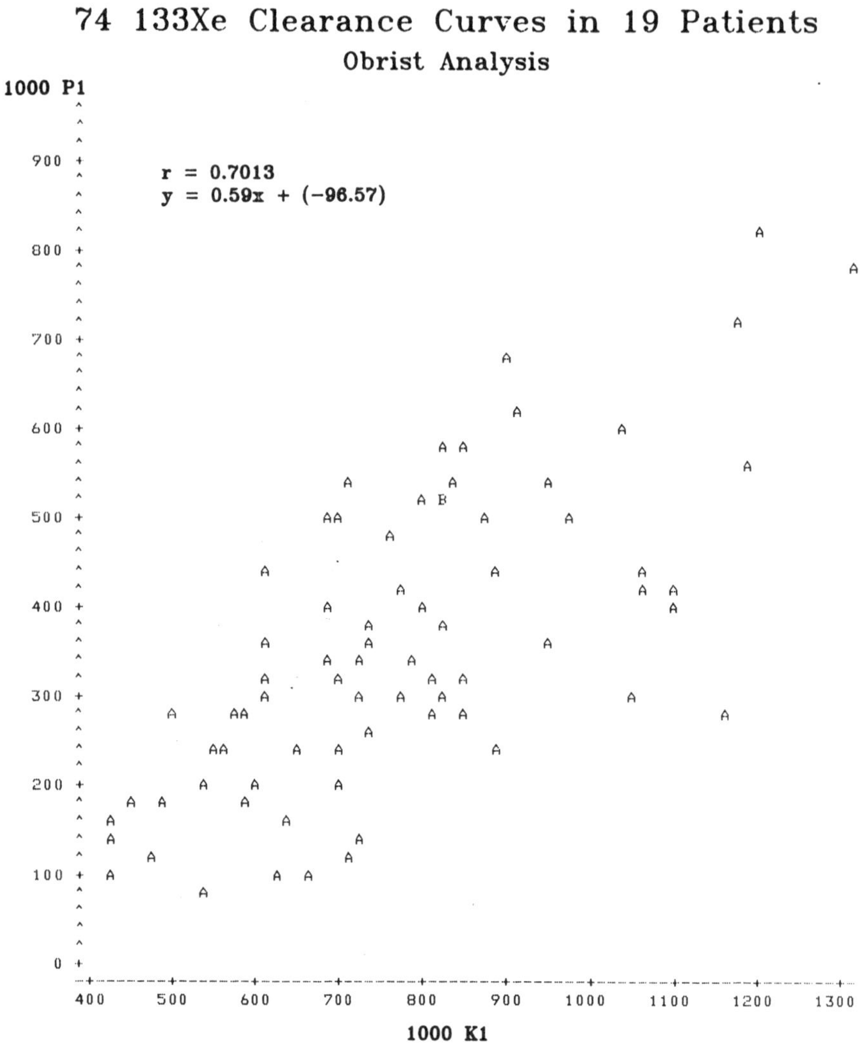

FIGURE 4.7. Within each compartment, clearance rate is correlated with compartmental magnitude. This is easily predicted from the basic equation, where $p = \alpha w \lambda k$; all else being equal, p should be proportional to k.

should occur when the clearance rates of the fast and slow compartments are very close to each other. No disease process is known to increase white-matter flow to levels comparable to gray-matter flow. The opposite, i.e., a depression of gray-matter flow to white-matter levels, can occur in severe pathological conditions such as deep coma, when flow and metabolism are still matched, or in ischemic conditions. It is important to realize that monoexponential solutions do not necessarily indicate the identical flows in both compartments, but only that the compartments cannot be distinguished by the program. A further complication is introduced by the fact that commercially available programs often branch to monoexponential solutions for other reasons, usually indicating degraded data, but the reason for the monoexponential solution is often not provided. It is left to the investigator to interpret the data.

Moreover, the precise setting of several parameters under those conditions is almost arbitrary. For example, given only one compartment, it can be called gray or white, fast or slow, although in fact it is neither but mean tissue perfusion. Depending on whether it is seen as fast or slow, the w_1 value may be set to zero or one; other parameters influenced by w_1, such as CBF_{15}, may then be artifactually increased or decreased. Similarly, either f_1 or k_2 may be set to zero, and the corresponding p value may be zero or nonzero. Under those conditions, the meaningful flow parameter would be some type of Initial Slope Index (ISI). Unfortunately, several commercial systems contain an inaccurate or undocumented version of an ISI, but it is still the best for monoexponential solutions. No flow interpretation should be made, however, until the investigator is confident that the monoexponential solution reflects low flows rather than some technical difficulty.

Slippage

One of the most interesting forms of data degradation is the so-called "slippage". As mentioned, there is normally a zero or weak negative relation between w_1 and f_1. This association is easily explained by considering the bicompartmental flow distribution. Since the fast compartment is rather large, and contains flows varying by at least a factor of two, there may be no clear point at which the "gray matter" ends, especially at the lower end of the range, where flow values may merge into the white-matter range. If the program places the cutoff point between the two compartments too high, so that the lower end of the fast distribution is interpreted as slow matter, the results will demonstrate underestimated w_1 and overestimated f_1, since the remaining gray-matter distribution is weighed by the higher end of the distribution. Thus, underestimating w_1 leads to an overestimated f_1, and therefore the negative correlation. Less often the opposite occurs, with overestimated w_1 and underestimated f_1.

In a preliminary attempt to characterize the occurrence of slippage, we have examined the results of 28 rCBF procedures in 3 elderly patients (underoing a course of electroconvulsive therapy for major depression). We defined slippage in each pair of homologous detectors as an f_1 asymmetry greater than 10% accompanied by reversed w_1 asymmetry of any magnitude. Using this criterion, we found in the 3 patients 3–6 pairs of detectors (out of 16) that evidenced slippage, as an average. In all 3 patients and in all measurements, the M2 analysis (to be discussed) yielded less slippage than the M1 (averages of 5.13, 3.40, and 3.80 pairs with the M2, compared with 5.75, 3.80, and 5.00 with M1). These figures represent approximately 20–30% incidence of this mild form of slippage. Within each patient there were consistent negative correlations between the number of slipped detector pairs and the peak count rates. These correlations ranged from −.14 to −.66 with the peak count rate of the end-tidal air curve, and from .09 to −.77 with the average cerebral peak count rate. However, the correlations were not always statistically significant, and the slipped pairs were not consistently the ones with lowest counts. The location of slipped pairs was also not highly informative. Both M1 and M2 models gave high slippage incidence in the F1 location (using the Novo 32c helmet), which is most anterior and is known to often suffer from leaks and scattered radiation. Other locations with high slippage incidence were more difficult to interpret: they included two other frontal locations (F3,F4), and two parietal ones (C1,P3).

These preliminary data indicate a weak relationship between count rates and slippage incidence, and somewhat better immunity of the M2 model. In clinical situations where slippage may interfere with interpretation of results it is recommended to use a less sensitive indicator (e.g., ISI) or to examine the relative compartment weight (w) along with flow.

Goodness of Fit

A good software package does not rely on the flow data alone, but provides additional indexes of data quality and more ways of examining and manipulating raw data. Perhaps the most important index of quality is an indicator of goodness of fit: the degree to which the least-squares solution has resulted in a fitted (reconstructed) function that really fits well the observed clearance curve. Note that the least-squares algorithm itself ensures, if properly implemented, that the solution found is the best one possible, within the constraints of the physiological model and additional requirements (such as a Start-Fit Time). However, the best solution found may not be good enough, usually due to degraded data. It serves, thus, as a warning to the investigator that there is a major discrepancy between the expectations of the model and the observed data. There are several such indexes that are implemented, with varying degrees of documentation, and several others that have been developed but not commercially implemented (e.g., Prohovnik & Risberg, 1982; Risberg, 1980; Risberg & Prohovnik, 1981).

The fit indexes are, to variable extents, affected by count rates. Count rates should also be independently examined, for reasons that have been outlined. Note, however, that during the measurement procedure only total count rates can be observed. Off-line, it is advisable to examine the different components of the peak count rate, e.g., for the different compartments. When complicated models are used that account for more than the usual two compartments, it is helpful to consider the peak cerebral flow count rate, and some measure of signal to noise, such as the relative magnitude of the cerebral flow compartments in relation to all other sources of counts. In the simple model (Obrist et al., 1975), where a SFT is used, it is important to verify whether the software provides the true peak count rate (reconstructed from the model) or the count rate at SFT. The previously mentioned criteria for peak counts (over 200 cps, preferably 400–1000 cps) refer to purely cerebral flow compartments, and to their true peak.

Graphic Evaluation of Data Quality

In our experience, there is no better way to evaluate data quality than direct examination of the graphic solutions. These consist of a plot of the observed data points, superimposed on the computed clearance functions, with each compartment being separated (see Fig. 4.4 for an illustration). This provides the most thorough evaluation of possible artifacts and their sources, as well as the possibility of correction.

This quality control method is rarely utilized, for several reasons. Some manufacturers do not provide it in commercial systems, or provide it with low quality or without the possibility of correcting errors. Some investigators do not use this method because they are inexperienced in the visual examination of exponential functions, or because it is extremely tedious: The generation and examination of 32 complex curves can be prohibitively time consuming. A solution for this problem has been developed, by the programming of a semi-intelligent routine into a noncommercial software system (Prohovnik & Risberg, 1982). This routine, a primitive expert system, uses several general criteria of quality control (most of which we have listed) to determine which curves were likely to contain problems. The routine then plots for visual examination only those suspected curves. This feature has been found to be highly useful: It is extremely efficient, and because conservative criteria are used, has yet to miss a bad curve.

INTERPRETATION

Parameters

Assuming that data quality has been found to be adequate, the next stage involves the interpretation of results, for a single clinical patient or for a research sample. The first question will probably involve the choice of parameters to be evaluated. Even the simplest physiological model (Obrist et al., 1975) yields 4 primary parameters, and at least 10 others can easily be generated. The f_1 parameter has the most straightforward physiological significance, but it is also highly sensitive to data degradation. There have been several attempts to investigate the utility of different parameters for different purposes and in various pathological populations (e.g., Halsey et al., 1981; Obrist & Wilkinson, 1979). No single parameter has yet emerged as superior under all circumstances, although some form of the ISI is generally considered to be the safest. It is recommended, especially for clinical purposes, to examine several parameters. The w_1 and k_2 parameters are probably most valuable as checks of data quality, although they may, in theory, be of diagnostic value. The f_1 is the most straightforward physiologically, and most sensitive under favorable conditions. Mean tissue perfusion parameters (e.g., CBF_{15}) probably provide the greatest stability, and ISI variants may provide the best combination of stability and sensitivity (see Obrist & Wilkinson, 1985; Prohovnik et al., 1985, for recent simulation tests of those parameters). For some purposes, such as revealing unperfused tissue (Blauenstein et al., 1978; Farrar, 1983) and arteriovenous malformations (Brawanski et al., 1985), the p values or their derivations must be considered.

Models

The choice and interpretation of flow calculations have recently become more complicated because several physiological and mathematical models are available. In addition to Obrist's classic four-unknown model, Hazelrig et al. (1981) and Prohovnik et al. (1981) have introduced six-unknown models. The first incorporates a version of the APA and the lung–brain circulation time, whereas the latter includes the APA and a vascular compartment. We have been using the simple model (M1) and the dual-artifact model (M2) in parallel for some time, and have collected results for comparison in more than 300 patients of different psychiatric and neurological diagnoses. In our experience, the two models are largely comparable, and their results are qualitatively similar in the great majority of cases. In research series, we usually find more reliable and sensitive results with the M2 (e.g., Bilder et al., 1985). In individual clinical cases we tend to place more confidence in the M2 results, as the M1 results often demonstrate substantial artifactual interference in frontotemporal locations. As mentioned, however, the differences are quantitative rather than qualitative. We have found a distinct difference in only one type of pathology so far. This involves the evaluation of arteriovenous malformations, where we find the vascular compartment estimate in the M2 model to be more useful than any other parameter. In other cases, the greatest differences between the models occur during low-flow conditions, and in particular areas more susceptible to blood artifacts, e.g., the anterior–inferior temporal pole. It is probably prudent to continue to use more than one model at the present time. A reasonable policy would be to suspect any case where two models yield conflicting results, until more data accumulate to definitely recommend one over the other. At the present time, our experience indicates that the M2 model is superior to the M1 under all conditions (Prohovnik et al., 1983b) except with severely degraded data, in which case the M1 model is more robust.

Arterial Carbon Dioxide Tension

Traditionally, arterial partial pressure of carbon dioxide ($PaCO_2$) has been known to exert a powerful influence on CBF. Its monitoring by end-tidal values ($PeCO_2$) has become routine in recent years, but has generated the question of the possibility and necessity of correcting CBF values to account for $PaCO_2$ variations.

There are several problems in the monitoring of $PeCO_2$. The first is concerned with the validity of assuming its faithful reproduction of arterial partial pressure. The method is generally assumed to be valid (Jaffe & Bernhart, 1982), in healthy, unanesthesized persons. Anesthesia and pulmonary ventilation-perfusion changes are known to change this relationship, but even under favorable conditions the confidence interval associated with the $PeCO_2$ estimate is unknown. We have obtained preliminary data (Prohovnik & Wolfson, 1984, unpublished data) that indicate a consistent underestimation of $PaCO_2$ and a substantial variance ($r = .66$) in a very small sample ($n = 5$) of unanesthetized surgical patients. We are now examining this more systematically in a larger sample of normal subjects.

Our computational models, deriving from Kety's original work, assume a constant flow (steady state) during the clearance period. To the extent that $PaCO_2$ varies, spontaneously or due to experimental manipulations, it may change CBF and thus violate this assumption. For example, the closed-loop inhalation minute may often be associated with changes in breathing that transiently change $PeCO_2$; gradual relaxation or occasional speech may also result in mild $PeCO_2$ shifts. Should a procedure be invalidated by such changes? And how does one compute average $PeCO_2$ for a measurement if it is not completely steady? How rapidly does CBF change in response to $PaCO_2$ changes?

Satisfactory answers to these questions are not yet available. It is unlikely, however, that procedures should be discarded due to small shifts, gradual or transient, in $PeCO_2$. The problem is sharpest during hypercapnic procedures in some commercial rCBF systems. Inhalation systems that only allow administration of hypercarbic air before and after, but not during, the Xenon inhalation minute generate measurements with abrupt and substantial changes of $PeCO_2$ at the beginning and end of the inhalation minute. We have examined the time constant of these changes, and found it to be rather slow. For example, a sudden change of inhaled air CO_2 concentration from normal to 4% will result in a gradual and relatively slow increase of exhaled concentrations; end-tidal levels will not stabilize at a higher level before 30 sec, and often as long as 40–50 sec. The change in $PaCO_2$ (as reflected by $PeCO_2$) is, thus, slow enough to ignore rapid transient changes of respiration. Even the 1-min inhalation period at normal inhaled CO_2 concentrations may be less of a problem than originally feared. This is supported by the results of transcranial Doppler flow measurements with similar rapid changes of inhaled CO_2 concentrations (Markwalder et al., 1984).

The blood flow changes are relatively slow, with time constants on a similar order of 30–60 sec (Markwalder, personal communication, 1984). It is possible, therefore, to administer hypercapnia before and after, but not during, the inhalation minute without invalidating the results. On the other hand, due to the relatively slow reaction of cerebral vessels to changes of inhaled CO_2 concentration, it is important to allow sufficient time for a dilatation to occur before administering the tracer. When hypercapnic flow values are sought, elevation of inspired CO_2 concentration should start at least 30 sec, and preferably 1 or 2 min before Xenon administration.

Finally, the question of PCO_2 correction often arises. Should individual or group data be corrected to some other PCO_2 value, and if so, to which value and by which correction factor? Such correction factors have been proposed (e.g., Maximilian et al., 1980; Olesen et al., 1971); although exact values are still controversial, the general order of magnitude is established. The practice of correction still differs widely, some investigators insisting on always correcting flow values to a standard PCO_2 value (commonly 40 mmHg), others stating that corrections should never be employed.

Part of the apparent disagreement may be clarified by a discussion of the rationale for PCO_2 corrections. The measurement of rCBF, if properly conducted and interpreted, always provides a valid estimate of cerebral perfusion for a particular time and condition. The results, however, are often employed to draw inferences about cerebral metabolism, or about cerebral perfusion under other conditions. PCO_2 corrections should never be employed to alter the conclusions about current perfusion; the results derived by the analysis of clearance curves, if properly interpreted, are the only possible conclusion about the level of perfusion during the measurement period. However, if inferences about metabolism are indicated, they may be affected by PCO_2 considerations. For example, amphetamine may be expected to raise cerebral metabolism, and therefore flow. However, it also causes hyperventilation, thus lowering $PaCO_2$ and decreasing flow; the observed CBF will reflect the net result of the two opposing mechanisms, and a PCO_2 correction may be necessary to estimate the purely metabolic effect. Similarly, the same low flow which may indicate dangerous ischemia in a normally breathing patient may reflect adequate perfusion in a patient who is severely hyperventilated. Thus, consideration of $PaCO_2$ is indicated for the purpose of inferring either metabolism or the flow-metabolism coupling.

COMMENT

There is a final consideration involved in CBF research that has not been mentioned so far, although it is highly relevant to considerations of data quality and interpretation. This final phase is concerned with the appropriate statistical tools and models for CBF analysis, and it has been left for this comment section mainly because it is still largely unresolved. There have been several sophisticated suggestions about the need for better experimental design and statistical analysis in the field of cerebral blood flow (e.g., Wood, 1980), but a solution is not yet in sight.

The issue of statistical inference does not only apply to those engaged in research. Any clinical impression of a single case is based on implicit, if not explicit, assumptions about the normal appearance of rCBF and the normal range of variation. What constitutes a significant hemispheric asymmetry? Is a 10% local asymmetry as significant in the anterior temporal lobe as in the inferior parietal lobe? Is it as significant in ISI as it is in CBF_{15}? Is gray-matter flow of 60 ml/100g/min normal or low for a 55-year-old male? For example, several authors adopted a strategy for rCBF interpretation that is based on relative flow distributions. The normal flow pattern consists of somewhat higher flow frontally (hyperfrontality) and lower flow temporally. Some authors interpret deviant patterns separately from absolute flow levels. In other words, a normal flow level in frontal regions that is lower than the hemispheric mean may be interpreted as abnormal because it is not hyperfrontal. Others claim that a flow deviation in any region of, e.g., 20% from the hemispheric mean is abnormal, even if the flow level by itself is within normal limits. Such practices are common, but authors rarely state an explicit reasoning or a thorough statistical justification.

There is some information available for purposes of clinical evaluation, but it is of limited value as normative standards vary somewhat as a function of models, parameters, administration routes and instruments. There is a lack of norms for females and for the extremes of the age range. There is also a lack of very detailed norms, which relate the level and variance of flow in a particular detector to other areas of the brain. This is also the area with the greatest need for sophisticated statistical tools for evaluation of group results. Developments in multivariate ANOVA or pattern-recognition algorithms have been mentioned as possible solutions to this most promising, yet most difficult aspect of rCBF data (e.g., Wood, 1980). Some recent attempts at correlational analysis (e.g., Metter et al., 1984) of similar data may also prove useful. This appears to be the next area of challenge for methodological development.

To conclude, this chapter has attempted to present a comprehensive discussion of quality-control aspects in rCBF. Data quality will steadily improve when investigators are made aware of the requirements for quality control, and when they demand such features from commercial manufacturers. It is hoped that this chapter will contribute to this goal.

ACKNOWLEDGMENT

Preparation of this chapter was partly aided by a grant from the Jean and Louis Dreyfus Foundation and by PHS grant AG 05433.

REFERENCES

Ackerman, R. H., Davis, S. M., Correia, J. A., Alpert, N. M., Kelley, R. E., Grotta, J. C., Merrill, E. W., & Rosner, B. (1983). Fibrosinen as a determinant of CBF in health and disease. In M. Reivich & H. I. Hurtis (Eds.), *Cerebrovascular diseases*. New York: Raven Press.

Atkins, H. L., Robertson, J. S., Croft, B. Y., Tsui, B., Susskind, H., Ellis, K., Loken, J., & Treves, S. (1980). Estimation of radiation absorbed doses from radioxenons in lung Imaging. *Journal of Nuclear Medicine, 21,* 459–465.

Baron, J. C., Ackerman, R. H., Correia, J. A., Nelson, C. N., & Taveras, J. M. (1979). Artifactual curves with 133-Xe inhalation rCBF measurement. *Acta Neurologica Scandinavica, 60*(Supp. 72), 238–239.

Berglund, M., & Risberg, J. (1981). Regional cerebral blood flow during alcohol withdrawal. *Archives of General Psychiatry, 38,* 351–355.

Bilder, R., Prohovnik, I., Mukherjee, S., Smith, G., Sackeim, H. A., Rieder, R., & Malitz, S. (1985). Cerebral blood flow in schizophrenia: Morphological and psychometric correlates. Paper presented at the 40th annual convention of the Society of Biological Psychiatry, Dallas.

Blauenstein, U. W., Halsey, J. H. J. R., Wilson, E. M., & Wills, E. L. (1978). 133-Xenon inhalation method: Significance of indicator maldistribution for distinguishing brain areas with impaired perfusion. *Stroke, 9,* 57–66.

Brawanski, A., Maximilian, V. A., & Prohovnik, I. (1985). Delineation of AVMs by arterial blood with noninvasive 133Xenon rCBF. Paper presented at the European Nuclear Medicine Congress, London.

Duckrow, R. B., Beard, D. C., & Brennan, R. W. (1985). Regional cerebral blood flow decreases during hyperglycemia. *Annals of Neurology, 17,* 267–272.

Dunn, W. L., Oswald, W. M., & Wahner, H. W. (1985). Performance evaluation of Xenon-133 inhalation rebreathing systems for regional blood flow measurements. *Journal of Nuclear Medicine, 26,* 783–789.

Farrar, J. K. A. (1981). Computerized technique for the display and comparison of regional cerebral blood flow data. *Stroke, 12,* 22–26.

———. (1983). Detection of cerebral ischemia using 133-Xenon. *Journal of Cerebral Blood Flow and Metabolism, 3*(Suppl. 1), 610–611.

Hall, G. H. (1972). Effects of nicotine, carbon monoxide and tobacco smoke on regional blood flow in the cerebral cortex. *European Journal of Pharmacology, 19,* 385–388.

Halsey, J. H., Kiyohiko, N., & Wariyar, B. (1981). Sensitivity of rCBF to focal lesions. *Stroke, 12,* 631–635.

Hazelrig, J. B., Katholi, C. R., Blauenstein, U. W., Halsey, J. H., JR, Wilson, E. M., & Wills, E. L. (1981). Total curve analysis of regional cerebral blood flow with 133 Xe inhalation. Description of method and values obtained with normal volunteers. *IEEE Transactions on Biomedical Engineering, 28,* 609–615.

Hoffer, P. B., Neumann, R., Quartararo, L., Lange, R., & Hernandez, T. (1984). Improved intrinsic resolution: Does it make a difference. *Journal of Nuclear Medicine, 25,* 230–236.

Jaffe, T. B., & Bernhart, J. (1982). CO_2 Monitoring during cardiopulmonary bypass. *Anesthesiology, 56,* 485.

Kee, D. B., & Wood, J. H. (1984). Rheology of the cerebral circulation. *Neurosurgery, 15,* 125–131.

Kety, S. S., & Schmidt, C. F. (1945). The determination of cerebral blood flow in man by the use of nitrous oxide in low concentrations. *American Journal of Physiology, 143,* 53–66.

Kubota, K., Yamaguchi, T., Abe, Y., Fujiwara, T., Hatazawa, & Matsuzawa, T. (1983). Effects of smoking on regional cerebral blood flow in neurologically normal subjects. *Stroke, 14,* 720–724.

Lassen, N. A., Hoedt–Rasmussen, K., Sorensen, S. C., Skinhoj, E., Cronquist, S., Bodforss, B., Eng, E., & Insvar, D. H. (1963). Regional cerebral blood flow in man determined by Krypton 85. *Neurology, 13,* 719–727.

Mallett, B. L., & Veall, N. (1985). The measurement of regional cerebral clearance rates in man using Xenon-133 inhalation and extracranial recording. *Clinical Science, 1965, 29,* 179–191.

Markwalder, T. M., Grolimund, P., Seiler, R. W., Roth, F., & Aaslid, R. (1984). Dependency of blood flow velocity in the middle cerebral artery on end-tidal carbon dioxide partial pressure—A transcranial ultrasound, doppler study. *Journal of Cerebral Blood Flow and Metabolism, 4,* 368–372.

Mathew, R. J., Barr, D. L., & Weinman, M. L. (1983). Caffeine and cerebral blood flow. *British Journal of Psychiatry, 143,* 604–608.

Maximilian, V. A., Prohovnik, I., & Risberg, J. (1980). Cerebral hemodynamic response to mental activation in normo- and hypercapnia. *Stroke, 11,* 342–347.

Mazziotta, J. C., Phelps, M. E., Carson, R. E., & Kuhl, D. E. (1982). Tomographic mapping of human cerebral metabolism: Sensory deprivation. *Annals of Neurology, 12,* 435–444.

Metter, E. J., Riege, W. H., Kameyama, M., Kuhl, D. E., & Phelps, M. E. (1984). Cerebral metabolic relationships for selected brain regions in Alzheimer's, Huntington's and Parkinson's diseases. *Journal of Cerebral Blood Flow and Metabolism, 4,* 500–506.

Obrist, W. D., Thompson, H. K., King, C. H., & Wang, H. S. (1967). Determination of regional cerebral blood flow by inhalation of 133-Xenon. *Circulation Research, 20,* 124–135.

Obrist, W. D., Thompson, H. K., Wang, H. S., & Wilkinson, W. E. (1975). Regional cerebral blood flow estimated by 133-Xenon inhalation. *Stroke, 6,* 245–256.

Obrist, W. D., & Wang, H. S. (1980). Comparison of 133-Xenon inhalation and IV-injection in regional CBF studies. Cerebral vascular disease. *Proceedings of the 10th International Salzburg Conference, 3,* 140–144.

Obrist, W. D., & Wilkinson, W. E. (1979). The non-invasive Xe-133 method: Evaluation of CBF indices. *Cerebral Circulation,* 119–124.

______. (1985). Stability and sensitivity of CBF indices in the noninvasive 133Xe method. In A. Hartmann & S. Hoyer (Eds.), *Cerebral Blood Flow and Metabolism Measurement.* Berlin: Springer–Verlag.

Olesen, J., Paulson, O. B., & Lassen, N. A. (1971). Regional cerebral blood flow in man determined by the initial slope of the clearance of intra-arterially injected 133Xe. *Stroke, 2,* 519–540.

Prohovnik, I. (1984). Regional cerebral blood flow in psychiatry: Methodological issues. In J. M. Morihisa (Ed.). *Brain imaging in Psychiatry.* Washington, DC: American Psychiatric Press.

Prohovnik, I., Espersen, J. O., & Christensen, F. K. (1983). Development and initial evaluation of a helmet for rCBF measurements. *rCBF Bulletin, 6,* 107–115.

Prohovnik, I., Knudsen, E., & Risberg, J. (1983). Accuracy models and algorithms for determination of fast-compartment flow by noninvasive 133 Xenon clearance. In P. L. Magistretti (Ed.). *Functional radionuclide imaging of the brain.* New York: Raven Press.

______. (1985). Theoretical evaluation and simulation test of the initial slope index for noninvasive rCBF. In A. Hartmann & S. Hoyer (Eds.). *Cerebral blood flow and metabolism measurement.* Berlin: Springer–Verlag.

Prohovnik, I., & Risberg, J. (1982). rCBF data analysis systems. *rCBF Bulletin,* 52–54.

Prohovnik, I., Risberg, J., Mubrin, Z., Bolmsjo, M., & Von Sabsay, E. (1981). Further improvements of the 133–Xe inhalation method. *Journal of Cerebral Blood Flow and Metabolism, 1*(Suppl. 1), 108–109.

Risberg, J. (1980). Regional cerebral blood flow measurements by 133Xe-inhalation: methodology and applications in neuropsychology and psychiatry. *Brain and Language, 9,* 9–34.

Risberg, J., Halsey, J. H., Wills, E. L., & Wilson, E. M. (1975). Hemispheric specialization in normal man studied by bilateral measurements of the regional cerebral blood flow—A study with the 133-Xe technique. *Brain, 98,* 511–524.

Risberg, J., & Prohovnik, I. (1981). RCBF measurements by Xenon 133 inhalation: Recent methodological advances. *Progress in nuclear medicine, 7,* 70–81.
Skinhoj, E., Oleson, J., & Paulson, O. B. (1973). Influence of smoking and nicotine on cerebral blood flow and metabolic rate of oxygen in man. *Journal of Applied Physiology, 35,* 820–822.
Wood, F. (1980). Theoretical, methodological, and statistical implications of the inhalation rCBF technique for the study of brain-behavior relationships. *Brain and Language, 9,* 1–8.

5 Functional and Vascular Challenge Procedures During Noninvasive rCBF Measurements

V. A. Maximilian,
A. Brawanski
Department of Neurosurgery, University of Würzburg, Federal Republic of Germany

Functional and vascular challenge procedures may increase the clinical utility of regional cerebral blood-flow (rCBF) measurements. This chapter is devoted to an analysis of the various activation procedures which have been implemented to date and attempts to assess their contribution to clinical decision making.

BASE-LINE rCBF MEASUREMENTS

Before appraising effects of supplementary activation procedures upon cerebral hemodynamics we must first discuss the conditions for accurate base-line rCBF measurements against which induced flow changes can be compared. Base-line, or "resting" rCBF measurements are ideally performed in a quiet, semidarkened laboratory where the supine patient, already familiarized with the measurement condition, keeps his eyes closed and breathes in a relaxed manner through a face mask. Due to the fact that we are measuring an *functional* parameter reflecting neuronal metabolism (Cooper et al., 1975; Raichle et al., 1976; Sokoloff, 1981), these are the only precautions we can take in order to approach a steady state condition. One may correct for pCO_2, Hb, Hct, and other variables influencing the cerebrovascular bed, but changes in ongoing mental processes throughout the CBF examination, which lasts several minutes, can not be controlled. We can, however, ensure a measurement procedure that excludes as many extraneous variables as possible. The reason why such emphasis is put on this issue is that only on the basis of reliable steady state measurements we can meaningfully interpret the blood-flow changes during activation.

Assessment of rCBF Results

For the clinical interpretation of a single rCBF measurement we should compare:

1. Perfusion level of one hemisphere vs. the other; in normal brains under normal conditions the hemispheric flow values are nearly identical,
2. Perfusion level in contralateral, homotopic detectors since rCBF is normally symmetrical and,
3. mean hemispheric values and regional flow distribution compared with normative values.

Cerebral blood-flow level has been shown to decrease with age (Hagstadius & Risberg, 1983, see Fig. 5.1; Meyer et al., 1978, see Fig. 5.8; Yamamoto et al., 1980, see Fig. 5.17), an important factor to consider when comparing individual CBF with a "normal" population.

The regional flow distribution obtained by noninvasive ^{133}Xe techniques is reproducible and correlates with the results obtained with the intra-arterial (IA) injection method. The rCBF pattern is characterized by what Ingvar (1976) has termed the "hyperfrontal distribution of the cerebral gray matter flow in resting wakefulness." As illustrated in Fig. 5.2, rCBF is normally 10–15% above the mean hemispheric flow level in frontal regions, at mean level centrally, and 5–10% below the mean postcentrally (see Fig. 5.27 for gray-matter rCBF distribu-

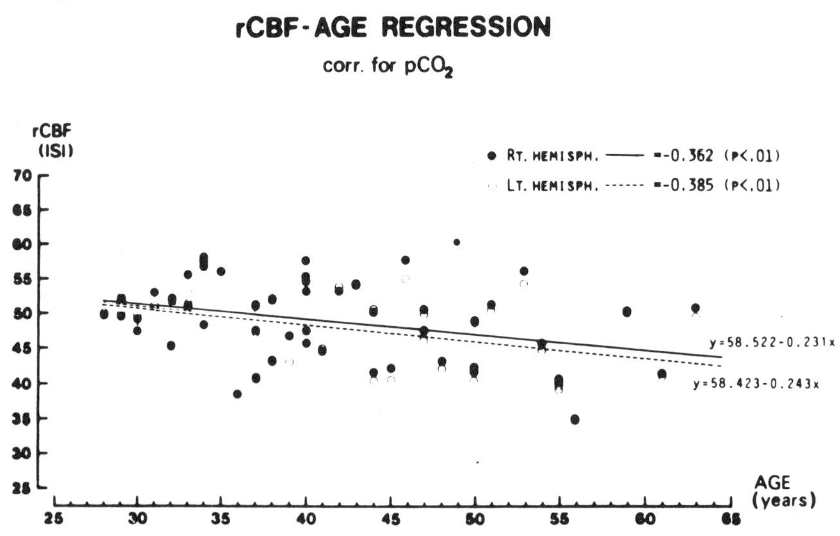

FIGURE 5.1. The regression lines for the right and left hemispheres respectively. The ISI values were corrected for PCO_2. (From Hagstadius & Risberg, 1983, with permission.)

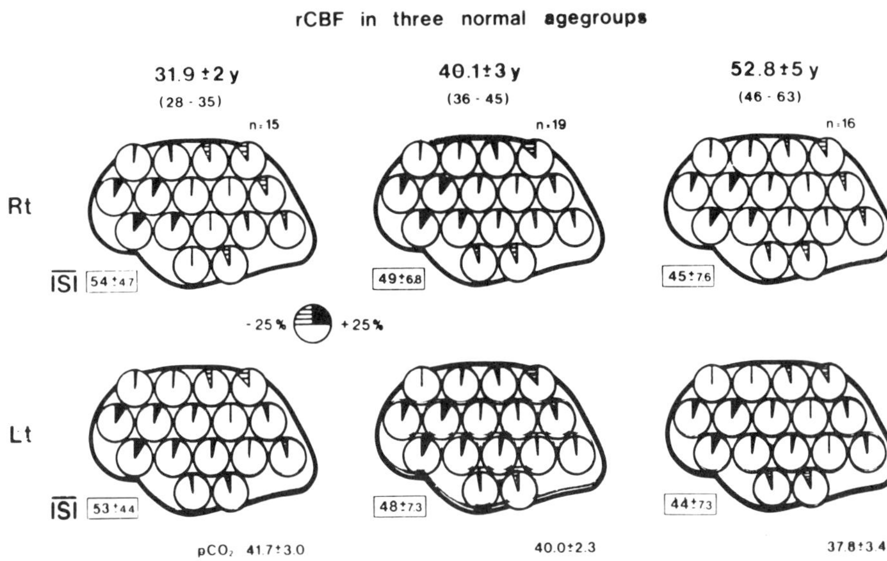

FIGURE 5.2. Base-line rCBF (ISI) in three normal age groups.

Left: × age 31.9 + 2y (28–35)
Middle: × age 40.1 + 3y (36–45)
Right: × age 52.8 + 5y (46–63)

Mean hemispheric flows (ISI) are shown in the boxes. Regional distribution flows are shown as deviations from the mean; black shadowing indicates a value higher than the mean, striped is lower than the mean. A 25% deviation from the mean is equal to 90° in the clock symbols. Average pCO_2 for each age group is shown at the bottom. (From Hagstadius & Risberg, 1983, with permission.)

tion pattern in ml/100 gr/min). This flow distribution appears not to change with advancing age. While there are no morphological determinants for this particular blood-flow landscape, a variety of functional explanations has been suggested (Prohovnik et al., 1980). The most practical interpretation of the typical base-line rCBF pattern is that it probably reflects normal ongoing mentation, general arousal, and control of behavior during the blood-flow examination; in other words no more and no less than "resting wakefulness" in a peculiar environment.

It should be emphasized, however, that even a thorough evaluation of base-line flow data according to the suggested criteria may not present an adequate assessment of the patient's hemodynamic status. Regional cerebral blood flow may be normal at rest but become abnormal when challenged under controlled stress conditions. Increasing evidence has emerged that more information can be obtained when base-line rCBF examinations are supplemented by flow measurements aimed at testing the hemodynamic response during specific cerebrovascular or functional activations.

FUNCTIONAL ACTIVATIONS

Functional activations in this context comprise what are variously referred to as behavioral, mental, psychological, or psychophysiological tests administered to the patient during the rCBF measurement. Sokoloff et al. (1955) were among the first to consider the possibility of activation when they measured oxygen uptake and blood flow with the Kety–Schmidt technique in a group of subjects performing mental arithmetic. Although no changes were found as a result of the activation procedure, Sokoloff and colleagues pointed out that flow redistributions in specific locations could have occurred and would probably not be detected by a method measuring global cerebral perfusion.

By means of a thermoelectrical technique, Cooper et al. (1975) lent support to Sokoloff's hypothesis by finding flow increases restricted to the occipital lobes during reading. However, already in 1965 Ingvar and Risberg (1965) commenced their prolific collaboration in the field of applied intrameasurement activation in clinical situations. They used the IA ^{133}-Xe injection technique for measuring flow during mental effort elicited by a digit-span-backward task. Placing four scintillation detectors over the left hemisphere (one per lobe), the authors were able to find not only a general flow increase during activation, but also a regional redistribution with the largest flow increases centrally and postcentrally, whereas perfusion decreased in the temporal region. This type of rCBF determinations developed by Ingvar and Risberg (Ingvar et al., 1975; Ingvar, 1976; Ingvar & Schwartz, 1974; Risberg & Ingvar, 1973) progressed to the well-known clinical research at Lassen's laboratory in Copenhagen (Larsen et al., 1977; Orgogozo & Larsen, 1979; Roland & Lassen, 1976). Using a high-resolution 254-detector system, Lassen and colleagues obtained functional rCBF landscapes of unparalleled sensitivity and specificity during a variety of activation tasks. In comparison, noninvasive blood-flow measurement techniques have a poorer resolution. The advantage of noninvasive rCBF techniques however, is that they can be used for repeated, bilateral assessments in normal as well as diseased subjects and as a result, it has given considerable insight into neuropsychological processes.

Functional Challenge in Healthy Subjects

Functional challenge procedures, which are usually performed after the base-line flow study, may comprise a variety of visual, auditory, tactile and stereognostic stimulation as well as arithmetic, verbal, and nonverbal, cognitive, mnestic, problem-solving, and other types of psychological performance tests. The activation procedure should be preferably designed in a manner engaging the subject throughout the rCBF measurement; this is not merely important for maintaining a stable measurement condition, but also to ensure that the hemodynamic response only represents the functional activity induced by the activation task per se.

HEMISPHERIC SPECIALIZATION

Risberg et al. (1975) were the first to use bilateral, noninvasive CBF measurements during functional activation. In a systematic study aimed at assessing hemispheric specialization in processing verbal and nonverbal material, the authors performed four rCBF measurements on each subject, two during base-line recordings, one during verbal (Miller Analogy Test) and one during a spatial test (Street-Test). In addition, they evaluated the effect of motivation upon the hemodynamic response to activation by dividing the subjects into two groups, one of which was promised a higher reward pending better test performance. In the more motivated group, flow increased 16% in the left and 13% in the right hemisphere during verbal task, and 7% and 10% in the left and right hemispheres respectively during spatial activation. Regional asymmetries were seen in the left occipital and parietal locations during the verbal activation with frontal and parietal asymmetries appearing during spatial processing. The rCBF data in the "poorly" motivated group showed a similar trend, but the results were not statistically significant. Risberg and coworkers thus confirmed the potential for distinguishing between two different types of mental activations, even with only seven detectors per hemisphere.

Similar results were also reported by Gur and Reivich (1980) and Gur et al. (1982), who found significant left–right rCBF differences, depending on whether the subjects performed a verbal or a spatial task during the flow investigation. These activation-induced asymmetries demonstrate that despite the "cross-talk" artifact which tends to diminish differences between homologous, contralateral detectors, in two-dimensional, noninvasive CBF techniques, significant interhemispheric differences may nevertheless emerge. In addition, the results of Risberg et al. (1975) indicated the influence of the motivational factors which have to be taken into consideration during functional activations requiring concentration and mental effort from the patient.

Encouraged by the results of Risberg et al. (1975), several CBF laboratories evaluated the implementation of various functional challenge procedures. The obvious implication was that if a specific neuropsychological activation could elicit significant flow increases in the healthy brain, such tests might be put as an objective parameter in assessing cerebral dysfunction. In this context significant flow increases are those induced and reproduced during a specific task associated with relatively well-localized cortical areas.

The issue of cortical localization had been addressed by Ingvar and Risberg, who in 1967 suggested that activation induced flow increases possibly represent a combination of well-localized task-specific response and diffuse general arousal components. Risberg and Ingvar (1973) found discrete frontal and postcentral flow increases in patients studied twice with the IA technique during performance of the reasoning test. This study was replicated by Risberg et al. (1977), using the ^{133}Xe inhalation technique with eight detectors covering the left cerebral hemisphere but this time the group comprised healthy volunteers. All subjects were studied four times over a 48-hour period in a counterbalanced rest–test design with daily rCBF measurements during base-line and activation by a visually presented problem-solving task (Raven's Advanced Progressive Matrices). On the first day, significant flow increases similar to those reported by Risberg and Ingvar (1973) were found in frontal and postcentral detectors. When rCBF measurements were repeated on the second day, however, the activation induced flow increases localized to postcentral areas. These results suggested that frontal regions were not specifically involved in the actual problem-solving process, but instead probably related to factors such as behavioral control or apprehension induced by the rCBF measurement conditions, to which the subjects subsequently habituated.

The extent of frontal lobe involvement during cognitive processes was further examined in Risberg's laboratory by Maximilian et al. (1978). Repeated rCBF measurements were performed during both learning and recalling lists of visually presented verbal material. During both mnestic activations, flow increased significantly in parieto-occipital regions. Reproducible frontal increases, however, were found solely during the learning task sessions (and not during recalling) which suggested that habituation of frontal activity is not a generalized phenomenon when all types of brain work are considered.

BRAIN-BEHAVIORAL RELATIONSHIP TO rCBF ACTIVATION RESPONSE

The degree of neurofunctional challenge is an important factor influencing the hemodynamic response. Monoaural left- or right-ear stimulation by a simple verbal listening task resulted in a small but significant temporo-parietal asymmetry, but not in a marked increase from base-line levels (Maximilian, 1982). Significant flow increases localized practically in the same cortical region were obtained, however, by Knopman et al. (1980, 1984) during a series of experiments using more demanding verbal and nonverbal auditory stimuli (Fig. 5.3). By comparison, during an aurally presented continuous verbal memorization activation procedure, where continuous attention and rapid memory operations switching between storage and retrieval of aurally presented word pairs are

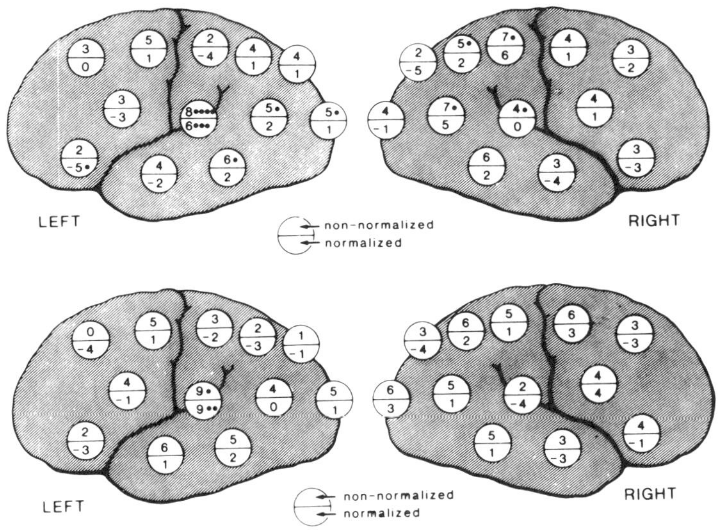

FIGURE 5.3. rCBF changes from base line during verbal (A) and nonverbal (B) auditory stimulation. Within the circles, the number above the line indicates absolute regional ISI values, the one below indicates the difference relative to the hemispheric mean. $+p.01 < p < .05$; $++.005 < p < .01$; $+++.001 < p < .005$; $++++p < .001$ (From Knopman et al., Permission granted by Academic Press, New York. *Brain and Language 9,* 93–112, 1980.

required, Prohovnik et al. (1983) obtained large and significant bihemispheric flow increases, especially in inferior left temporal regions (Fig. 5.4).

The relation between functional demand and hemodynamic response in terms of regional distribution and magnitude was further evidenced by Risberg and Prohovnik (1983). A group of eight healthy subjects was asked to look through the eyepiece of a Spiral-After-Effect (SAE) apparatus, first at a stationary and then at a rotating spiral with no further instructions other than to relax. During the third rCBF measurement, subjects were required to concentrate and report the visual illusion induced by the SAE test. Consequently, the experimental design included three similar conditions of visual perception, yet all differing in visual processing complexity. As can be seen in Fig. 5.5, rCBF was higher during the rotating as compared with the stationary spiral perception session and further, significant increases in cerebral perfusion were obtained during the SAE task.

A subsequent experiment involved repeated rCBF measurements during tactile stimulation of the left and right hand. Here subjects were either instructed to relax and ignore the weak stimulation which was automatically applied by a device with nine small pins moved by compressed air (sensation condition), or carefully attend and report when only one of the pins actually touched the hand.

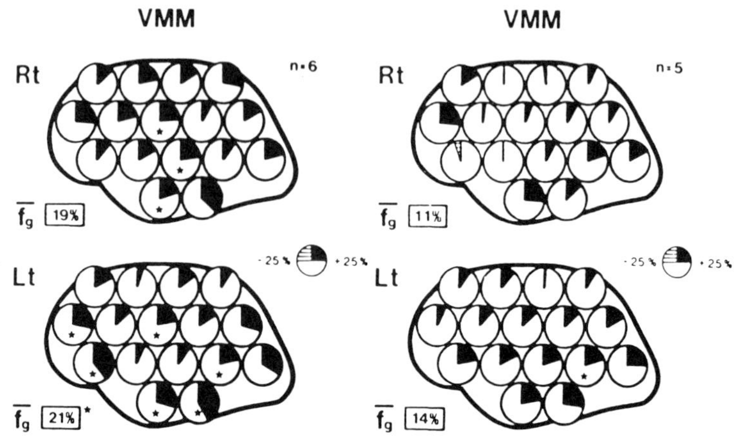

FIGURE 5.4. Flow increases during (A) Continuous verbal report of retrieved word pairs, (B) Infrequent verbal response. (From Prohovnik et al.; permission granted by Raven Press, New York; temporal lobe activation by verbal memorization studied with ^{133}Xenon inhalation rCBF; *J. of Cerebral Blood Flow and Metabolism 3,* (Suppl. 1), S276–277, 1983.)

The clearly divergent hemodynamic responses obtained with this experimental design are illustrated in Fig. 5.6. Interesting to note were the marked activation induced differences between the left- and right-hand tactile attention measurements, which were probably related to increased cognitive effort during selective attention to the left hand in strictly right-handed subjects. Similar results were

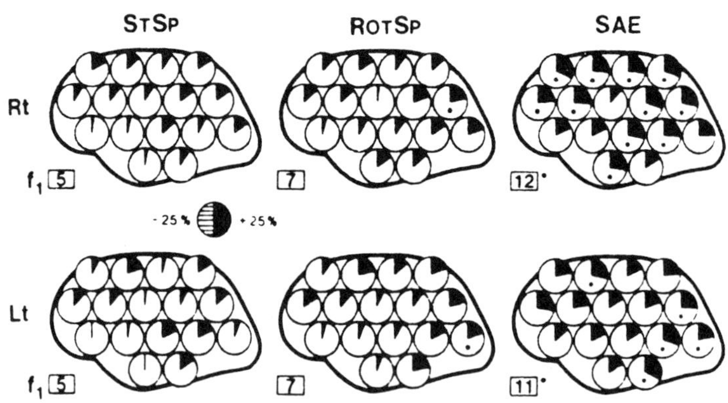

FIGURE 5.5. rCBF increases from base-line level during three visual stimulation conditions: stationary spiral (left), rotating spiral (middle) and Spiral-After-Effect (right). $p < .05$. (From Risberg & Prohovnik; Permission granted by Springer-Verlag, New York; *Human Neurobiology 2,* 5–10, 1983.)

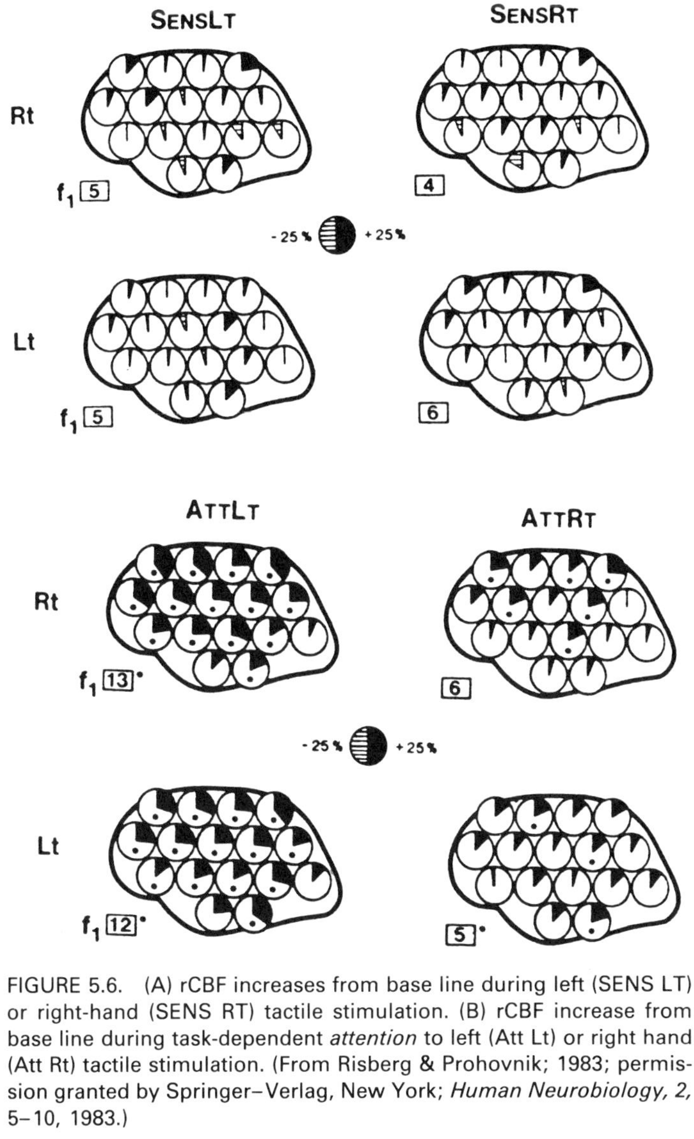

FIGURE 5.6. (A) rCBF increases from base line during left (SENS LT) or right-hand (SENS RT) tactile stimulation. (B) rCBF increase from base line during task-dependent *attention* to left (Att Lt) or right hand (Att Rt) tactile stimulation. (From Risberg & Prohovnik; 1983; permission granted by Springer–Verlag, New York; *Human Neurobiology, 2,* 5–10, 1983.)

obtained by Halsey et al. (1979, 1980), who measured rCBF in a group of right-handed subjects during a task consisting of repeatedly opposing in succession the thumb to each finger of either the right or left hand; while the flow increases were most prominent in the rolandic region contralateral to the active hand, the largest response was again found in the right hemisphere during the left-hand finger movement task (Fig. 5.7).

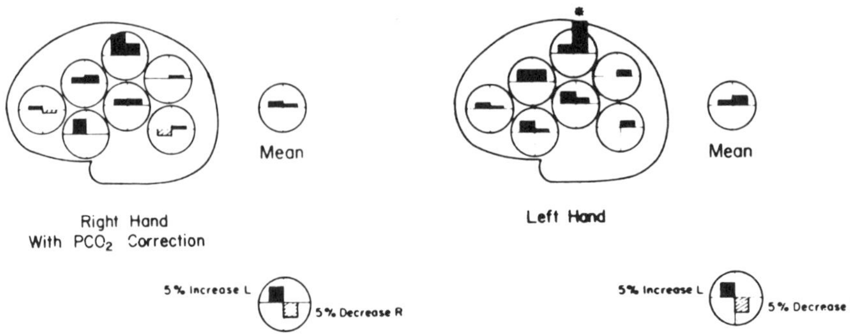

FIGURE 5.7. Right- and left-hand finger movement in right-handed healthy volunteers. (From Halsey et al.; Permission granted by Academic Press, New York; *Brain and Language 9,* 47–60, 1980.)

Wood et al. (1980) were among the first to study divergence of rCBF response between two different cognitive tasks which were based on an identical stimulation input. Subjects were instructed to perform a recognition test and a semantic classification task based on the same list of aurally presented words. The authors found significantly larger flow increases in the left hemisphere during the semantic classification task in comparison with recognition of the words.

Leli et al. (1984) have shown that it is possible to deconfound the rCBF response induced by a complex cognitive task from its sensory–motor components. During a visually presented right–left discrimination task, the subjects were asked to push a button for the correct response. In the sensory–motor control task, the subjects had to push the button each time a blank slide appeared on the screen. Whereas significant flow changes were obtained during both activations, significantly higher flow increases were found during the right–left discrimination task in comparison with the sensory–motor control study in the a priori hypothesized parieto-occipital regions. In a recent report Leli et al. (1984) have shown that even the sensory–motor task components may significantly alter the hemodynamic response to a specific activation procedure. Significantly divergent rCBF distribution patterns were reported during performance of identical visually presented number recognition tasks to which the subjects had to respond orally in one study and manually in the other. It consequently emerges that rCBF increases, during neurobehavioral challenge, are not only related to the nature of the task, but also to its sensori-motor components and effort required during its performance.

FUNCTIONAL HEMODYNAMIC RESPONSE AND AGING

Meyer et al. (1978) reported significant differences between mean base-line CBF and mean CBF values during a "multiple psychophysiological activation procedure'' (a task combing motor, sensory, speech, arithmetic, and audiovisual stimulation) in a group of 14 healthy controls aged 24 to 62 ($\bar{x}$ age 42 +/− 14). Whereas both mean hemispheric base-line and activation flow levels decreased with age, the *hemodynamic response* to functional challenge was very similar in younger and older subjects (Fig. 5.8). This suggests that the cerebral functional reserve is not impaired in elderly, healthy subjects.

That capacity to increase CBF during mental activity is preserved with age although base-line rCBF values were lower in the older age groups was also shown by Hagstadius and Risberg (1983). Aging did not impair the rCBF response to a visual-spatial constructive task (puzzle test), indeed older healthy subjects actually presented higher increases that the younger controls (Fig. 5.9). Test performance, however, was significantly lower in the oldest subjects when compared with the younger groups and significant negative correlations were found between both age and performance, as well as performance and activation induced flow increases. The author proposed that the larger flow increments seen in the senior subjects reflected the greater effort demanded by the task and the increased frontal rCBF, seen only in this group, was attributed to higher levels of arousal. Similar results were obtained by Risberg and Hagstadius (1984) in a study assessing effects of exposure to a mixture of neurotoxic organic solvents (e.g., ketones, aromatic hydrocarbons, ethers, alcohols, etc.) in occupationally exposed factory workers; the group of workers with the higher exposure levels performed worse on the activation task, but demonstrated larger flow increases.

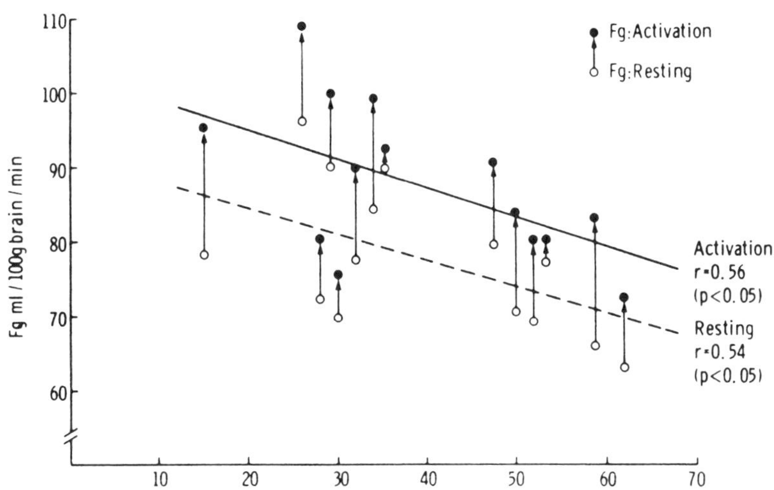

FIGURE 5.8. Correlation of hemispheric mean gray-matter flow (Fg) values with advancing age for both resting values (quiet, dark) and during multiple psychophysiological activation (motor speech and audiovisual stimulation) in normal volunteers (*n.* = 14), aged 40 ± 14 years. (From Meyer et al., *Archives of Neurology, 35,* 350–359, 1978; with permission.)

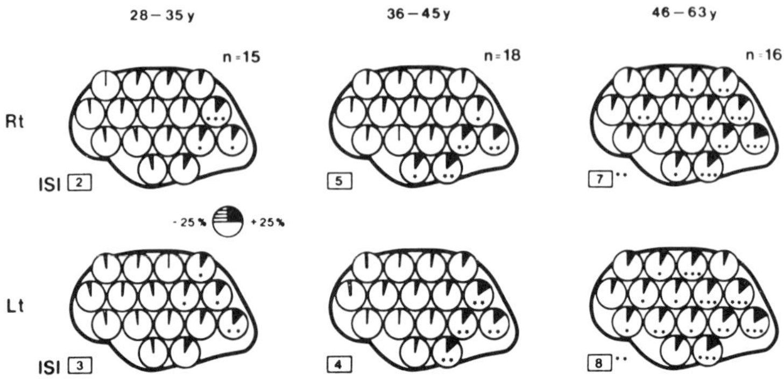

FIGURE 5.9. Changes of ISI% in three age groups of healthy volunteers during a visually presented visuospatial constructive task (Puzzle test). Left: 28–35 years, Middle: 36–45 years, Right: 46–63 years. (From Hagstadius & Risberg, 1983; with permission.)

CBF AND PERFORMANCE

The previous findings bring to mind the issue addressed by Lassen during the seventh international CBF and Metabolism Symposium 1977, in Copenhagen. During a discussion pertaining to the significance of flow increases during cerebral activity, Lassen wondered if the better chess player comfortably winning his game would have a higher or lower rCBF than his less gifted opponent. In view of the preceding results, it appears that the losing chess player would have been the one with the higher perfusion. The exact reason remains obscure: Several interplaying factors, such as motivation, stress, increased effort, or simply harder "brain work," could have necessitated activation of more extensive cortical areas. Further examples in the following section will also show that mildly impaired patients may demonstrate higher hemodynamic responses during functional activation than either those more severely damaged, or even normal controls.

The combination of a low rCBF response to a specific mental task and poor performance could be used as an indication of neurofunctional impairment. This is illustrated in the following example. Maximilian et al. (1982) studied the effects of long-term exposure to neurotoxic organic solvents on CBF in 32 industrial workers. These workers differed from the group investigated by Risberg and Hagstadius in that they were symptomatic patients who sought medical aid for a variety of symptoms such as tiredness, memory disturbance, dizziness, and headache. They had been exposed to organic solvents for an average time of 24.5 years. All patients were studied during base-line and verbal memory activation. Compared with the normative data of Maximilian et al.

(1978), during the performance of an identical task (learning of word pairs), only minor activation was seen in left-hemispheric postcentral regions, and no frontal flow response was demonstrated. Recall performance, tested after the verbal learning activation, was significantly lower than that found in healthy subjects (30 vs. 50 recalled word pairs). Significant negative correlations were obtained between age and CBF, and length of exposure and CBF. Recall performance was also significantly inversely related to length of exposure, but not with age. To control for the effect of aging per se, patients were divided in two age-matched subgroups consisting of a "shorter exposed" (SE) group ($\bar{x}$ age 50, $\bar{x}$ exposure

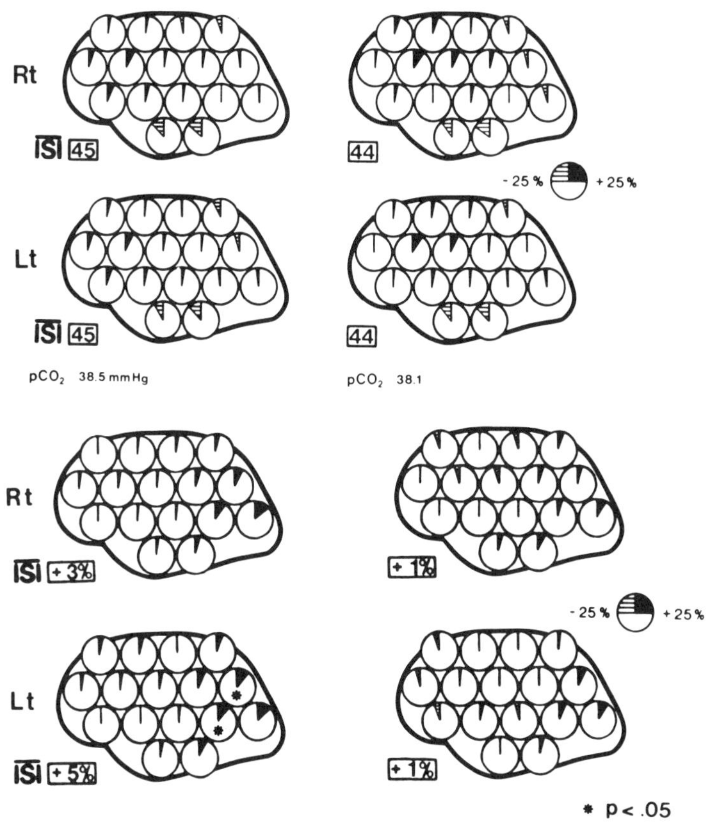

FIGURE 5.10. (A) rCBF distribution in age-matched symptomatic industrial workers exposed to toxic solvents. Left: Short exposed group ($\bar{x}$ 13 y), $N = 10$, × age 50. Right: Long exposed group ($\bar{x}$ 31 y), $N = 10$, × age 49. (B) rCBF changes from base line during a visually presented verbal memory test. Left: Short exposed subjects. Right: Long exposed subjects. (From Maximilian et al.; Permission granted by Academic Press, New York; *Brain and Cognition 1,* 196–205, 1982.)

length 13 years) and a "longer exposed" (LE) group ($\bar{x}$ age 49, $\bar{x}$ exposure length 31 years). As evident from Fig. 5.10a, there were practically no differences between the bihemispheric base-line landscape and flow levels.

During challenge by the learning task, however, small, but statistically significant differences were found between groups, both in mean hemispheric levels (especially in the left), as well as significant regional flow increases localized postcentrally and displayed only by the shorter exposed patients (Fig. 5.10b). Performance was also significantly higher in the SE group (35 vs. 21 recalled items). Significant negative correlations between age, CBF and exposure variables were found only in the longer exposed patients on this occasion. These results were interpreted as a combined effect of aging and prolonged exposure to neurotoxic agents in the LE group, perhaps attributable to the gradually evolving organic brain syndrome reported in occupationally exposed workers (Münchinger, 1963).

CLINICAL APPLICATIONS OF NEUROFUNCTIONAL ACTIVATIONS

Meyer et al. (1978) tested differences in cerebrovascular functional reserve between a group of healthy subjects and patients with left carotid occlusion. Healthy controls demonstrated a 14% CBF increase in the left hemisphere and 11% in the right during activation but only minimal flow changes were evident in patients with multi-infarct dementia (Fig. 5.11a). Patients with left-carotid occlusion displayed reduced flows on the affected side with relatively well-preserved functional reserve in the right hemisphere (Fig. 5.11b). By comparison, 11 patients with mild to moderate Alzheimer's disease displayed no flow increases whatsoever during the same activation procedure (Fig. 12; Meyer et al. 1980).

Largen et al. (1981) reported that patients with early putative Alzheimer's disease had significant bihemispheric mean CBF response of 18% during Raven matrices problem solving with diffusely spread regional flow increases between 10% to 29%, although base-line flows were lower than normal, the increase in flow which occurred during activation meant that "activated" flow values were nearly the same as in controls, in whom only a 2% increase from base line was measured. The authors attributed the patient's excessive flow increases to the considerable effort demanded in solving what appeared to be a simple task for controls, and suggested that the similarity in mean CBF levels during activation may indicate that task performance is related to a typical flow level (see also Risberg et al., 1977 and Maximilian et al., 1980). Here again we see an example of low base line flow levels coupled to high flow increases.

Similar results were reported in normal elderly subjects by Hagstadius and Risberg (1983), who found that in the oldest poorer performing individuals (see

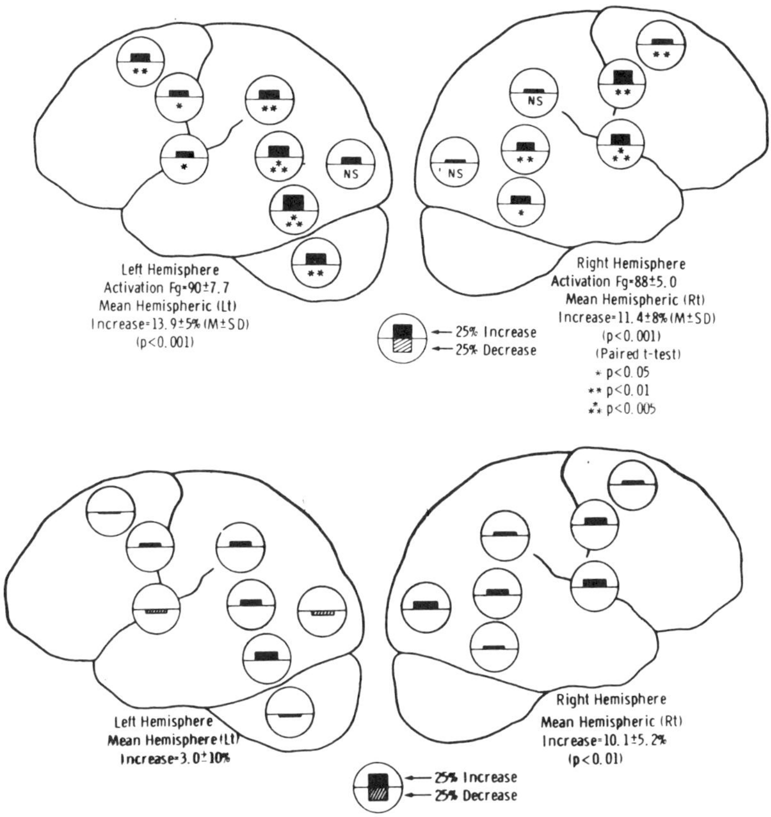

FIGURE 5.11. (A) Regional increases of gray-matter flow (Fg) during cerebral activation (motor speech and audiovisual stimulation) compared with values at rest in quiet darkness in normal volunteers $N = 14$ aged 40 ± 14 years. Resting: MABP = 89.7 mm Hg $PECO_2$ = 37.5 mm Hg, activation: MABP = 90.1 mm Hg. (B) Regional gray-matter flow (Fg) changes during multiple psychophysiological activation (motor speech and audiovisual stimulation compared with values at rest (quiet, dark) in patients with left carotid occlusion ($N = 4$), aged 56 to 70 years. Resting: MABP = 96.2 mm Hg, $PECO_2$ = 38.2 mm Hg; activation: MABP = 97.0 mm Hg, $PECO_2$ = 37.6 mm Hg. (From Meyer et al., *Archives of Neurology 35,* 350–359, (1978; with permission.))

Fig. 5.9), increased effort induced a nonlocalized, excessive flow response. This functionally determined excessive perfusion may be ascribed to the involvement of larger parts of the cortex during the task performance. The discrepancy in the activation induced flow changes between the patient group of Largen et al. (1981) and lack of response in those studied by Meyer et al. (1980) could partly be explained by differences in clinical condition but also by the employed func-

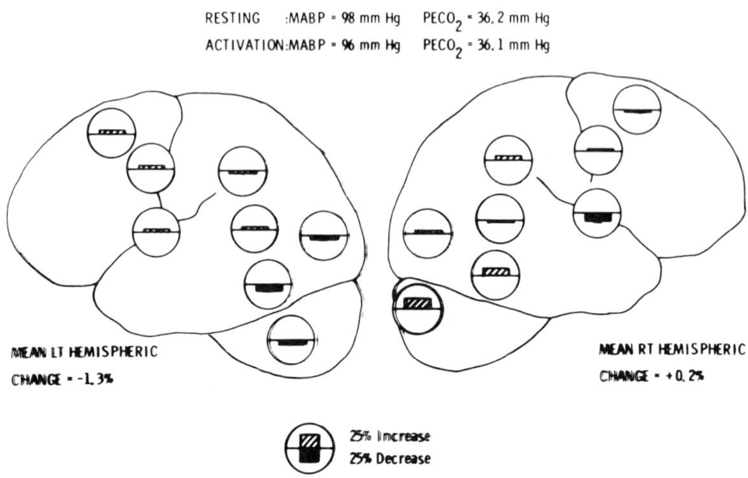

FIGURE 5.12. Schematic diagram to show changes during behavioral activation in regional F1 values over both cerebral hemispheres and brain stem-cerebellar regions in 11 right-handed patients with mild to moderate dementia due to Alzheimer's disease. The mean age was 65 + 10 years. There was no significant change in mean blood pressure or $PECO_2$ between the two measurements. There is a diffuse failure of regional F1 increases (compared with normals) over both cerebral hemispheres and the brain stem-cerebellar regions. (From Meyer et al.; Permission granted by Academic Press, New York; *Brain and Language 9,* 61–77, 1980.)

tional activation procedure which demanded divergent cognitive processing and motivational involvement from the patient. Raven's matrices problem solving require both concentration and employment of specific strategies for their solution. The multiple psychophysiological activation on the other hand is a relatively uncontrolled behavioral challenge during which the patients, while listening to music, watching laboratory personel moving around, and occasionally answering questions related to their well-being, as well as performing some simple arithmetic. Consequently, the two functional challenge procedures cannot be compared by stringent scientific criteria.

Gur et al. (1983) compared flow during base line and activation by both verbal (verbal analogies) as well as spatial (Benton Line Orientation Test) tasks in schizophrenics and age-matched controls. Controls could not be distinguished from patients on the basis of base-line rCBF values. During task performance, however, significant differences emerged between the groups. Whereas controls presented the usual left-verbal, right-spatial flow increase, schizophrenic subjects showed no interhemispheric asymmetry during the verbal task and paradoxical left-hemispheric flow increases during the spatial task. These findings confirmed the author's hypothesis of an excessive left-hemispheric activation in schizophrenics during spatial cognition. Gur et al. (1982) used the same experimental design in patients with stroke or TIAs. The authors reported that while patients could not be discerned from the neurologically normal controls solely on the base-line flow data, marked differences between controls and patients became apparent in the hemodynamic response to the activation procedures that have been mentioned.

The value of functional challenge in patients with cerebral ischemia was reported by several other authors. Analogous to the findings of Gur et al. (1982, 1983), resting rCBF measurements have been shown to have little prognostic value in aphasic stroke patients, except in those with total aphasia. Functional challenge by a verbal expression task, however, suggests that those aphasics who have the largest response to activation also have the most favorable prognosis, particularly so in patients with Broca's aphasia (Demeurisse et al., 1983). Similar to results reported by Ott et al. (1979), Demeurisse and colleagues (1982, 1983) found that less disabled aphasic patients had significantly larger hemodynamic response to activation compared with both more severely impaired patients, and even controls.

Knopman et al. (1984) also used serial CBF measurements to study the recovery process in patients with aphasia after left-hemispheric ischemic infarction. While base-line CBF measurements could not distinguish between those patients who would make a nearly complete recovery from those who would not, functional activation by an aurally presented language comprehension task demonstrated an initial involvement of the right hemisphere in recovering aphasics, which was followed by a gradual takeover of previously impaired left-hemispheric regions.

Reversibility of function was also found in patients with alcohol dementia (Berglund & Risberg, 1980). Within the initial 24 days of withdrawal, the hemodynamic response to a visually presented mnestic task (Thurstone Memory Test) was characterized by transient large and diffuse rCBF increases, which subsequently normalized to the localized, postcentral cortical activation, as seen in healthy subjects.

DISCUSSION

In comparison with the vascular challenge procedures which will be discussed next, evaluation of rCBF results obtained during functional activations requires a neuropsychologically meaningful evaluation. Fortunately, not all activation tasks necessitate expatiated inferences regarding complex cognitive processes. Ackermann et al. (1979) reported 17% flow increases in left-hemispheric sensory-motor regions during submaximal right-hand movement. Knezevic et al. (1982) measured rCBF in patients following postconcussion syndrome and minor head trauma and found that squeezing a rubber ball failed to elicit the significant

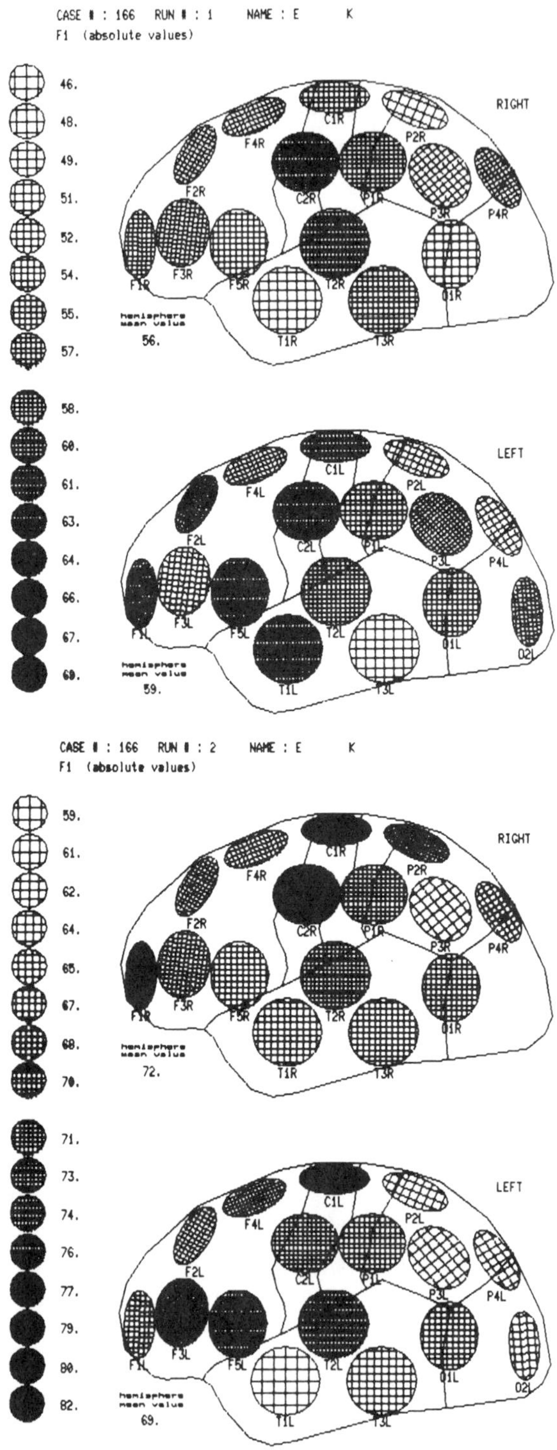
CASE # : 166 RUN # : 1 NAME : E K
F1 (absolute values)
46.
48.
49.
51.
52.
54.
55.
57.
58.
60.
61.
63.
64.
66.
67.
69.
RIGHT
C1R
F4R
P2R
F2R
C2R
P1R
P3R
P4R
F1R
F3R
F5R
T2R
O1R
T1R
T3R
hemisphere mean value
56.
LEFT
C1L
F4L
P2L
F2L
C2L
P1L
P3L
P4L
F1L
F3L
F5L
T2L
O1L
O2L
T1L
T3L
hemisphere mean value
59.
CASE # : 166 RUN # : 2 NAME : E K
F1 (absolute values)
59.
61.
62.
64.
65.
67.
68.
70.
71.
73.
74.
76.
77.
79.
80.
82.
RIGHT
C1R
F4R
P2R
F2R
C2R
P1R
P3R
P4R
F1R
F3R
F5R
T2R
O1R
T1R
T3R
hemisphere mean value
72.
LEFT
C1L
F4L
P2L
F2L
C2L
P1L
P3L
P4L
F1L
F3L
F5L
T2L
O1L
O2L
T1L
T3L
hemisphere mean value
69.

FIGURE 5.13.

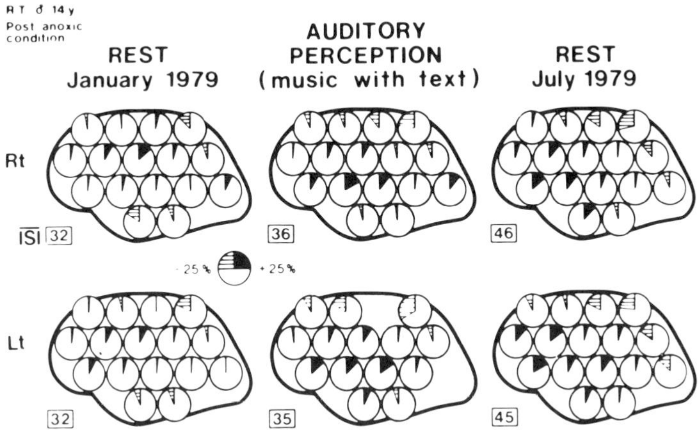

FIGURE 5.14. Postanoxic prognostic evaluation of brain function. Left: Base-line rCBF in a 14-year-old boy with hereditary cardiomyopathy in coma (degree 5–6) after respiratory and circulatory arrest. Middle: rCBF changes during auditory perception (music with text). Right: Base-line rCBF 6 months later. (From Hagstadius et al., paper presented at the eighth annual meeting of the International Neurophysiological Society, San Francisco, 1980; with permission.)

hemodynamic response displayed by age-matched controls. Figure 5.13 illustrates a case study from our laboratory in which the rCBF results during rigorous arm movement provided evidence against the preliminary clinical diagnosis of a subclavian steal.

During visual stimulation by a silent movie, Hartmann and von Kummer (1982) found that patients with homonymous hemianopsias secondary to occipital lobe infarctions, demonstrated 16% flow increases in the healthy hemisphere, as compared with only 8.5% on the side of the infarction. Finally, Hagstadius et al. (1980) examined a 14-year-old boy with hereditary hypertrophic cardiomyopathy, comatose after respiratory and cardiac arrest and who 2 weeks before the CBF study showed no cortical EEG activity. Base-line flow levels were in fact severely reduced but auditory stimulation by a familiar tape

---

FIGURE 5.13. (Top) Run 1: Base-line rCBF in a 60-year-old male patient presenting clinical signs suggesting a left-sided subclavian steal (pCO_2 44 mm Hg). (Bottom) rCBF during vigorous left-arm movement throughout the duration of the flow study. Flow increased bihemispherically (probably due to the displayed effort), accompanied by an evident hemodynamic response to the task in the right hemisphere. The indication vs. subclavian steal was subsequently confirmed by angiography. (From Brawanski & Maximilian, 1984; unpublished data.)

recording, induced marked bihemispheric temporal and fronto-temporal flow increases (Fig. 5.14). The authors interpreted the preserved hemodynamic response as an indication of maintained cortical function. A follow-up measurement 6 months later showed a normalized rCBF, in good agreement with the patient's partial recovery. The last example illustrated an assessment of cerebral function without the patient's active participation during activation. Generally, three issues must be considered before a rCBF functional challenge investigation:

1. What particular aspect of the patient's neurological status warrants further elucidation?
2. Can a selective activation procedure be derived?
3. Is the activation procedure appropriate to the patient's overall clinical condition?

VASOACTIVE CHALLENGE PROCEDURES

Vasoactive challenge procedures are designed to assess the cerebrovascular response to induced changes in various parameters which influence vascular resistance. Changes in cerebral circulation can be induced by manipulating arterial pCO_2 or pO_2 levels during the blood-flow measurement. The most effective CBF stimulant is CO_2. During inhalation of this potent vasodilator, CBF in the normal brain may significantly increase from base-line levels between 30–240% (Herrschaft & Schmidt, 1973; Harper & Glass, 1965; Kety & Schmidt, 1948; Reivich, 1964; Shapiro et al., 1966; Waltz, 1970; Yamaguchi et al., 1971). Cerebral blood flow can also be reduced during vasoactive challenge procedures by hyperventilation or increasing the pO_2 levels through inhalation of 100% O_2. The magnitude of change in cerebral perfusion from normal levels is not as large as during hypercapnia, with reported values ranging from 10% to maximally 43% (Juge et al., 1979; Kety & Schmidt, 1946; Lambertsen et al. 1953; Wasserman & Patterson, 1961).

A definite advantage of such "cerebrovascular activators" is that the resultant vasodilation (e.g., hypercapnia) or vasoconstriction (e.g., during hyperoxia) occurs reflexively and requires no active cooperation from the patient (except of course in voluntary hyperventilation tests). The change in CBF is independent of, and not interfering with, local metabolic activity (Carlsson et al., 1977; Folbergrova et al., 1972; Kety & Schmidt, 1946; Wasserman & Patterson, 1961); what is actually being altered by changes in cerebrovascular resistence is the cerebral blood volume, irrespective of the nutritional needs of the tissue (Maximilian et al., 1980).

In clinical practice, usually following an initial base-line CBF measurement, cerebrovascular reserve is tested in a subsequent examination where the patient, instead of breathing ambient room air, either voluntarily hyperventilates, or is administered 5–7% CO_2 or 100% O_2 through a face mask. Such interventions pose a definite challenge to the cerebrovascular system, of which compliance (or lack of) can be quantified by rCBF measurements.

It should be remembered that rCBF measurements predominantly quantify the responsiveness of the smaller intraparenchymal vessels. Those are most important in the regulation of tissue perfusion and also most affected by the challenge procedure. This has been demonstrated by Huber and Handa (1967) who angiographically measured changes in arterial caliber following CO_2 inhalation and hyperventilation. Arteries with a diameter of 25 mm or more showed no significant changes during hypercapnia, whereby those in the range of 2.5 to 1 mm dilated between 4–8%, respectively. The smallest measurable vessels between 0.5–1 mm showed, however, the largest response (22%) and the authors suggested that arteries smaller than 0.5 mm dilate even more. The vasoconstrictory response to hyperventilation showed the same trend, however, of a lesser magnitude.

By comparison to behavioral activation, the results yielded by cerebrovascular challenge studies are easier to evaluate: depending on the chosen procedure,

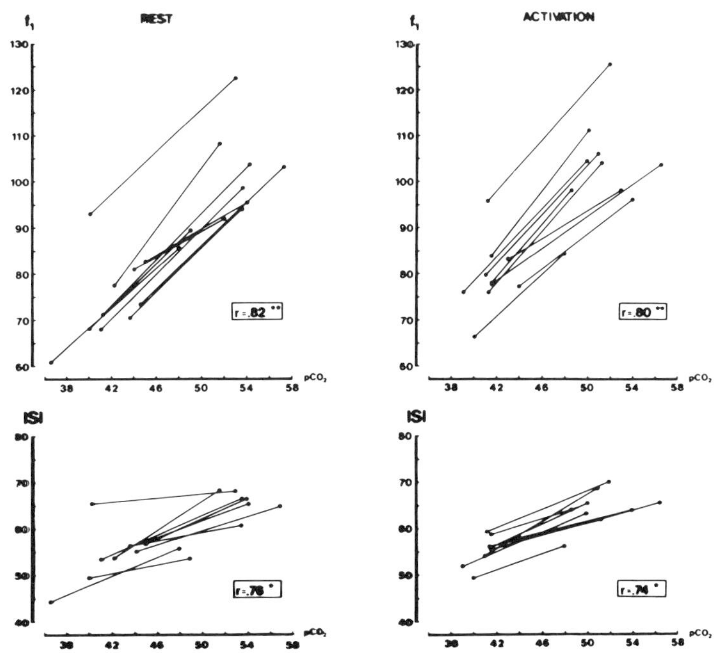

FIGURE 5.15. CBF reactivity to CO_2. Above, gray-matter flow (F1 in m1 100gr/min), and below ISI are on the ordinata, pCO_2 (in mm Hg) on the abscissa. Product moment correlations between base-line F1 and CO_2 induced increases are shown with their respective significance levels. Note the lower, but nevertheless statistically significant ISI response to hypercapnia (14%). (From: Maximilian et al.; permission granted by American Heart Association, Dallas; Mental activation in normo- and hypercapnia; *Stroke, 11,* 342–347, 1980.)

flow should normally either *increase* or *decrease* in all measured cortical regions.

CEREBROVASCULAR RESPONSIVENESS IN THE NORMAL BRAIN

In 10 healthy volunteers, Juge et al. (1979) found that during relaxed voluntary hyperventilation a 9 mm Hg reduction in pCO_2 (from 37 to 27 mm Hg) decreased

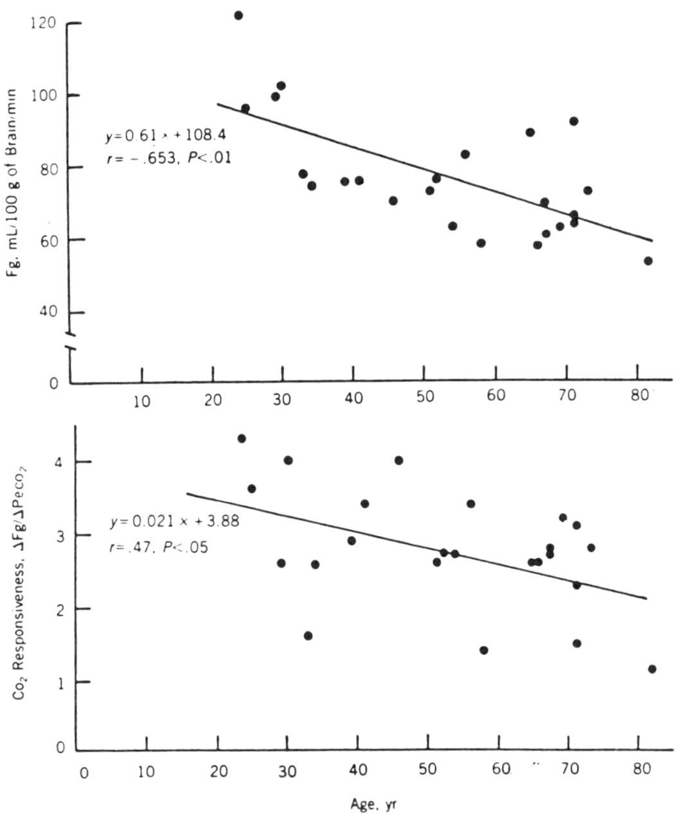

FIGURE 5.16. Top: Correlation between mean steady state hemispheric flow (fg) values and advancing age in normal, healthy volunteers (N = 24). Mean fg in steady state is progressively reduced with advancing age ($p < .01$). Bottom: Absolute cerebral vasodilation response to hypercarbia is correlated with age in normal, healthy volunteers (N = 24). / Fg is change in Fg; / $PeCO_2$, change in end-tidal partial pressure for CO_2. There is significant reduction of vasodilation response to hypercarbia with advancing age that parallels decline of Fg values with advancing age in steady state. (From Yamamoto et al.; *Archives of Neurology, 37,* 489–496, 1980; with permission.)

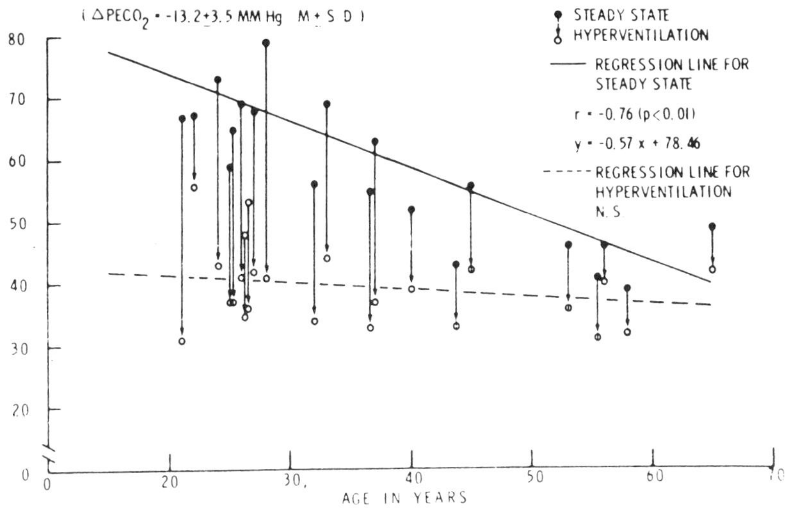

FIGURE 5.17. ISI value before and during hyperventilation correlated with age in normal volunteers ($N = 22$). (From Yamaguchi et al.; permission granted by Biomedical Press, Elsevier/North–Holland; *Journal of the Neurological Sciences 44,* 87–94, 1979.)

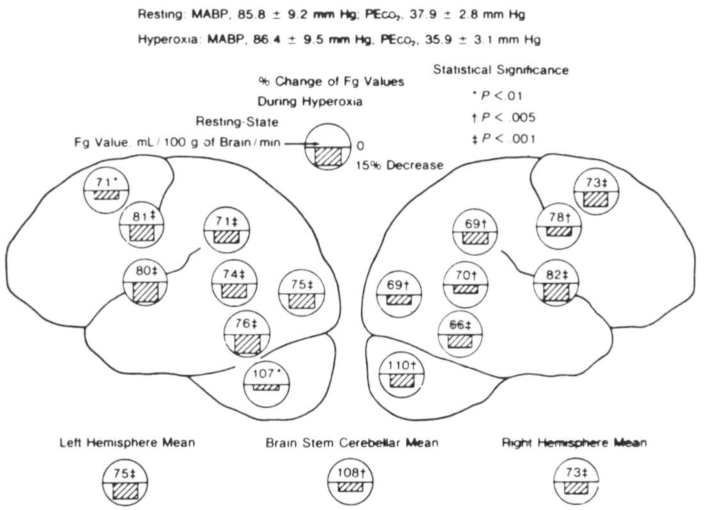

FIGURE 5.18. Percentage reductions in gray-matter flow (fg) before and during 100% oxygen inhalation in 49 normal healthy volunteers (mean age 60,2 ± 15.0 years). Decrease is symmetrical and statistically significant for all regions (paired t-test). MABP indicates mean arterial BP; $PECO_2$, end-tidal carbon dioxide tension. (From Nakajima et al.; *Archives of Neurology, 40,* 271–276, 1983; with permission.)

mean hemispheric CBF values by 37%. Maximilian et al. (1980) reported that an increase in pCO_2 of 11 mm Hg (from 42 to 53) induced by inhalation of 6% CO_2, significantly increased the global perfusion by 33% (Fig. 5.15).

These findings indicate that flow changes 3–4% for every mm Hg change in pCO_2, which closely agrees with results reported by other authors (cf. Obrist et al., 1975; Olesen, 1974).

Yamamoto et al. (1980) have shown that cerebrovascular responsiveness to hypercarbia declines with advancing age (Fig. 5.16). Similar results were also obtained during hypocapnia by Yamaguchi et al. (1979), who attributed this reduced compliance to either subclinical atherosclerosis or diminished vessel elasticity in elder subjects. As illustrated in Fig. 5.17, it is interesting to note that across all age groups, ISI did not decrease during hyperventilation below a level of 30 units, possibly an ischemic threshold beyond which flow will not further decrease. Finally, Nakajima et al. (1983) found in a group of healthy controls ranging in age between 25–86 ($\bar{x}$ 60) 11% CBF reductions during a rise in pO_2 (128–634 mm Hg) induced by 100% O_2 inhalation (Fig. 5.18).

Subjects below the age of 50 had, however, a 16% decrease in CBF, and the authors concluded that responsiveness to hyperoxia also diminishes with advancing age.

CLINICAL TESTS OF CEREBROVASCULAR RESERVE

Several studies in a variety of clinical situations have documented the utility of cerebrovascular challenge procedures implemented during the CBF measurement. Hoedt–Rasmussen et al. (1967), using the intracarotid ^{133}Xenon injection technique, were among the first to show a focally impaired response to hypercapnia. In patients with acute strokes, administration of 10% CO_2 did not cause further vasodilation in hyperemic focuses, as compared with surrounding regions. Similar results were also found by Fieschi (1968), and Fieschi et al. (1969). McHenry et al. (1972) reported that while hypercapnia causes flow increases in healthy controls, vascular compliance may be globally reduced in patients with diffuse cerebrovascular disorders and, as in the preceding reports, only regionally impaired in patients with focal CVD.

Noninvasive ^{133}Xenon clearance techniques considerably facilitated serial rCBF measurements supplemented by tests of cerebrovascular compliance across a wider range of patients. Yamamoto et al. (1980) compared CBF reactivity with induced hypercapnia between normal subjects with no history of risk factors for cerebral atherosclerosis, volunteers with risk factors for atherosclerotic stroke (e.g., arterosclerotic heart disease, hypertension, diabetes mellitus, hyperlipidemia) and patients with either vertebrobasilar insufficiency (VBI) or chronic CVD (e.g., hemispheric infarction or ischemia coupled with TIA). As illustrated in Fig. 5.19, the response to hypercapnia was slightly reduced in the volunteers

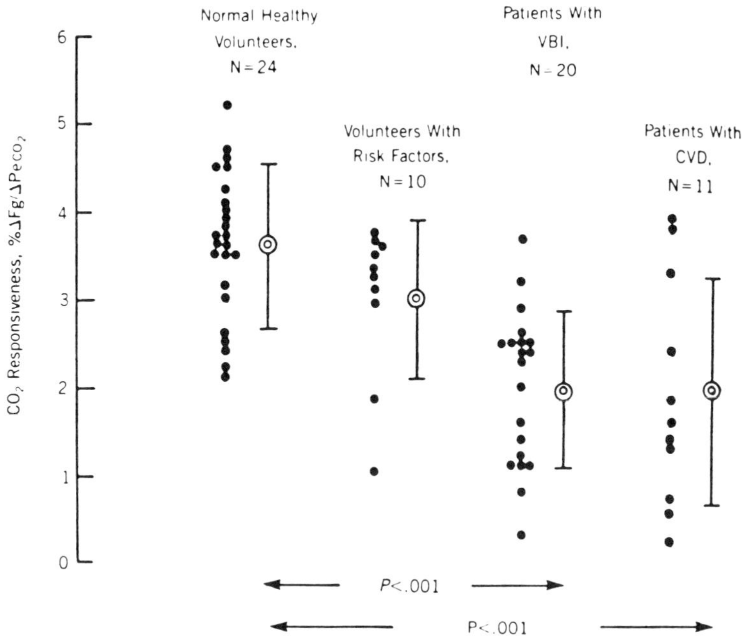

FIGURE 5.19. Mean relative reduction of hemispheric response to hypercarbia in volunteers with risk factors, patients with vertebrobasilar arterial insufficiency (VBI), and patients with hemispheric ischemia or infarction (CVD) compared with normal, healthy volunteers. CO_2 responsiveness is significantly less in patients with VBI or CVD compared with volunteers. Percentage of Fg indicates percentage of change in hemispheric flow and $PECO_2$ indicates change in end-tidal partial pressure for CO_2. (From Yamamoto et al.; *Archives of Neurology, 37,* 489–496, 1980; with permission.)

with risk factors. Additionally, the authors found bilateral, regionally reduced vasodilation in locations corresponding to the territory supplied by the middle cerebral artery (MCA). Yamamoto and coworkers consequently suggested that beside the use of CBF measurements in conjunction with cerebrovascular challenge for evaluating CVD patients, serial base-line/CO_2 activation studies may be useful as a screening procedure for asymptomatic patients suspected to be at risk from stroke. The CO_2 response was found to be significantly diminished in both VBI and chronic CVD patients, regionally manifested by a diffuse loss of vascular compliance most pronounced, however, in the ischemic hemisphere, which led the authors to suggest that, even in patients with domumented regional disorders, there is also evidence of diffuse atherosclerosis.

A similar study was conducted by Nakajima et al. (1983), who compared cerebral vasomotor responsiveness to hyperoxia between healthy volunteers,

volunteers with risk factors, patients with VBI, and patients with either chronic or acute hemispheric infarctions. As illustrated in Fig. 5.20, all groups showed a significant vasoconstrictive response to hyperoxia, except patients with acute hemispheric infarctions, where a paradoxical increase of flow was found, predominantly in those regions previously assessed as ischemic by CT scan, a combination of clinical signs, and base-line measurements. Differences in re-

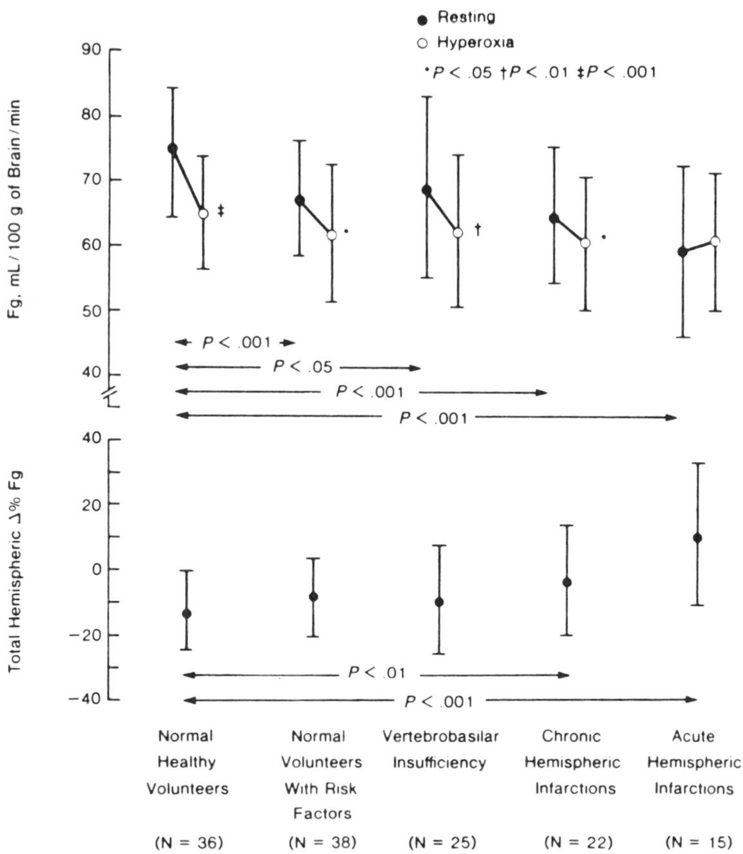

FIGURE 5.20. Comparison of total hemispheric gray-matter flow (fg) changes and vasomotor responsiveness to 100% oxygen inhalation in normal volunteers and patients with ischemic episodes. Top: Comparison between groups for total hemispheric fast component of flow values before and after 100% oxygen inhalation. Bottom: Vasomotor responsiveness expressed as a percentage of change in fg. Vasoconstrictor response is significantly reduced in chronic hemispheric infarction and becomes paradoxically vasodilatory in acute infarction. (From Nakajima et al.; *Archives of Neurology, 40,* 271–276, 1983; with permission.)

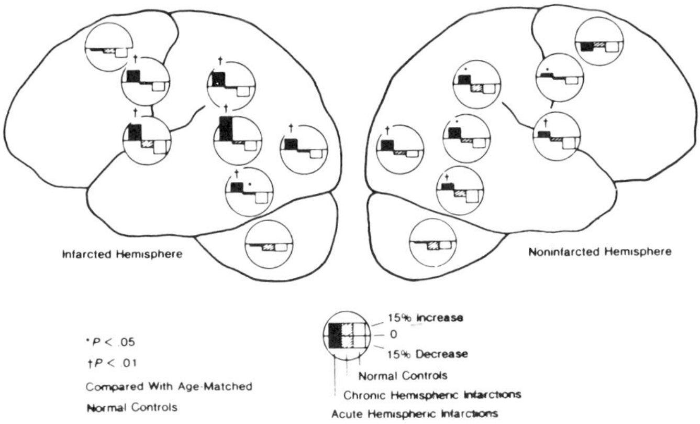

FIGURE 5.21. Regional changes (vasomotor responses) during 100% oxygen inhalation in patients with acute ($N = 15$) or chronic ($N = 22$) hemispheric infarction and in age-matched normal controls ($N = 36$). During acute stages of infarction, there are bilateral paradoxical increases primarily involving infarcted hemisphere. In chronic stage, vasoconstrictive responses are more reduced in infarcted hemisphere. (From Nakajima et al.; *Archives of Neurology, 40,* 271–276, 1983; with permission.)

gional responsiveness to 100% O_2 between healthy controls and patients with chronic and acute infarction are shown in Fig. 5.21. Nakajima and colleagues also reported a trend toward a normalized vasoconstrictory response in patients measured during subacute to chronic stages of cerebral infarction.

Halsey et al. (1982) found in 19 patients with ICA occlusion a significant negative correlation between preoperative response to hypercarbia and reactivity after the STA-MCA bypass; in other words, the poorer the preoperative vascular compliance, the greater the reactivity after the surgical intervention. The authors interpreted these results as an indication of vascular surgery having improved cerbrovascular capacitance, but not base-line perfusion.

Studying 39 patients with unilateral carotid occlusion in subacute and chronic stage Norrving et al. (1982) found preserved vasodilatory response to CO_2 inhalation in patients with adequate collateral flow via the circle of Willis. The authors proposed that these patients have a hemodynamically adequate vascular supply and may not profit from bypass surgery. Impaired responsiveness to CO_2 was found, however, in the hemisphere on the side of the occlusion if collateral supply via the circle of Willis was compromised by contralateral IC stenosis, particularly when hemispheric perfusion was only maintained by retrograde ophthalmic flow. The subgroup presenting this type of vascular insufficiency may benefit from EC/IC bypass, and Norrving et al. (1982) proposed that serial CBF measurements in conjunction with a cerebrovascular challenge such as hypercapnia, may help identify those patients in whom the hemodynamic reserve is exhausted.

Meyer (1981) and Meyer et al. (1982) found vascular challenge during rCBF determinations to improve identification of the infarcted regions and proposed its implementation as a routine screening procedure for patients with reduced cerebrovascular reserve. Jarrett et al. (1982) compared the clinical relevance of rCBF results during base-line and hypercapnia in a group of 92 patients with TIA, infarction, VBI and other cerebrovascular abnormalities documented by arteriography, CT scan and Doppler ultrasound. The authors claimed that delineation of cerebrovascular abnormalities *not* detected during base-line flow measurements increased significantly from 30% (normocapnia) to 90% (hypercapnia) in 20 TIA patients examined before carotid endarterectomy. Similar results were found in the remaining 72 patients with other varieties of CVD (40% base line vs. 82% hypercapnia). Unfortunately, no regional flow data were presented in this publication.

A poor response to either 5% CO_2 inhalation or hyperventilation was found in patients with severe neurological deficits and vasospasm as a consequence of

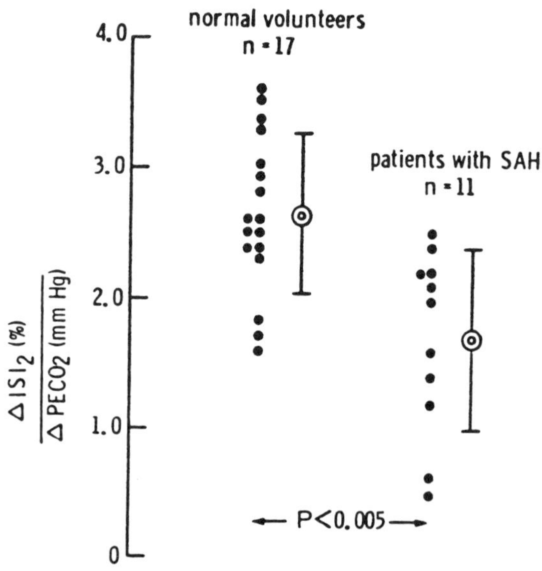

FIGURE 5.22. Cerebrovascular responsiveness during hypocapnia expressed as a percentage of change of IS12 per mm Hg $PECO_2$ in patients with SAH compared with normal volunteers. CO_2 responsiveness in patients with SAH was significantly reduced compared with normal volunteers. (From Yamamoto et al.; permission granted by Biomedical Press, Elsevier/North-Holland; *Journal of the Neurological Sciences, 43,* 301–311, 1979.)

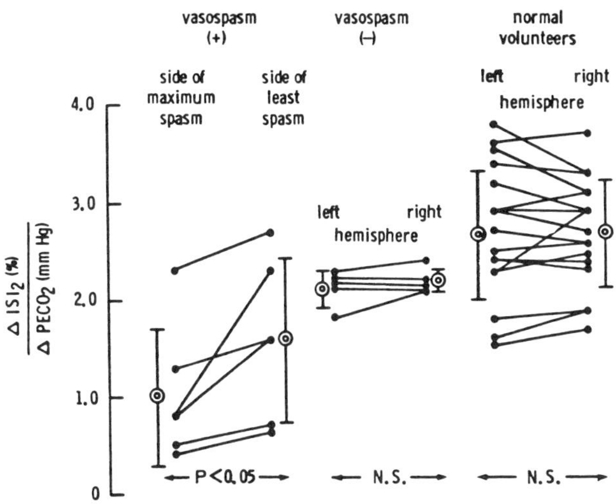

FIGURE 5.23. Hemispheric vasomotor responsiveness during hypocapnia correlated with presence or absence of vasospasm. CO_2 responsiveness on the side of maximum spasm was significantly reduced compared with the side of least spasm demonstrated by angiography. In patients without spasm and in normal volunteers, there is no significant difference of CO_2 responsiveness between the two hemispheres. (From Yamamoto et al.; permission granted by Biomedical Press, Elsevier/North–Holland; *Journal of the Neurological Sciences, 43,* 301–311, 1979.)

ruptured intracranial aneurysm, and Ishii (1979) reported good clinical results by delaying surgery in patients with low CBF and impaired vasomotor responsiveness. Yamamoto et al. (1980) measured CBF in patients with subarachnoid hemorrhage (SAH) and found clear correlation between both F1 and ISI and severity of neurological deficit. SAH patients also had a significantly lower response to hyperventilation in comparison with healthy controls (Fig. 5.22); vascular reactivity was maximally reduced within the first 10 days after the bleeding, but subsequently recovered. While no interhemispheric difference in reactivity was found in patients without spasm, this was clearly displayed by SAH patients examined during vasospasm (Fig. 5.23). The authors concluded that such a procedure paradigm can predict presence and course of vasospasm, offering a definite aid for determining the optimal time for the surgical intervention.

Obrist et al. (1984) found a preserved vasoconstrictory response to hyperventilation in most comatose patients examined following acute head injury, most evident, however, in those presenting cerebral hyperemia. Impaired vascular compliance indicated an unfavorable prognosis. Hyperventilation is commonly used to control ICP in patients with acute head injury and the authors proposed that "knowledge of hemodynamic variables could contribute to decisions regarding the appropriateness, magnitude and timing of therapy".

Cerebrovascular reserve measurements have not been exclusively applied to patients with CVD and major head trauma. Dandona et al. (1978, 1979) found, for example, an impaired response to CO_2 in patients with diabetes mellitus and in a subgroup of insulin-dependent diabetics, suggesting that reduced vascular compliance may indicate a new vascular complication of diabetes (Dandona et al., 1981). In a study designed to determine the relation between hyperviscosity and vascular compliance, Wade (1981) examined CO_2 reactivity before and after venesection in patients with primary high hematocrit. While base-line CBF increased by 30% following venesection, the lack of significant changes in reactivity conclusively demonstrated that cerebrovascular reserve is not compromised by hyperviscosity. A variable response to hypercapnia was found in patients with migraine and cluster headache (Sakai & Meyer, 1979). From 79 patients examined during normo- and hypercapnia, 21 migraineurs had an excessive response to CO_2 during the headache-free interval in the affected, as compared with the nonaffected hemisphere. During the headache phase, however, 5 migraineurs and two cluster headache patients had a reduced vasodilatory response, which then improved 24 hours after the pain subsided. Administration of 100% O_2 to 77 patients with various headache disorders induced the expected CBF decreases in all patients, except in migraineurs during the headache phase (Amano & Meyer, 1981). Additionally, the authors found that while aspirin treatment only minimally affected base-line flow and did not alter reactivity to CO_2, indomethacin considerably reduced both base-line and reactivity values.

Further examples of cerebrovascular challenge during pharmacological interventions have been demonstrated by Forster et al. (1983) and Traub et al. (1982). A new water-soluble benzodiazepine (midazolam) was shown to decrease resting flow values but increase CBF reactivity to hypercarbia and Forster et al., proposed that midazolam could be safely used for induction of anesthesia and sedation, and as a thiopental substitute for patients with intracranial hypertension. An impaired CO_2 response in elderly patients with systolic hypertension was found by Traub and colleagues (1982). The reduced vascular compliance did not improve after diuretic therapy with hydrochlorothiazide, which could indicate that these patients may be prone to cerebral ischemia during more aggressive treatment.

DISCUSSION

Evidently, detection of hemodynamic pathophysiology is substantially enhanced by vasomotor challenge determinations. It is noteworthy, however, that no consensus has emerged about which challenge procedure is most appropriate for a particular clinical condition, or which is most practical when implemented in conjunction with noninvasive rCBF measurements. There are a number of advantages, as well as disadvantages, associated with either hypercapnia, hyperoxia, or hyperventilation, which merit further consideration.

In cases with impaired perfusion CO_2 administration may be more desirable than either 100% CO_2 or hyperventilation because it specifically examines the vasodilatory reserve, which may be of crucial significance when evaluating patients in whom surgery designed to improve flow, is contemplated. Hypercapnia is evidently of questionable value in patients with hyperemia when hyperventilation proved to be an excellent test of cerebrovascular reserve Obrist et al., (1984) and Nakajima et al. (1983) recommended hyperoxia as a safe procedure in patients with stroke and cerebral edema, hypertension, and cardiac arythmias because it does not affect heart rate, ICP and blood pressure as hypercapnia may.

Addressing some procedural questions pertaining to cerebrovascular challenge, one should bear in mind that despite inherent advantages, the noninvasive CBF measurement is methodologically more complex than the IA injection technique. During the 1-minute equilibrium phase, the patient inhales the ^{133}Xenon/oxygen mixture from a closed loop system. While CO_2 and O_2 administration is relatively simple during both the preceding background registration and subsequent clearance measurement, this is not easily accomplished during the 1-minute tracer inhalation interval. Cerebrovascular challenge usually begins 2–3 minutes prior ^{133}Xenon inhalation, is then discontinued for 60 seconds, and recommended immediately after equilibrium. Consequently, there is for 1 minute following and preceding a hyper-/or hypocapnic condition, a sudden interval of normocapnia. Whereas this may not significantly affect flow results calculated with a delayed Start-Fit Time, valuable data pertaining rapidly perfused tissues could be lost in studies using full-curve analysis models (cf. Prohovnik, chapter 4 in this volume). Moreover, it should be remembered that the induced cerebral vasodilation is not instantaneous and a steady state may take up to 25 seconds (Shapiro et al., 1966).

Consequently, regardless of the calculation model, and despite valid clinical results obtained with this less-than-perfect modus operandi, one cannot ignore the fact that the patient is categorically *not* in the aspired steady state condition throughout the blood-flow examination. This, however, does not affect measurements performed with the IV technique, where the patient continuously inhales ambient room air. In this case, administration of vasoactive gases is more practical and requires no discontinuation during the equilibrium phase. CBF measurements during hyperventilation are of course methodologically simpler, requiring only a change in the patient's breathing rate. On the other hand, keeping a stable end-tidal CO_2 throughout the CBF measurement is not an easy accomplishment. Moreover, while CO_2 and O_2 can be administered to nearly all spontaneously breathing, as well as ventilated patients, hyperventilation requires a certain effort and constant patient cooperation (except in mechanically ventilated patients). Some of these problems appear to be alleviated by a more prac-

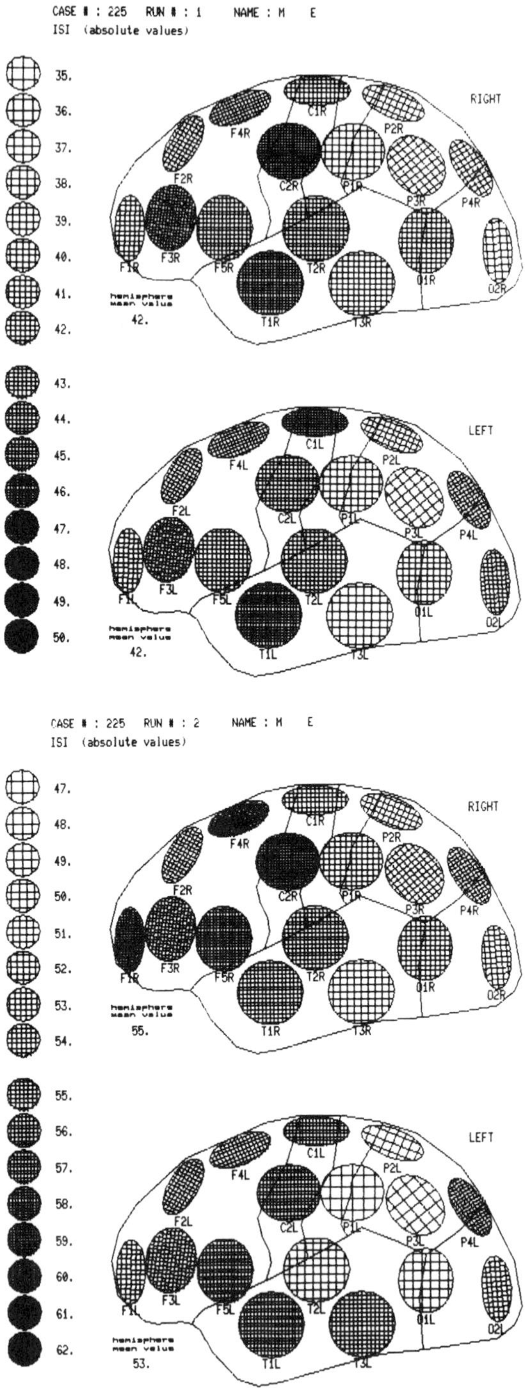
CASE # : 225 RUN # : 1 NAME : M E
ISI (absolute values)
35.
36.
37.
38.
39.
40.
41.
42.
43.
44.
45.
46.
47.
48.
49.
50.
RIGHT
C1R
F4R
P2R
F2R
C2R
P1R
P3R
P4R
F1R
F3R
F5R
T2R
O1R
O2R
T1R
T3R
hemisphere mean value
42.
LEFT
C1L
F4L
P2L
F2L
C2L
P1L
P3L
P4L
F1L
F3L
F5L
T2L
O1L
O2L
T1L
T3L
hemisphere mean value
42.
CASE # : 225 RUN # : 2 NAME : M E
ISI (absolute values)
47.
48.
49.
50.
51.
52.
53.
54.
55.
56.
57.
58.
59.
60.
61.
62.
RIGHT
hemisphere mean value
55.
LEFT
hemisphere mean value
53.

FIGURE 5.24.

tical vasomotor challenge procedure described in the study of Vorstrup et al. (in press).

Using the IA [133]Xenon injection technique, the Danish group studied the effects of acetazolamide (Diamox ®), a selective carbonic anhydrase inhibitor upon CBF and cerebral metabolic rate for oxygen ($CMRO_2$) in six normally perfused patients. By retained CO_2 in the tissue, Diamox mimics the effects of CO_2 upon cerebral perfusion. CBF increased significantly by 55% at 3 minutes and 70% at 20 minutes after IV injection of 1 gr. Diamox. A significant increase of venous O_2 saturation percent of 17% and 21% was registered after the 3- and 20-minute intervals respectively, but no significant changes were found in $CMRO_2$ arterial O_2 saturation, $paCO_2$, $pyCO_2$, and arterial and venous pH. These results suggest several advantages of cerebrovascular challenge by injection of azetolamide: (1) There is a significant vasodilatory response (with no change in cerebral metabolic activity, (2) It requires no patient cooperation, and no additional apparative manipulation and monitoring during the induced hypercapnia, and (3) It enables de facto a steady state during vascular challenge measurements when performed 20–30 minutes after the administration of acetazolamide. On the other hand, in comparison with the vascular challenge procedures that have been discussed, this intervention cannot be discontinued if the patient becomes symptomatic. In our laboratory we have tested the efficacy of acetazolamide for vascular challenge in more than 30 candidates for reconstructive surgery who tolerated the procedure very well. In conjunction with ^{133}Xe inhalation-flow studies this test of vascular compliance is considerably easier to perform than CO_2 administration.

Our preliminary findings have shown that in comparison with base-line studies, rCBF measurements during cerebrovascular challenge significantly improve delineation of regions with impaired autoregulation. This is illustrated by the following examples of a well-localized impaired hemodynamic response (Fig. 5.24) and a case with compromised compliance in nearly the entire supply area of the right ICA (Fig. 5.25). In general, the working hypothesis behind such measurements is to evaluate whether the revascularization procedure may improve the patients' *cerebrovascular reserve* instead of causing a perfunctory increase of CBF per se. Consequently serial measurements comparing cere-

FIGURE 5.24. rCBF measurements in a 45-year-old male presenting signs of agraphia, mixed aphasia and slight apraxia following isolated occlusions of the left arteria gyri angularis and arteria temporalis posterior. Top: Base-line rCBF measurement showed a relatively normal regional flow distribution with slight asymmetries in left parieto-posterior temporal areas. Bottom: A markedly reduced hemodynamic response during vascular challenge isolated in left-hemispheric posterior regions was evidenced by a subsequent flow study 30 min after I.V. injection of 1 gr. acetazolamide. (From Brawanski & Maximilian, 1984; unpublished data.)

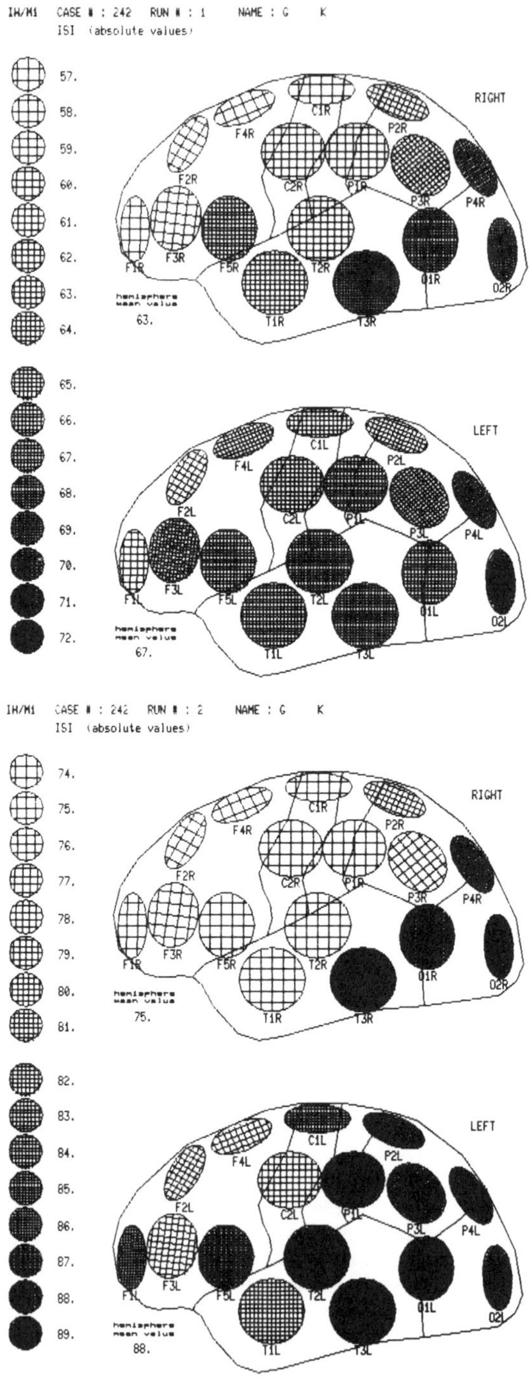

IH/M1 CASE # : 242 RUN # : 1 NAME : G K
ISI (absolute values)
57.
58.
59.
60.
61.
62.
63.
64.
65.
66.
67.
68.
69.
70.
71.
72.
RIGHT
C1R
F4R
P2R
F2R
C2R
P1R
P3R
P4R
F1R
F3R
F5R
T2R
O1R
O2R
T1R
T3R
hemisphere mean value
63.
LEFT
C1L
F4L
P2L
F2L
C2L
P1L
P3L
P4L
F1L
F3L
F5L
T2L
O1L
O2L
T1L
T3L
hemisphere mean value
67.
IH/M1 CASE # : 242 RUN # : 2 NAME : G K
ISI (absolute values)
74.
75.
76.
77.
78.
79.
80.
81.
82.
83.
84.
85.
86.
87.
88.
89.
RIGHT
hemisphere mean value
75.
LEFT
hemisphere mean value
88.

FIGURE 5.25.

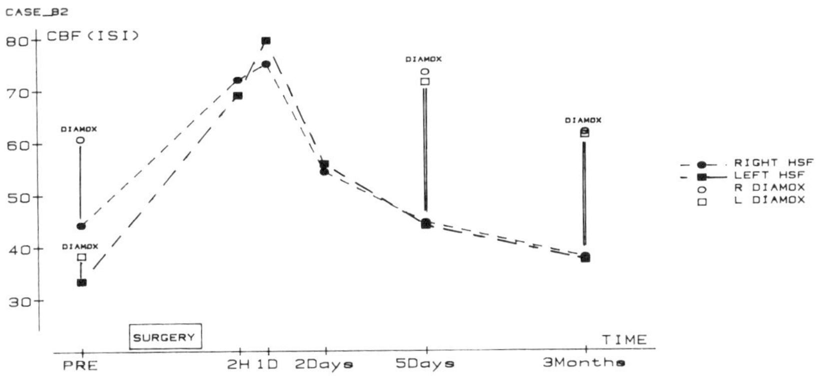

FIGURE 5.26. Serial bedside CBF measurements (^{133}Xe I.V. technique) during base-line and acetazolamide reactivity studies before and after left-carotid endarterectomy. (From Schroeder et al., unpublished data, 1984; with permission.)

brovascular reserve before and after surgery are of considerable value as shown by Schroeder et al. (1984, personal communication), who tested reactivity to acetazolamide before and after carotid endarterectomy (Fig. 5.26).

CONCLUSION

We contend that rCBF measurements supplemented by challenge procedures provide a greater clinical yield. McHenry et al. (1972) proposed that the severity

---

FIGURE 5.25. rCBF measurements in a 55-year-old woman with occlusion of the right internal carotid artery (ICA) and stenosis by the left-ICA. Six months prior to the rCBF study angiography revealed bilateral ICA stenoses (right 80%/left 85%). Ten days following left-carotid endarterectomy the patient developed a left-sided hemiparesis. At this time we performed the first rCBF examination (base line) which showed clear left-right asymmetries with reduced perfusion in several right hemispheric frontal, superior-frontal and central regions (Top). Additionally, an abnormal rCBF distribution pattern was observed in the better perfused left hemisphere. Bottom: Cerebrovascular responsiveness was tested in a subsequent examination 30 min following I.V. injection of 1 gr. acetazolamide. The hemodynamic response was significantly reduced in the entire supply area of the right ICA. A compromised compliance was also seen in few left-hemispheric locations but not of the same magnitude as on the right side. Angiography taken shortly after the rCBF measurements showed a right ICA occlusion and mild stenosis of the left ICA (Brawanski & Maximilian, 1984; unpublished data).

and extent of cerebrovascular abnormalities may be reflected by the magnitude or absence of vascular compliance, to which the studies by Nakajima et al. (1983), Yamamoto et al. (1979) and Norrving et al. (1982) have provided supportive evidence. Additionally, the studies of Meyer et al. (1978), Demeurisse et al. (1982, 1983) and Knopman et al. (1984) have suggested that functional challenge may work in the same manner for parenchymal disorders.

Because CBF reflects both metabolic demand and purely vascular components, Maximilian and Prohovnik (1984) suggested that by selecting the appropriate activation paradigm it may be possible to infer extent of pathology in either metabolic-flow coupling or in the vascular bed itself. Measuring CBF in healthy subjects under normocapnic and hypercapnic conditions during both resting and functional activation by a problem-solving task, Maximilian et al. (1980) demonstrated that vascular and metabolic flow increases are additive and do not interact. As illustrated in Fig. 5.27, both the resting flow pattern and task-induced hemodynamic response were clearly preserved during hypercapnia. More importantly, these results show, that even with available procedures both CBF components can be differentiated and combined by mapping flow changes during either vascular or functional challenge, or both. Although such a paradigm may help in differentiating between patients with vascular and for parenchymal disorders, some problems need further consideration.

With reference to the perspicuity of results obtained during cerebrovascular challenge, the responsiveness we are looking for affects the entire cortex, and thus inter-, as well as intrahemispheric divergences can be detected with relative ease. As for type of challenge procedure, acetazolamide, pending further clinical evaluation, offers at the moment exciting possibilities.

The hemodynamic response to functional activation is, by comparison, complex, and demands a more sophisticated evaluation of the results. As opposed to vascular challenge procedures, the choice regarding functional activations is more idiosyncratic, often based on trial-and-error experimentation. It may be that activation tasks used for patients with neurological or behavioral deficits are inappropriate for assessing another specific clinical condition. Consequently, generalizations are not possible and proper choice of specific intrameasuremental activations should be carefully considered. Additionally, functional tests must be implemented in accordance with their distinctive suitability in assessing different cerebral processes such as hemispheric specialization, functional reorganization, or localization of the rCBF response. Consequently, the activation technique used will vary and requires a priori knowledge of specific neuropsychologic postulates. Ideally, we should develop for parenchymal activation an analog to CO_2 for vascular compliance. This could either be a potent, stimulating task, or even better, an exogenous agent reliably inducing global, uniform increases in neuronal activity. Particularly, the latter solution may allow an objective assessment of the hemodynamic response which would follow the same straightforward criteria applied during vascular challenge. It would evidently have the same

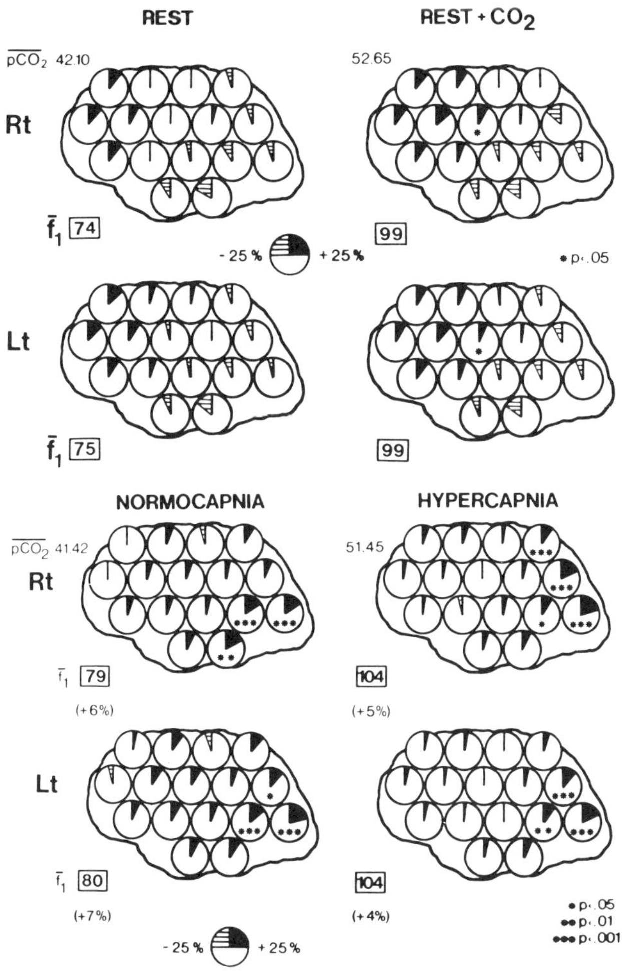

FIGURE 5.27. Top: Resting rCBF pattern during normo- and hypercapnia. Bottom: rCBF changes from base-line levels during a visually presented problem solving test. Left: Under normal conditions. Right: During hypercarbia. Note that the comparatively small hemodynamic response to functional activation was detected on top of the globally CO_2 induced hyperemia. (From Maximilian et al.; permission granted by the American Heart Association, Dallas; Cerebral hemodynamic response to mental activation in normo-and hypercapnia, *Stroke, 11,* 342–347, 1980.)

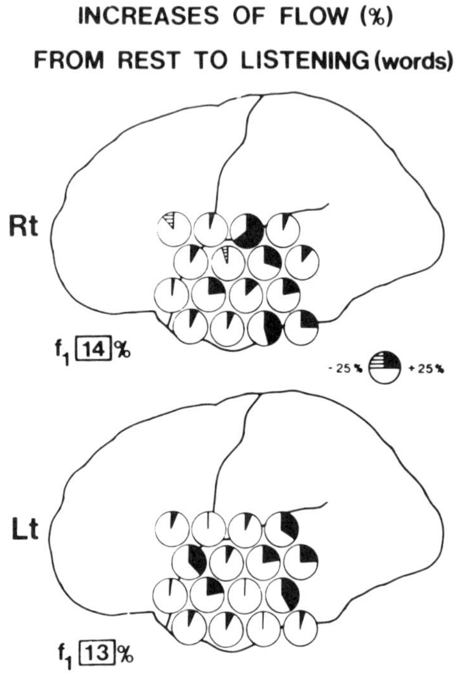

FIGURE 5.28. rCBF increases from base line during passive listening using high-resolution miniature scintillation detectors. By comparison, Maximilian (1982) using an identical activation procedure found no regional flow increases with standard detectors. (From Risberg & Hagstadius, 1984; with permission.)

advantages as, for example, hypercapnia, during which patient alertness, effort, performance, motivation, etc., are not instrumental to the adequate interpretation of the results. Unfortunately, we have no such compound, and a safe ''metabolic activator'' remains a grail yet to be discovered.

The clinical relevance of functional challenge procedures used so far may increase with better delineation of areas displaying pathologic functional activity. (In this context it is necessary to remember the precise topographical localization of activation induced rCBF response using the IA technique and a 254-detector system by e.g., Larsen et al., 1977.) Most noninvasive rCBF measurement systems to date have detectors with a diameter of approximately 2.5 cm. Risberg and Hagstadius (1984) recently presented promising results regarding the feasibility of high-resolution flow measurements with ^{133}Xenon inhalation. Two newly developed detector blocks, each containing 16 miniature detectors of 1 cm diameter were placed bihemispherically over the temporal cortex and the authors found marked asymmetrical focal increases during passive listening (Fig. 5.28). Nevertheless, based on our experience, considering the state of the art, consistency of results, and prognostic value of functional vs. vascular challenge procedures, it is our impression that the latter has shown the greater yield in clinical practice.

ACKNOWLEDGMENT

Part of this work was supported by DFG grant Bra–84312-1.

REFERENCES

Ackermann, R. H., Baron, J. C., & Correia, J. A. (1979). Comparison of two methods for monitoring cerebral activity: 133-Xenon inhalation blood flow studies and compressed spatial analysis of EEG. *Acta Neurologica Scandinavica, 60*(Suppl. 72), 22–23.

Amano, T., & Meyer, J. S. (1981). Prostaglandins and human CBF control: Effect of aspirin and indomethacin. *Journal of Cerebral Blood Flow and Metabolism, 1*(Suppl. 1), S403–404.

Berglund, M., & Risberg. (1980). Reversibility of alcoholics dementia. *Advances in Experimental Medicine and Biology*, 787–790.

Berne, R. M., Winn, H. R., & Rubio, R. (1981). The local regulation of cerebral blood flow. *Progress in Cardiovascular Disease, 24*, 243–260.

Buchsbaum, M. S., Holcomb, H. H., Johnson, J., King, A. C., & Kessler, R. (1983). Cerebral metabolic consequences of electrical cutaneous stimulation in normal individuals. *Human Neurobiology, 2*, 35–38.

Carlsson, A., Holmin, T., Lindqvist, M., et al. (1977). Effect of hypercapnia and hypocapnia on tryptophan and tyrosine hydroxylation in rat brain. *Acta Neurologica Scandinavica, 99*, 503–509.

Cooper, R., Papakostopoulos, D., & Crow, H. (1975). Rapid changes of cortical oxygen associated with motor and cognitive functions in man. In M. Harper (Ed.), *Blood flow and metabolism in the brain* Edinburgh: Churchill Livingstone.

Dandona, P., James, I. M., & Beckett, A. G. (1981). Vascular reactivity in diabetes. Letter to the Editor. *Lancet, 26*, 694.

Dandona, P., James, I. M., Woolard, M. L., Newbury, P., & Beckett, A. G. (1978). Cerebral blood flow in diabetes mellitus: evidence of abnormal cerebrovascular reactivity. *British Medical Journal, ii*, 325–327.

———. (1979). Instability of cerebral blood flow in insulin dependent diabetics. *Lancet, ii*, 1203–1205.

Demeurisse, G., Capon, A., & Verhas, M. (1983). Clinical and rCBF sequential study during the recovery from aphasia. *Journal of Cerebral Blood Flow and Metabolism, 3*(Suppl. 1), 282–283.

Demeurisse, G., Verhas, M., Capon, A., & Demol, O. (1982). Regional cortical activation during a naming test in aphasia: A rCBF study with 133-Xenon inhalation method. In C. Reynaud (Ed.). *Nuclear medicine and biology* (pp. 116–119). Paris: Pergamon.

Fieschi, C. (1968). Regional cerebral blood flow in acute apoplexy, including pharmacodynamic studies. *Scandinavian Journal of Laboratory and Clinical Investigation*, (Suppl. 102), *16*, E.

Fieschi, C., Agnoli, A., Battisti, N., Bozzao, L., & Prencipe, M. (1969). Derangement of regional cerebral blood flow and of its regulatory mechanisms in acute cerebrovascular lesions. *Neurology, 18*, 1166–1179.

Fieschi, C., Agnoli, A., & Prencipe, M. (1969). Impairment of the regional vasomotor response to hypercarbia in vascular disease. *European Journal of Neurology, 2*, 13–30.

Folbergrova, J., MacMillan, V., & Siesjö, B. K. (1972). The effect of moderate and marked hypercapnia upon the energy state and upon the cytoplasmic NADH/NAD+ ratio of the rat brain. *Journal of Neurochemistry, 19*, 2497–2505.

Forster, A., Juge, O., & Morel, D. (1983). Effects of Midazolam on cerebral hemodynamics and cerebral vasomotor responsiveness to carbon dioxide. *Journal of Cerebral Blood Flow and Metabolism, 3*, 246–249.

Frost, E. A. M. (1984). Some inquiries in neuroanesthesia and neurological supportive care. *Journal of Neurosurgery, 60,* 673–686.

Gur, R. C., Gur, R. E., Obrist, W. D., Hungerbuhler, J. P., Younkin, L., Rosen, A. D., Skolnick, B. E., & Reivich, M. (1982). Sex and handedness differences in cerebral blood flow during rest and cognitive activity. *Science, 217,* 654–660.

Gur, R. C., & Reivich, M. (1980). Cognitive task effects on hemispheric blood flow in humans: Evidence for individual differences in hemispheric activation. *Brain and Language, 9,* 78–92.

Gur, E. G., Skolnick, B. E., Gur, R. C., Caroff, S., Rieger, W., Obrist, W. D., Younkin, D., & Reivich, M. (1983). Brain function is psychiatric disorders. I. Regional cerebral blood flow in medicated schizophrenics. *Archives of General Psychiatry, 40,* 1250–1254.

Hagstadius, S., & Risberg, J. (1983). The effects of normal aging on the rCBF during resting and functional activation. *rCBF Bulletin, 6,* 116–120.

Hagstadius, S., Risberg, J., & Prohovnik, I. (1980). The prognostic value of regional cerebral blood flow measurements in a case of cerebral anoxia. *Paper presented at the eighth annual meeting of the International Neurophysiological Society, San Francisco.*

Halsey, J. H., Blauenstein, U. W., Wilson, E. M., & Wills, E. H. (1979). Regional cerebral blood flow comparism of right and left hand movement. *Neurology, 29,* 21–28.

———. (1980). Brain activation in the presence of brain damage. *Brain and Language, 9,* 47–60.

Halsey, J. H., Morawetz, R. B., & Blauenstein, U. W. (1982). The hemodynamic effect of STA–MCA bypass. *Stroke, 13,* 163–167.

Harper, A. M., & Glass, H. I. (1965). Effect of alterations in the arterial carbon dioxide tension on the blood flow through the cerebral cortex at normal and low arterial blood pressures. *Journal of Neurology, Neurosurgery and Psychiatry, 28,* 449–452.

Hartmann, A., & von Kummer, R. (1982). Atraumatic measurement of regional cerebral blood flow: Methods and reliability test. *rCBF Bulletin, 5,* 85–96.

Herrschaft, H., & Schmidt, H. (1973). Die quantitative Messung der örtlichen Hirndurchblutung in Allgemeinnarkose unter Normo-, Hypo- und Hypercapnie. *Anaesthesist, 22,* 442–456.

Hoedt–Rasmussen, K., Skinhoj, E., Paulson, O., Ewald, J., Bjerrum, J. K., Fahrenkrug, A., & Lassen, N. A. (1967). Regional cerebral blood flow in acute apoplexy: The "luxury perfusion syndrome" of brain tissue. *Archives of Neurology, 17,* 271–281.

Huber, P., & Handa, J. (1967). Effect of contrast material, hypercapnia, hyperventilation, hypertonic glucose and papaverine on the diameter of the cerebral arteries. *Investigative Radiology, 2,* 17–32.

Ingvar, D. J. (1976). Functional landscapes of the dominant hemisphere. *Brain Research, 107,* 181–197.

———. (1979). Hyperfrontal distribution of the cerebral gray matter flow in resting wakefulness; on the functional anatomy of the conscious state. *Acta Neurologica Scandinavica, 60,* 12–25.

Ingvar, D. H., & Risberg, J. (1965). Influence of mental activity upon regional cerebral blood flow in man. In D. H. Ingvar & N. A. Lassen (Eds.). Regional cerebral blood flow, an international symposium. *Acta Neurologica Scandinavica,* (Suppl. 14).

Ingvar, D. H., Risberg, J., & Schwartz, M. S. (1975). Evidence of subnormal function of association cortext in presenile dementia. *Neurology, 25,* 964–974.

Ingvar, D. H., & Schwartz, M. (1974). Blood flow patterns induced in the dominant hemisphere by reading. *Brain, 97,* 274–288.

Ishii, R. (1979). Regional cerebral blood flow in patients with ruptured aneurysms. *Journal of Neurosurgery, 50,* 587–594.

Jarrett, F., Polcyn, R., Levin, A., & McCormick, D. (1982). The use of hypercapnia in the study or regional cerebral blood flow abnormalities with 133-Xenon. *Journal of Surgical Research, 32,* 104–110.

Juge, O., Meyer, J. S., Sakai, F., Yamaguchi, F., Yamamoto, M., & Shaw, T. (1979). Critical appraisal of cerebral blood flow measured from brain stem and cerebellar regions after 133-Xenon inhalation in man. *Stroke, 10,* 428–437.

Kety, S. S., & Schmidt, C. F. (1946). The effects of active and passive hyperventilation on cerebral blood flow, cerebral oxygen consumption, cardiac output, and blood pressure of normal young men. *Journal of Clinical Investigation, 15,* 107–119.

———. (1948). Effects of arterial tensions of carbon dioxide and oxygen on cerebral blood flow and cerebral oxygen consumption of normal young men. *Journal of Clinical Investigation, 27,* 484–492.

Knezevic, S., Zurak, N., & Gubarev, N. (1982). Regional cerebral blood flow in patients following post concussion syndrome and minor head trauma. *rCBF Bulletin, 5,* 101–103.

Knopman, D. S., Rubens, A. B., Klassen, A. C., & Meyer, M. W. (1982). Regional cerebral blood flow correlates of auditory processing. *Archives of Neurology, 39,* 487–493.

Knopman, D. S., Rubens, A. B., Klassen, A. C., Meyer, M. W., & Niccum, W. (1980). Regional cerebral blood flow patterns during verbal and nonverbal auditory activation. *Brain and Language, 9,* 93–112.

Knopman, D. S., Rubens, A. B., Selness, O. A., Klassen, A. C., Meyer, M. W. (1984). Mechanisms of recovery from aphasia; evidence from serial 133-Xenon cerebral blood flow studies. *Annals of Neurology, 15,* 530–535.

Lambertsen, C. J., Kough, R. H., & Cooper, D. Y. (1953). Oxygen toxity: Effects in man of oxygen inhalation at 1 and 3,5 atmospheres upon blood gas transport, cerebral circulation and cerebral metabolism. *Journal of Applied Physiology, 5,* 471–486.

Largen, J. W., Shaw, T., Weinman, M., & Meyer, J. S. (1981). Order effects and responsiveness of regional cerebral blood flow in early Putative Alzheimer's Disease. *Journal of Cerebral Blood Flow and Metabolism, 1*(Suppl. 1), S483–S484.

Larsen, B., Skinhoj, E., Soh, K., Endo, H., and Lassen, N. A. (1977). The pattern of cortical activity provoked by listening and speech revealed by rCBF measurements. *Acta Neurologica Scandinavica, 56,* 208–209.

Lassen, N. A. (1959). Cerebral blood flow and oxygen consumption in man. *Physiology Revue, 39,* 183–238.

Mathew, R. J., Largen, J. W., Dobbins, K., Meyer, J. S., Sakai, F., & Claghorn, J. L. (1980). Biofeedback control of skin temperature and cerebral blood flow in migraine. *Headache, 20,* 19–28.

Maximilian, V. A. (1982). Cortical blood flow asymmetries during monoaural verbal stimulation. *Brain and Language, 15,* 1–11.

Maximilian, V. A., & Prohovnik, I. (1984). A historical perspective of non-invasive rCBF measurements: The method's development, present status and future prognosis. Libelli Medici . . .

Maximilian, V. A., Prohovnik, I., & Risberg, J. (1980). Cerebral hemodynamic response to mental activation in normo- and hypercapnia. *Stroke, 11,* 342–347.

Maximilian, V. A., Prohovnik, I., Risberg, J., & Hakansson, K. (1978). Regional blood flow changes in the left cerebral hemisphere during word pair learning and recall. *Brain and Language, 6,* 22–31.

Maximilian, V. A., Risberg, J., Prohovnik, I., & Rehnström, S. (1982). Regional cerebral blood flow and verbal memory after chronic exposure to organic solvents. *Brain and Cognition, 1,* 196–205.

Mazziota, J. C., Phelps, M. E., Carson, R. E., & Kuhl, D. B. (1982). Tomographic mapping of the human cerebral metabolism: auditory stimulation. *Neurology, 32,* 921–937.

McHenry, L. C., Goldberg, H. I., Jaffe, M. E., Kenton, E. J., West, J. W., & Cooper, E. S. (1972). Regional cerebral blood flow: Response to carbon dioxide inhalation in cerebrovascular disease. *Archives of Neurology, 27,* 403–412.

Meyer, J. S. (1981). Applications of studies of cerebral blood flow: Ischemic cerebrovascular disease. In J. Moosy & D. M. Reinmuth, (Eds.). *Cerebrovascular diseases.* New York: Raven Press.

Meyer, J. S., Nakajima, S., Okabe, T., Centeno, R., Lee, Y. Y., Levine, J., Levinthal, R., & Rose, J. (1982). Redistribution of cerebral blood flow following STA–MCA bypass in patients with hemispheric ischemia. *Stroke, 13,* 774–784.

Meyer, J. S., Sakai, F., Naritomi, H., & Grant, P. (1978). Normal and abnormal patterns of cerebrovascular reserve tested by 133-Xenon inhalation. *Archives of Neurology, 35,* 350–359.

Meyer, J. S., Sakai, F., Yamaguchi, F., Yamamoto, M., & Shaw, T. (1980). Regional changes in cerebral blood flow during standard behavioral activation in patients with disorders of speech and mentation compared to normal volunteers. *Brain and Language, 9,* 61–77.

Münchinger, R. (1963). Der Nachweis zentralnervöser Störungen bei Lösungsmittel-exponierten Arbeitern. In *Proceedings of the International Congress of Occupational Health,* Madrid, 687–689.

Nakajima, S., Meyer, J. S., Amano, T., Shaw, T., Okabe, T., & Mortel, K. F. (1983). Cerebral vasomotor responsiveness during 100% oxygen inhalation in cerebral ischemia. *Archives of Neurology, 40,* 271–276.

Norrving, B., Nilsson, B., & Risberg, J. (1982). rCBF in patients with carotid occlusion. Resting and hypercapnic flow related to collateral pattern. *Stroke, 13,* 155–162.

Obrist, W. D., Thompson, H. K., Wang, H. S., & Wilkinson, W. E. (1975). Regional cerebral blood flow estimated by 133-Xenon inhalation. *Stroke, 6,* 245–256.

Obrist, W. D., Langfitt, T. W., Jaggi, J. L., Cruz, J., & Gennarelli, T. (1984). Cerebral blood flow and metabolism in comatose patients with acute head injury. *Journal of Neurosurgery, 61,* 241–253.

Olesen, J. (1974). *Cerebral blood flow methods for measurement regulation, effects of days and changes in disease.* Copenhagen: Fadl's Forlag.

Orgogozo, J. M., & Larsen, B. (1979). Activation of the supplementary motor area during voluntary movement in man suggests it works as a supramotor area. *Science, 206,* 847–850.

Ott, E., Marguc, K., Lechner, H., & Bertha, G. (1979). Patterns of regional cerebral blood flow induced by speech in acute, subacute and chronic stages of expressive aphasia. In A. Bes & G. Geraud (Eds.), *Circulation cerebrale,* Toulouse, France.

Paulson, O. B., Olesen, J., Christensen, M. S. (1972). Restauration of autoregulation of cerebral blood flow by hypocapnia. *Neurology, 22,* 286–293.

Prohovnik, I. (1983). Clinical studies of rCBF by two-dimensional non-invasive 133-Xenon clearance: Review of applications and methodological comments. In R. P. Spencer (Ed.). *Interventional nuclear medicine.* New York: Grune & Stratton.

Prohovnik, I., Hakansson, K., & Risberg, J. (1980). Observations of the functional significance of regional cerebral blood flow in "resting" normal subjects. *Neuropsychologia, 18,* 203–217.

Prohovnik, I., Risberg, J., & Hagstadius, S. (1983). Temporal lobe activation by verbal memorization studied with 133-Xenon inhalation rCBF. *Journal of Cerebral Blood Flow and Metabolism,3*(Suppl. 1), S276–277.

Raichle, M. E., Grubb, R. L., Gado, M. H., Eichling, J. O., & Ter–Pogossian, M. M. (1976). Correlation between regional cerebral blood flow and oxidative metabolism. *Archives of Neurology, 33,* 523–526.

Reivich, M. (1964). Arterial PCO_2 and cerebral hemodynamics. *American Journal of Physiology, 206,* 25–35.

Risberg, J. (1980). Regional cerebral blood flow measurements by 133-Xenon inhalation: Methodology and applications in neuropsychology and psychiatry. *Brain and Language, 9,* 9–34.

Risberg, J., & Hagstadius, S. (1983). Effects on the regional cerebral blood flow of long-term exposure to organic solvents. *Acta Psychiatrica Scandinavica, 67*(Suppl. 303).

Risberg, J., & Hagstadius, S. (1984). *Pilot experiments with high-resolution rCBF-technique.* Abstract. Paper presented at the Nordic meeting in neuropsychology, August 14–18, Lund, Sweden.

Risberg, J., Halsey, J. H., Wills, E. L., & Wilson, E. N. (1975). Hemispheric specialization in normal man studied by bilateral measurements of the regional cerebral blood flow. *Brain, 98,* 511–524.

Risberg, J., & Ingvar, D. H. (1973). Patterns of activation in the gray matter of the dominant hemisphere during memorizing and reasoning. *Brain, 96,* 737–756.

Risberg, J., Maximilian, V. A., & Prohovnik, I. (1977). Changes of cortical activity patterns during habituation to a reasoning test. *Neuropsychologia, 15,* 793–798.

Risberg, J., & Prohovnik, I. (1983). Cortical processing of visual and tactile stimuli studied by nonyinvasive rCBF measurements. *Human Neurobiology, 2,* 5–10.
Roland, P. E., & Larsen, B. (1976). Focal increase of cerebral blood flow during stereognostic testing in man. *Archives of Neurology, 33,* 551–558.
Rozenfeld, D., & Wolfson, L. I. (1981). The effects of activation procedures on regional cerebral blood flow in humans. *Seminars on Nuclear Medicine, 11,* 172–185.
Sakai, F., & Meyer, J. S. (1979). Abnormal cerebrovascular reactivity in patients with migraine and cluster headache. *Headache, 19,* 257–266.
Shapiro, W., Wasserman, A. J., & Patterson, J. L. (1965). Human cerebrovascular response time to elevation of arterial carbon dioxide tension. *Archives of Neurology, 13,* 130–138.
Shapiro, W., Wasserman, A. J., & Patterson, J. L. (1966). Mechanism and pattern of human cerebrovascular regulation after rapid changes in blood CO_2 tension. *Journal of Clinical investigation, 45,* 913–922.
Sokoloff, L. (1960). The effects of carbon dioxide on the cerebral circulation. *Anesthesiology, 21,* 664–673.
Sokoloff, L. (1981). Relationship among functional activity, energy metabolism, and blood flow in the central nervous system. *Federation Proceedings, 40,* 2311–2316.
Sokoloff, L., Mangold, R., Wechsler, R. L., and Kety, S. S. (1955). The effect of mental arithmetic on cerebral circulation and metabolism. *Journal of Clinical Investigation, 34,* 1101–1108.
Traub, M., Shapiro, A., Dujovny, M., & Nelson, D. (1982). Cerebral blood flow changes with diuretic therapy in elderly subjects with systolic hypertension. *Clinical and Experimental Hypertension—Theory and Practice, A4 (7),* 1193–1201.
Vorstrup, S., Engell, H. C., Lindewald, H., & Lassen, N. A. (1984). Hemodynamically significant stenosis of the internal carotid artery treated with endarterectomy. *Journal of Neurology, 60,* 1070–1075.
Vorstrup, S., Henriksen, L., & Paulson, O. B. (1985). The effect of azetazolamide on cerebral blood flow and cerebral metabolic rate for oxygen. in press
Wade, J. H. P. (1981). Reactivity of the cerebrovascular bed to carbon dioxide in patients with primary high hematocrit before and after venesection. *Acta Neurologica Scandinavica, 63,* 306–314.
Waltz, A. G. (1970). Effect of $ApCO_2$ on blood flow and microvasculature of ischemic and nonischemic cerebral cortex. *Stroke, 1,* 27–37.
Wasserman, A. J., & Patterson, J. L. (1961). The cerebral vascular response to reduction in arterial carbon dioxide tension. *Journal of Clinical Investigation, 40,* 1297–1303.
Wood, F., Taylor, B., Penny, R., & Stump, D. (1980). Regional cerebral blood flow response to recognition memory versus semantic classification tasks. *Brain and Language, 9,* 113–122.
Yamaguchi, F., Meyer, J. S., Sakai, F., & Yamamoto, M. (1979). Normal human ageing and cerebral vasoconstrictive responses to hypocapnia. *Journal of the Neurological Sciences, 44,* 87–94.
Yamaguchi, F., Meyer, J. S., Sakai, F., & Yamamoto, M. (1980). Case reports of three dysphasic patients to illustrate rCBF responses during behavioral activation. *Brain and Language, 9,* 145–149.
Yamaguchi, F., Meyer, J. S., Yamamoto, M., Sakai, F., & Shaw, T. (1980). Noninvasive regional cerebral blood flow measurements in dementia. *Archives of Neurology, 37,* 410–418.
Yamaguchi, T., Regli, F., & Waltz, A. G. (1971). Effect of $PaCO_2$ on hyperemia and ischemia in experimental cerebral infarction. *Stroke, 2,* 139–147.
———. (1972). Effects of hyperventilation with and without carbon dioxide on experimental cerebral ischemia and infarction. *Brain, 95,* 123–132.
Yamamoto, M., Meyer, J. S., Naritomi, H., Sakai, F., Yamaguchi, F., & Shaw, T. (1979). Noninvasive measurement of cerebral vasospasm in patients with subarachnoid hemorrhage. *Journal of the Neurological Sciences, 43,* 301–311.
Yamamoto, M., Meyer, J. S., Sakai, F., & Yamaguchi, F. (1980). Aging and cerebral vasodilator response to hypercarbia. *Archives of Neurology, 37,* 489–496.

6 Utility of Regional Cerebral Blood-Flow Measurements in Clinical Pharmacology

Zdenko Mubrin
Stevo Knežević
Pliva Research Institute and Department of Neurology, University Hospital Center, Zagreb, Yugoslavia

GENERAL CONSIDERATIONS

One of the avis of clinical pharmacology is to decide whether a particular substance which has passed a long and exhausting set of preclinical and toxicological tests is both suitable and effective in the treatment of a certain disease. The method chosen for the evaluation of a drug treatment must be relevant to the clinical deficit, the disordered physiological mechanisms and the pharmacology of the employed substance. Furthermore, the evaluation must be reasonably economical with patient's time so that numerous subjects can be studied on many occasions. This repetition is necessary to reduce the impact of fluctuations in the severity of deficit. The process of evaluation must bear little risk to the patient. In addition, reproducibility of results, high sensitivity, and repeatability are important criteria by which the method of evaluation is assessed (Calne, 1980).

The principal users of "cerebroactive" drugs, mainly elderly people, pose serious clinical problems with their cohort of ill-definable or unpredictable neurological and mental symptoms which are frequently attributed to the cerebrovascular disease. Almost certainly, cerebrovascular disease is overdiagnosed as a cause of mental deterioration in the elderly but the pressure on physicians to prescribe vasoactive drugs is considerable.

Some progress has been made in assessing cerebral blood flow, its interaction with basic metabolic events, the brain's electrical activity and certain morphological aspects. However, the whole field of behavioral and psychometric assessment must be regarded with extreme caution because of the lack of satisfactory base-line data and comparative criteria for assessment of outcome (Spagnoli & Tognoni, 1983).

Since the introduction of the method for measuring cerebral blood flow (Kety & Schmidt, 1948), a great number of investigations have been done in order to test the effects of various drugs on the cerebral circulation. Measurements of change of CBF are not restricted to the effects of "vasoactive drugs," but also to a large group of pharmaceuticals used in the treatment of neurological and psychiatric diseases which can alter brain functions in different and often poorly understood ways. This chapter, primarily concerns itself with data derived from human subjects and experimental studies in animals where necessary.

Basic Principles and Classification of Drugs Acting on Cerebral Circulation

In order to exert its effects, a drug must reach the target site. Getting to the site of action normally involves two separate processes; absorption into the blood stream and movement from the blood into the tissue. Blood vessels supplying the central nervous system differ from the systemic vessels because of the blood-brain barrier. The blood-brain barrier is of considerable importance in determining the extent of penetration and hence the neuropharmacological action of many drugs.

Blood-brain Barrier

A detailed description of the anatomy and physiology of the blood-brain barrier is beyond the scope of this chapter, but some basic features should be mentioned. The blood-brain barrier comprises the major membrane system segregating brain extracellular space from the systemic one. Its primary function is to protect the brain from disturbing and potentially noxious exogenous and endogenous agents circulating in the blood. It is located within the endothelium of brain capillaries, which are devoid of fenestration and rarely exhibit pynocytosis. Only lipid soluble molecules pass the blood-brain barrier freely while the lipid insoluble substances are transferred via various other mechanisms, e.g., carrier mediated systems, active transport, etc. (See Bradbury, 1984; Hertz & Paulson, 1983; Weindl, 1983).

In certain pathological situations the blood-brain barrier changes its characteristics and becomes more permeable to various water-soluble substances, including drugs, which may otherwise not pass into the brain tissue. Acute hypertension can cause the barrier to open, probably due to a direct mechanical effect on cerebral vessels with consequent widening of tight junctions (Ziylan, 1984). Reversible opening of the blood-brain barrier has been observed after the administration of a number of hyperosmolar solutions (Rapoport et al., 1971) and no gross neurological deficits have been seen in monkeys subjected to such a procedure (Rapoport & Thompson, 1973).

The blood-brain barrier is not the only factor influencing the distribution of drugs within the brain. Blood vessel density and consequently the level of regional blood flow, will also influence drug distribution (Kety, 1974). Since vascular diameter and blood flow may be altered by different drugs, this may have bearing on the subsequent distribution of the substance in the tissue of a particular region.

Basic Mechanisms of Drug Action on the Brain

Drugs can influence neurochemical pathways by mechanisms involved in energy production, formation of structural components and the maintenance of ionic concentration gradients across cell membranes. These biochemical mechanisms are probably similar throughout the brain so the effect can be considered unselective. However, drugs can act selectively if they effect synaptic transmission in specific pathways utilizing particular transmitter chemicals (Eadie & Tyrer, 1980).

Cerebral Blood-flow Changes Induced by Drugs

Until recently, only a few methods have given quantitative information about blood flow in the human brain. By and large, indicator methods still constitute the most widely used techniques. Most data on the effects of various drugs on cerebral blood flow have been obtained by ^{133}Xe methods using both intra-arterial and noninvasive techniques. More sophisticated methods, particularly positron emission tomography have great potential but are so expensive that their use will be limited to a few centers.

The relatively old classification of drugs acting on cerebral circulation proposed by Carpi (1972) remains acceptable and helpful.

1. Drugs related to natural agents and possessing vascular activity; e.g., substances that interfere with endogenous mediators (catecholamines), local hormones and autocoids (histamine, prostaglandins, etc.).
2. Drugs acting directly on peripheral vessels through myogenic receptors other than those involved in the reaction of the first group (papaverine, xanthines, etc.).
3. Drugs acting primarily on the metabolic activity of the central nervous system and subdivided into central depressants and stimulants.
4. Miscellaneous agents which effect CBF by different means from the foregoing, or poorly understood mechanisms.

DRUGS RELATED TO NATURAL AGENTS

Sympathomimetic Drugs

The action of substances related to neurotransmitters on CBF in humans is relatively rarely studied and results vary according to the method of blood-flow measurement employed, patient selection, the route of administration and the dosage used. Pharmacological effects of different catecholamines on the cerebral vascular smooth muscle were comprehensively reviewed by Purves in 1972 and only newer data will be described here.

Using the invasive ^{133}Xe technique for regional cerebral blood-flow measurement it has been shown that intra-arterial administration of epinephrine or norepinephrine does not cause changes either in mean hemispheric or in regional blood flow. The intravenous administration of norepinephrine induces a moderate increase of CBF in some patients while in others, a slight decrease was observed. Comparing the results of intravenous and intracarotid administration of norepinephrine, it was concluded that an increase in cerebrovascular resistance was secondary to blood pressure changes and due to a direct effect on cerebral vessels (Olesen, 1972). We would not expect epinephrine or norepinephrine to modify cerebral metabolism except after opening of the blood-brain barrier. However, large doses of norepinephrine can open the blood-brain barrier as a result of the sudden increase in arterial blood pressure. Animal experiments suggest that for a given metabolic rate, a higher blood flow is needed to perfuse a brain structure during norepinephrine infusion than in control conditions. It was explained as indirect effect of inhibitory transmitters released through activation of baroreceptor reflex (Kuschinsky et al., 1983).

No effects on CBF or cerebral oxygen consumption was observed after intravenous infusion in normotensive subjects (Fazekas et al., 1960a), while in severe hypotension the response of CBF is unpredictable (Fazekas et al., 1960b).

The role of dopamine in CBF regulation remains controversial. In Parkinson's disease, where a defect in dopamine accounts for the clinical signs and symptoms, no change in CBF was noted despite decreased metabolism in the parietal cortex (Lenzi et al., 1979). Using the ^{133}Xe inhalation technique in a group of patients suffering from Parkinson's disease established on oral levodopa (a drug known to cross blood-brain barrier) combined with a peripheral dopa-decarboxylase inhibitor, no significant changes in CBF were found (Melamed et al., 1978). When dopamine was administered by infusion to patients with postoperative cerebral vasospasm, following the successful clipping of the aneurysm of internal carotid artery, an increase in CBF was noted. This was explained by increased perfusion pressure across a spastic blood vessel caused by increase in systemic arterial pressure (Montgomery et al., 1981).

Recently published data show that in vitro, dopamine has a direct vasodilating action on human cerebral arteries and that the response is mediated via dopaminergic receptors (Toda, 1983). Dopamine does not cross the blood-brain barrier but a similar effect might occur in vivo if the barrier is disrupted.

Drugs Acting on Adrenoreceptors

Drugs which exert their effect through adrenergic receptors influence norepinephrine release in the synaptic cleft resulting in altered postsynaptic activity as schematically shown in Fig. 6.1.

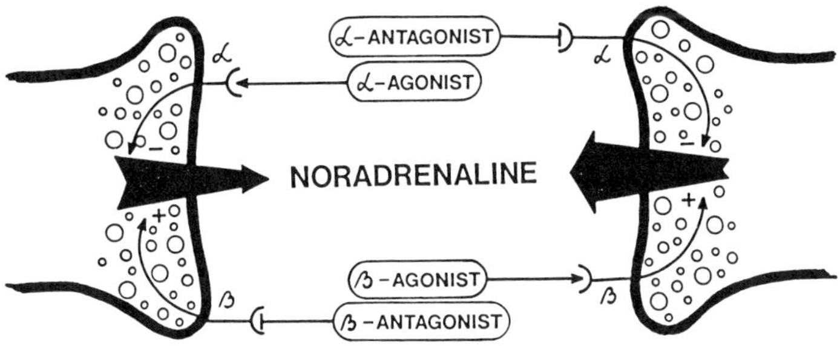

FIGURE 6.1. Basic mechanism of noradrenaline release from the presynaptic nerve endings. Various drugs, acting on pre- and post-synaptic alpha- or beta-receptors influence release of noradrenaline from the presynaptic nerve endings in different, sometimes completely opposite way, generally depending on the type of receptor occupied.

α-adrenergic Receptor-blocking Drugs. Isoxsuprine, a phenylethylamine derivative of epinephrine, is an alpha-adrenoreceptor antagonist with beta-adrenoreceptor stimulating properties (Cook & James, 1981b). In high doses it may also normalize platelet hyperaggregability and lower blood viscosity (Weber et al., 1980). After intravenous administration in patients with chronic cerebrovascular disease, CBF was reported either to decrease (Fazekas & Alman, 1964) or to show no difference from control subjects (Gottstein, 1965; Heiss, 1973; Heiss & Podreka, 1979). Regional impairment has been shown in ischemic areas (Heiss, 1973; Heiss & Podreka, 1979) which makes it theoretically unsuitable for clinical use in acute stroke.

Phenoxybenzamine is closely related to the drugs of the nitrogen mustard group and is powerful α-adrenoreceptor blocker but with a slow onset of action even after intravenous injection. Its effect on CBF and metabolism has been measured by means of hydrogen clearance method in patients with acute and subacute cerebral ischemia. Hemispheric blood flow did not change. Metabolic changes were observed however, with diminished hemispheric oxygen consumption and carbon dioxide production, explained on the basis of a possible recoupling of oxidative phosphorilation in damaged areas (Meyer et al., 1974b).

Ergot Alkaloids. Ergotamine is a selective alpha-adrenoreceptor blocker used in the treatment of migraine. No changes in CBF were observed after intramuscular injection (Hachinski et al., 1978). Similar results were reported previously where ergotamine was administered intravenously (Simard & Paulson, 1973). When ergotamine was given during the headache phase of migraine no changes in CBF were seen in spite of subjective improvement reported by patient (Norris et al., 1975).

Dihydroergotoxine. An equal mixture of ergocornine, ergocristine and ergocryptine, dihydroergotoxine is devoid of the vasoconstrictor properties of ergotoxine alkaloids and possesses alpha-adrenoreceptor blocking and weak dopaminergic activity. Data on its effect on CBF are somewhat contradictory. In patients with symptoms of "cerebrovascular insufficiency" CBF measured by a modificated Kety–Schmidt technique, remained essentially the same as before drug administration (Gottstein, 1965). A similar lack of effect was obtained with ^{133}Xe invasive technique after single intramuscular injection of dihydroergotoxine. Regional changes were also unremarkable except when a focal abnormality was influenced as a result of changes in systemic arterial pressure (McHenry et al., 1971). Reduced cerebral blood flow has also been reported, accompanied by focal decreases in areas with impaired autoregulation (Olesen & Skinhøj, 1972). According to all the studies, the drug appears not to affect blood flow unless autoregulation is impaired.

Nicergoline is found to improve hemodynamic, metabolic, and behavioral sequelae in a model of cerebral ischemia in aged rats (Le Poncin–Lafitte et al., 1984) but in humans contradictory results have been obtained. No effect was seen in a group of patients suffering from cerebral ischemia studied by Herrschaft (1976) but higher doses given to a similar group of patients by other investigators, caused an "inverse steal" effect. Even larger doses led to blood-flow increases in ischemic areas although mean hemispheric flow was unaltered (Philippon et al., 1982).

β-adrenergic Receptor-stimulating Drugs. Nylidrin is structurally similar to isoxsuprine acts as a beta-adrenoreceptor stimulant. Its effect on CBF is similar to isoxsuprine, namely slight hemispheric decrease resembling those seen in controls, but accompanied by regional deterioration of blood flow in ischemic areas (Heiss, 1979).

Isoprotenerol has a very powerful β-action but is almost devoid of α-adrenoreceptor activity. When given intraarterially, regional cerebral blood flow was significantly reduced and accompanied by a decrease in arterial pCO_2. After correction of this concomitant change in arterial gas tension, the change was no longer significant (Olesen et al., 1978).

β-adrenergic Receptor-blocking Drugs. Propranolol has a prolonged competitive blocking action and has been widely used to treat angina pectoris by blocking the effects of the increased sympathic drive during exercise. Its effect on CBF and some pathological conditions of the central nervous system has been investigated by several authors. Animal experiments indicate that CBF and $CMRO_2$ are reduced by pharmacological beta-adrenergic blockade (Aoyagi et al., 1976). In patients with cerebral ischemia reduced CBF followed when estimated by the hydrogen clearance technique. No effect of propranolol was seen on the 7% CO_2 and air inhalation (Meyer et al., 1974a). When ^{133}Xe intra-arterial method was employed for the assessment of changes of CBF after intra-arterial propranolol administration, significant decreases were found but only after pCO_2 correction. After propranolol, the rCBF changes caused by alterations in the arterial pCO_2 were normal and the focal flow increase during the activation procedure was not influenced by simultaneous propranolol injection in the carotid artery (Olesen et al., 1978). In hypertensive patients, long-term therapy with low doses of propranolol did not influence regional CBF. When higher doses were administered, CBF increased significantly. The effect is unlikely to be solely due to the specific blockade of adrenergic receptors and was attributed, at least partly, to a direct vasodilating effect on cerebral blood vessels (Globus et al., 1983). Experiments where propranolol has been used for the treatment of acute focal cerebral ischemia failed to find any protective effect (Capraro et al., 1984) although such an effect has been reported in animal models but with a shorter duration of ischemic brain damage (Little et al., 1982). On the basis of previous reports, the effect of beta-adrenergic blockers on regional CBF remains unsettled both in physiological and in pathological conditions.

Histamine and its Agonists

Intravenous infusion of histamine does not affect CBF when measured either with Kety–Schmidt technique (Alman et al., 1952) or ^{133}Xenon invasive method (Krabbe & Olesen, 1982). This is to be expected in patients with a normal blood-brain barrier. When the barrier was opened experimentally in rats, a highly significant increase in CBF was observed after histamine (Gross et al., 1981).

Betahistine. An analog of histamine, it acts as a relatively pure histamine–1–receptor agonist. One week of the oral treatment caused CBF to increase, but in some cases with cerebrovascular disease, a minor "steal-effect" was revealed (Meyer et al., 1974c). Only a small increase in CBF was observed in a group of young healthy volunteers (Hughes et al., 1981).

Prostaglandins and Inhibitors of Their Synthesis

Although discovered some 20 years ago, prostaglandins have only been intensively studied in the last decade. The term prostaglandins refers to a group of endogenously formed substances whose action on blood vessels is sometimes quite different. It is generally accepted that prostacyclin acts as a vasodilator whereas other prostaglandins and thromboxanes constrict blood vessels (Moncada, 1983; Moskowitz & Coughlin, 1981; Siesjö & Wieloch, 1983). Labile metabolites of archidonic acid, e.g., thromboxanes and prostacyclin, formed by the cyclo-oxygenase pathway, have potent albeit opposing pharmacological actions, perhaps reflecting an interactive modulation between these two substances. An imbalance in this modulatory influence, resulting from dysfunction of the cell, tissue or organ may be an important mechanism underlying the development of pathological processes (Whittle & Moncada, 1983). This may be the reason why many conflicting results have been observed in different experimental conditions. Besides its cerebrovascular action (see White & Hagen, 1982) it is suggested that at least some prostaglandins primarily act on brain metabolism, producing a secondary change in CBF (Pappius & Wolfe, 1983; Siesjö & Wieloch, 1983). There are at least four possible mechanisms by which prostaglandins can modify the function of cerebral vessels; mediating platelet-vessel wall interaction, altering smooth muscle contractility, modifying neural transmission, and by modifying or mediating the activity of other vasoactive substances (Moskowitz & Coughlin, 1981).

Several experimental studies have failed to show any significant effect of exogenously administered prostacyclin on CBF or its regulation following global cerebral ischemia (Van den Kerchkoff et al., 1983). In an experiment where focal cerebral ischemia were induced by middle cerebral artery occlusion in cats, intravenously administered prostacyclin appeared to protect against blood-brain barrier breakdown. However, the systemic hemodynamic influence of prostacyclin may compromise CBF in areas of impaired autoregulation and offset any direct beneficial effect (Awad et al., 1983). Cyclo-oxygenase inhibition does not reduce postischemic reactive hyperemia in the rat brain following an ischemic insult (Kågström et al., 1983). Other investigators found that inhibition of cyclo-oxygenase and lypoxygenase with eicosapentaenoic acid which is structurally similar to arachidonic acid, prevents postischemic cerebral edema and hyperperfusion in ischemic gerbils without affecting the levels of brain prostaglandins and thromboxane (Black et al., 1984).

The effect of prostaglandins on CBF has also been studied in humans with variable results. No significant changes in CBF were observed after injection of prostaglandin E_1 in patients with angiographic evidence of cerebral vasospasm following subarachnoid hemorrhage (Steiner et al., 1972), while a mild increase in blood flow in all regions followed intracarotid administration of prostaglandin E_1 in ''cerebrovascular'' patients (Olesen, 1976). Flushing of the skin was observed in both studies. In a small number of patients with acute cerebral ischemia, infusion of prostacyclin appeared beneficial only in patients with no CT evidence of infarction (Miller et al., 1984).

In healthy volunteers, using aspirin, indomethacin and naproxen, all inhibitors of cyclo-oxygenase, only indomethacin affected basal CBF and the cerebrovascular response to hypercapnia to any appreciable extent. The effect was short-lasting and disappeared after 1 week of continued treatment, indicating that the intact formation of prostaglandins is not a prerequisite for the maintenance and regulation of CBF in normal humans (Uyama et al., 1983). The administration of diclofenac, a drug with better prostaglandin inhibitory properties than indomethacin failed to effect base-line CBF and did not attenuate the response to hypercapnia (Hougaard et al., 1983). Similarly, in patients with cerebrovascular disease, mild hypercapnia did not alter endogenous prostacyclin formation and CBF went up appropriately suggesting that endogenous PGI_2 are not the mediator for the CBF response to CO_2 (Wennmalm et al., 1983).

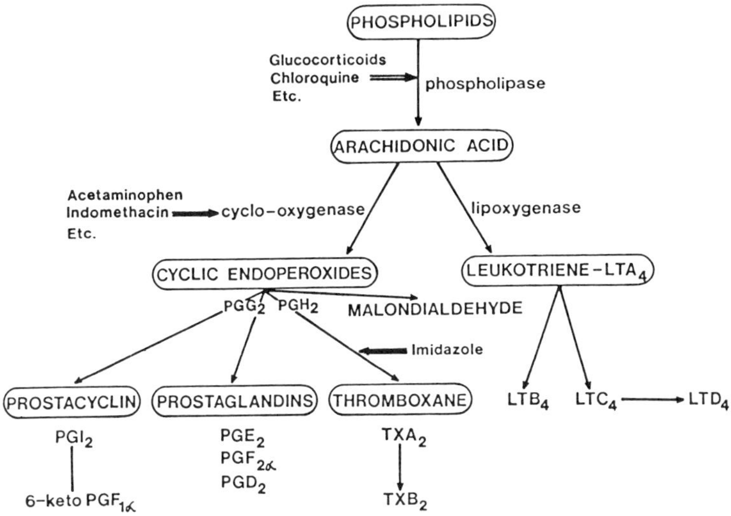

FIGURE 6.2. Arachidonic acid metabolic cascade. Various drugs can alter pathway of arachidonic acid metabolism by different mechanisms. Drugs can decrease arachidonate availability (open arrowhead) or to inhibit specific enzymatic system (arrowhead) essential for normal metabolism. Sometimes the mechanism of action is dose dependent.

Experimental animal data are also conflicting. It has been suggested that hypoxia but not hypercapnia appears to produce cerebral vasodilation by increasing prostacyclin production (McCalden et al., 1984a) but conflicting results have also been published (Siesjö & Wieloch, 1983). Experiments performed in rats suggest that prostaglandins do not contribute signficantly to regulation of cerebral circulation during normo- and hypercapnia (Busija, 1983). Also, the steady-state cerebral vasodilation induced by hypercapnia is largely preserved after inhibition of prostaglandin synthesis by indomethacin (Busija & Heistad, 1983).

High dose salicylates appear to have an effect on the CBF response to CO_2 in normal volunteers (Pickard et al., 1977). In patients with acute stroke, internal jugular prostaglandin concentration correlates significantly with the degree of CBF autoregulation disturbance (Oiwa et al., 1984). When hemodynamic studies were performed using ultrasound techniques, indomethacin treatment in patients with the Shy-Drager Syndrome, clearly limited the postural depression of blood pressure, an effect which was attributed to the inhibition of prostaglandin synthesis (Tsuda et al., 1983).

The role of prostaglandins and other eicosanoids in the control of CBF in health and after an acute cerebrovascular event has been recently reviewed by Pickard and Walker (1984), but many of the controversies mentioned here remained unsettled.

DRUGS ACTING DIRECTLY ON PERIPHERAL VESSELS

Papaverine and Papaverine-like-acting Drugs

Papaverine, once popular for the treatment of cerebrovascular disease, has been studied by several workers in order to evaluate its effect on CBF, using invasive (Capon et al., 1977; Gottstein, 1965; Herrschaft, 1976; Mankovsky et al., 1979; Melamed & Lavy, 1979; Olesen & Paulson, 1971) and noninvasive techniques (McHenry et al., 1983; Shaw & Meyer, 1978; Vasileva, 1981). The results of the CBF response vary from increases (Herrschaft, 1976; McHenry et al., 1983; Olesen & Paulson, 1971; Shaw & Meyer, 1978, Vasileva, 1981), unpredictable responses but more often decreases in infarcted (Capon et al., 1977) as well as in contralateral noninfarcted regions (Melamed & Lavy, 1979). Some investigators demonstrated a decrease only in ischemic regions (Mankovsky et al., 1979). Their results were similar to those obtained with global CBF measurement using Kety–Schmidt technique, where no effect was observed on already altered blood flow in patients with atheroschlerotic brain disease (Gottstein, 1965). More recently, the inhalation technique for regional CBF measurement has been used in normal subjects following a single dose of papaverine. Both single oral dose or IV administration of the drug were equally effective in increasing CBF (McHenry et al., 1983). Long-term treatment of patients suffering from chronic cerebrovascular ischemia with oral papaverine, revealed significant increase of blood flow in regions supplied by the vertebrobasilar system, and zones of severe, remote cerebral infarction appeared refractory to the drug (Shaw & Meyer, 1978). The response may be diminished by simultaneous cigarette smoking or alcohol consumption (Vasileva, 1981).

A few authors consider papaverine beneficial for the treatment of cerebrovascular disease (Herrschaft, 1976; Vasileva, 1981) but most conclude that vasodilators, such as papaverine, should be avoided in the treatment of stroke (Capon et al., 1977; Mankovsky et al., 1979; Melamed & Lavy, 1979). Cyclandelate, which possesses some structural similarities to papaverine, significantly increases CBF without influencing pCO_2 or blood pressure. No improvement has been reported in any patients with cerebrovascular disease, but the response was measured after a single dose (O'Brien & Veall, 1966). Naftidrofuryl, a papaverine-like vasodilator, may reduce CBF marginally and large doses may induce a greater reduction in cerebrovascular patients (Heiss, 1973; Heiss & Zeiler, 1978). Another study revealed significant CBF reduction after a dose of 100 mg without appreciable changes in arterial pCO_2 or mean arterial blood pressure (Herrschaft, 1976). Chronic oral treatment with naftidrofuryl did not have any significant effect on CBF in patients with chronic cerebrovascular disease (James et al., 1978). Completely different results were found in the acute and subacute stages of cerebral ischemia where significant increases in the affected regions were found after 1–2 weeks of treatment (Kobayashi et al.,

1984a). Hexobendine is a derivative of 3-methoxybenzoic acid and is derived from alkaloid reserpine. When given intravenously, it caused slight but significant increase in CBF, while oral treatment was ineffective. In regions with severe flow impairment due to vascular disease, improvement followed administration of the drug (Heiss, 1973).

Another study on the effects of hexobendine on CBF failed to reveal significant changes (Herrschaft, 1976). In patients with ischemic cerebrovascular disease, increased hemispheric blood flow and metabolism were found when the drug was given orally or intravenously in spite of a slight decrease in mean arterial blood pressure. Increased CBF has been observed in both the noninfarcted and ischemic hemisphere after single dose administration (Meyer et al., 1971). Increased brain blood flow is also found in hypertensive stroke patients after the single intravenous application of hexobendine. The drug may increase blood flow in localized as well as in diffuse intracranial vascular disease but cerebral metabolism and systemic cardiovascular hemodynamics remained unaltered in this study (McHenry et al., 1972).

Xanthines

Caffeine. The effect on CBF was examined in two groups of normal volunteers after single dosage of 250 or 500 mg given orally. Mean hemispheric blood flow decreased significantly, regardless of the dosage, while the regional pattern remained unaltered (Mathew et al., 1983). The results of this study confirm a previous one where invasive methods for the assessment of CBF changes were used (Shenkin, 1951). These results are different from those reported in animal experiments where caffeine and theophylline have been shown not to have a global effect on the utilization of glucose in the rat brain (Grome & Stefanovich, 1984) where normal coupling between blood flow and glucose utilization is expected.

Theophylline derivatives have been shown to reduce cerebral blood flow (Gottstein & Paulson, 1972; Herrschaft, 1976; Magnussen et al., 1977; Skinhøj & Paulson, 1970) although no effect was reported in one study (Gottstein, 1965). The reduction in CBF has been observed after intracarotid (Gottstein & Paulson, 1972) and intravenous (Magnussen et al., 1977; Skinhøj & Paulson, 1970) administration of aminophylline.

Pentoxyphylline possesses different properties than other xanthine derivatives with respect to CBF. Its effect on phosphodiesterase is similar to the other xanthines. Besides this effect, its main action is to increase red cell deformability (Marcel & George, 1983). Increased CBF has been reported in chronic cerebrovascular patients after treatment with pentoxyphylline and acute treatment with oral and parenteral forms of the drug respectively (Passero et al., 1981). In a group of patients with cerebrovascular disease, the effect of the drug was more pronounced in regions with low flow (Hartmann, 1983).

DRUGS ACTING ON CNS METABOLIC ACTIVITY

Due to the impossibility of defining the mechanism of their cerebrovascular action, these substances are subdivided into depressants and stimulants on the basis of their main pharmacological actions.

Central Nervous System Depressants

Anesthetics have been frequently studied with respect to their effects on cerebral circulation. All anesthetic agents and procedures alter intracranial dynamics and the importance of maintaining CBF, especially when it is compromised with neurological damage, is of great importance (Frost, 1984). As expected, CBF is usually decreased but the degree and duration of the flow response differs, depending on the type of anesthetics used.

Intravenous Anesthetic Agents

Barbiturates. A copious literature concerning the effect of these type of drugs on CBF is available. The main reason for this is the fact that barbiturates exert beneficial effects in ischemic brain damage (Nemoto et al., 1977; Simeone et al., 1979; Smith et al., 1975), ameliorate postischemic encephalopathy in experimental animals (Bleyaert et al., 1977), stop further reduction in blood flow and $CMRO_2$ during the recirculation period after brain ischemia (Nordström et al., 1977) and prevent the rise of potassium ions in ischemic rat brain (Astrup et al., 1977). In humans, their effect on CBF has received less attention. Following a single intravenous injection of sodium-thiopental, CBF decreased uniformly to about 45 % of initial values when measured with ^{133}Xe intra-arterial technique. The reduction lasted more than 10 minutes after termination of injection (Herrschaft & Schmidt, 1973). Metohexital also induces a reduction in CBF similar in extent to the one obtained with thiopental, but the effect is short-lasting and is not visible after 10 minutes (Herrschaft & Schmidt, 1974); in patients comatose as a result of head injury, pentobarbital produced a 20% decrease in CBF accompanied by an 18% decrease in $CMRO_2$. With hyperventilation and pentobarbital treatment, the reduction in CBF was even more pronounced at 43.7% while $CMRO_2$ diminished less dramatically by 23%. These cumulative effects of hyperventilation and CNS depressants might protect the brain in patients with brain injury (Escuret et al., 1977).

Besides its effect on cerebral metabolism there have recently appeared two reports concerning possible mechanisms of barbiturate action on cerebral blood vessels. When pentobarbital was administered to the dog, after inhalation of CO_2, reduced CBF and $CMRO_2$ was found, with the conclusion that there is no direct effect of barbiturate on blood vessels (Chin et al., 1983). But there is also an evidence that barbiturates, given in anesthetic concentrations, may exert direct vasodilator actions on cerebral arterial smooth muscle. The relaxation appears to be related to the inhibition of calcium ion influx in cerebral vessels which may be important in the salutary actions of barbiturates in brain ischemia, vascular spasm, or trauma (Altura & Altura, 1984). In patients with cerebral ischemia, thiopenthal and alfatesine-etomidate diminished CBF, except in ischemic areas where the response was abolished or even reversed, which could be of diagnostic and prognostic value (Bidabe–Renou et al., 1978). In patients with brain tumor where CBF and $CMRO_2$ were already reduced by pentobarbital-induced and halothane-maintained anesthesia, a significant further drop was observed during thiopental loading accompanied by an almost equivalent reduction in brain metabolism (Astrup et al., 1984).

Propanidid is an intravenous, short-acting anesthetic which reduces cerebral blood flow to 45% of resting values, but the effect disappears after 10 minutes (Herrschaft & Schmidt, 1973; Herrschaft et al., 1971–72).

Ketamine produces a state of dissociation from the environment with analgesia, amnesia, and light sleep. It is quite frequently used as an anesthetic. Its mechanism of action is not clear but experimental data show a relative increase of deoxyglucose labeling in limbic regions at various doses. By contrast, in superficial brain regions, ketamine induced a relative decrease of deoxyglucose uptake. Metabolic changes, reflected by the alteration of deoxyglucose uptake in various cortical regions, might be a consequence of a ketamine-induced activation of specific neuronal pathways with special neurochemical features (Hammer & Herkenham, 1983). Experiments, performed in vitro with slices of cerebral cortex, revealed a decreased stimulatory effect of norepinephrine on cyclic AMP formation under the influence of anesthetic concentrations of ketamine (Okuda et al., 1984). Apart from these effects, ketamine was found to exert a spasmogenic action on cerebral arteries (Altura & Altura, 1984), which may explain some of the CBF changes during anesthesia with this agent. In normal subjects, ketamine produced a reduction of CBF by 28% but the effect was short-lasting and 5 minutes after completing the IV injection, blood flow returned to the normal values (Herrschaft & Schmidt, 1973; Herrschaft et al., 1971–72). Measured 2–4 minutes after IV injection, CBF showed a variable response with marked regional increases in the frontotemporal and parieto-occipital regions, suggesting that the alteration in rCBF is secondary to changes in regional neuronal activity (Hougaard et al., 1974).

Althesin is a short-acting steroidal anesthetic. The only empirical study was an abstract and the data are insufficiently documented but an inverse "steal" syndrome was apparently observed in some patients with cerebrovascular disease although not in others (Renou et al., 1977).

Inhalation Anesthetic Agents

Halothane, a halogenated hydrocarbon, is used more often than any other volatile anesthetic agent. Its vasodilating properties lead to increased CBF. Decreased cerebral vascular resistance has been seen in experimental settings

(Gelman et al., 1984; Todd & Drummond, 1984) and in clinical practice (Brodersen et al., 1977; Wollman et al., 1969a). Experimental evidence suggests that the blood-flow increase associated with halothane inhalation is a transient phenomenon after which cerebral blood flow gradually returns to control levels over a protracted period of time (Albrecht et al., 1983). In man, light anesthesia leads to a decrease in CBF which is followed by an increase as anesthesia deepens (Wollman et al., 1969a). Halothane leads to an increase in CBF in anesthetic concentration and this change was accompanied by a decrease in $CMRO_2$ (Wollman et al., 1969a). Changes in CBF correlate poorly with arterial halothane concentrations, suggesting that if a direct cerebral vasodilation does occur, the effect is modest in intensity and can be modified by metabolic activity (Smith, 1975). Unlike phenobarbitone, halothane does not exert a protective effect in experimental ischemia (Smith et al., 1975). When the effect of halothane was studied in patients with brain tumors, where CBF remained reduced during hypocapnic halothane anesthesia, a further drop in cerebral perfusion pressure indicated that halothane produced vasodilation despite maintained hypocapnia. Hypocapnic halothane anesthesia may therefore be a safe compromise between preventing intracranial pressure rise and lowering CBF in neurosurgical patients (Brodersen et al., 1977).

Halogenated Ethers. Although each possesses some distinctive pharmacological properties with respect to CBF, their action is generally similar. Experimentally, increased CBF has been reported by one group of investigators (Gelman et al., 1984) but not by another (Todd & Drummond, 1984). Decreased cerebral vascular resistance was found to be dose-related although not to such an extent as during halothane anesthesia (Todd & Drummond, 1984). In humans, during moderately deep ethrane anesthesia, CBF remains normal in spite of decreased cerebral perfusion pressure and decreased brain metabolism (Wollman et al., 1969b). Only a small and in two regions significant decrease in rCBF was seen in spite of a significant decrease of mean arterial pressure which, however, remained within autoregulatory limits (Rolly & Van Aken, 1979). When similar concentrations of enflurane were employed by other workers, the results were similar but increasing the concentration led to a rise in CBF and a drop in $CMRO_2$ suggesting direct vasodilating properties (Sakabe et al., 1983). Generally, halogenated ethers and halothane reduces cerebral vascular resistance but the changes are drug-specific, organ-specific, and often dose-related (Lognecker, 1984).

Alcohol

Although not strictly regarded as therapeutic, alcohol has also been studied with respect to its effect on CBF. Alcohol possesses anesthetic properties but the action on the central nervous system depends greatly on the amount ingested as well as the duration and regularity of its use. The effect of alcohol on CBF is of particular interest because of its widespread recreational use all over the world. Occasional ethanol intoxication and regular heavy drinking both seem to carry an increased risk of ischemic brain infarction (Hillbom & Kaste, 1983) so it is interesting to examine its effects on cerebral blood flow.

In normal, social drinkers, intake of a moderate dose of alcohol produces increased flow in cortical gray matter. Regional changes are symmetrical in posterior areas, but flow increased more in the right than left frontal areas. Besides the direct vasodilatory effect of alcohol, these findings can be explained by an asymmetrical effect on metabolism (Newlin et al., 1982). Changes in autoregulatory limits have been observed during acute alcohol intoxication in the rat, with a downward shift of the lower threshold (Barry & Hemmingsen, 1984). Effects of long-term alcohol abuse have also been studied. In chronic alcoholics and patients with Korsakoff's psychosis, decreased CBF has been found, reflecting reduced cerebral metabolism. Regional reduction appears more pronounced in anterior temporal and frontal areas. Patients with Korsakoff's psychosis revealed higher CBF than the other alcoholics (Berglund & Ingvar, 1976). Alcohol withdrawal was also accompanied by reduced blood flow while the regional distribution was dependent on the level of consciousness and the presence of other psychopathological symptoms (Berglund & Risberg, 1981).

Other Central Nervous System Depressants

Midazolam. A new, water soluble, short-acting benzodiazepine is recommended for the introduction of anesthesia. In normal volunteers, it leads to a fall in CBF despite an increase in $PaCO_2$ secondary to its respiratory depressant activity (Forster et al., 1982). Under hypercapnic conditions, reduction of CBF was less pronounced than during normocapnic states, suggesting that it should be used cautiously in patients with intracranial hypertension due to its effect on arterial pCO_2 (Forster et al., 1983).

Haloperidol was studied in patients with paranoid symptomatology using the noninvasive ^{133}Xe inhalation technique. Decrease of mean hemispheric flow was observed together with a "deactivating" effect on frontotemporal areas where regional blood flow was increased prior to treatment (Nilsson et al., 1977). In experiments performed on rats, haloperidol significantly reduced glucose utilization in the majority of brain regions studied (Pizzolato et al., 1984), indicating that the effect on CBF is a secondary event.

Another neuroleptic, *thiothixene,* was studied with positron emission tomography in schizophrenic patients. Frontal hypometabolism remained unchanged after treatment but an increase in metabolic rate was observed in basal ganglia (Brodie et al., 1984).

Bromides have a general depressant action on the central nervous system with anticonvulsant activity and are no longer used. Markedly subnormal CBF was reported in one patient with bromide psychosis. After dialysis, CBF increased and regional changes normalized (Berglund et al., 1977).

Lithium has an established role in the treatment of recurrent manic–depressive psychosis and more recently it has found use in certain types of vascular headaches. It has no effect on CBF in patients with cluster headache and the CO_2 responsiveness remains unaltered (Okayashu et al., 1984). Studies on animals have provided similar results (Preskorn et al., 1981).

Central Nervous System Stimulants

Nicotine is the most important pharmacological constituent of tobacco and the smoke from an average-sized cigarette may contain 6–8 mg nicotine. It causes escitation, followed by inhibition at all sympathetic and parasympathetic ganglia, and it acts on central nervous system in a similar fashion.

Cigarette smoking represents an important risk factor for atherosclerotic vascular disease. The acute effect of cigarette smoking in healthy volunteers is a decrease in cerebral vascular resistance and a rise in CBF, probably due to increased cerebral oxygen consumption (Wennmalm, 1982). Cigarette smoking may improve attention, memory (Peeke & Peeke, 1984) and rapid information-processing performance (Wesnes & Warburton, 1983) perhaps as a result of an influence on central cholinergic systems.

But chronic cigarette smoking leads to a decrease in CBF probably because it enhances cerebral atherosclerosis (Rogers et al., 1983). In addition, an exaggerated reduction of CBF with advancing age has been observed (Kubota et al., 1983). Chronic cigarette smoking influences cerebrovascular reactivity to oxygen and carbon dioxide. Reduced vasodilator and vasoconstrictor responses were found in smokers when compared with age-matched nonsmokers (Rogers et al., 1984).

Amphetamine is rarely employed in clinical therapy but as a drug of abuse it deserves attention. Experimental investigations have shown a dose-dependent increase in CBF (Berntman et al., 1978; Rovere et al., 1977). The greatest regional increase was confined to the frontotemporal regions while other cortical or subcortical areas showed moderate hyperemia. CBF changes were accompanied by an increase in $CMRO_2$ (Berntman et al., 1978). It has also been shown that increased blood flow is prevented by atropine or chlorpromazine (Rovere et al., 1977). Decreased blood flow was observed in basal ganglia but pretreatment with haloperidol prevented these changes (Lavyne et al., 1977). When CBF was measured during amphetamine intoxication in a young addict, it was found to be elevated 30% above values in nonintoxicated state. The most marked augmentation was found in the frontal regions and in the left hemisphere (Berglund & Risberg, 1980) which corresponds to the findings obtained experimentally in animals (Berntman et al., 1978).

MISCELLANEOUS AGENTS WHICH AFFECT CBF

Drugs used to Treat Cerebrovascular Disorders

Calcium Antagonists

Calcium antagonists are a group of drugs recently introduced in the treatment of cerebrovascular disorders. Their potential effects on hypoxic tissue are related to the prevention of the exaggerated entry of calcium ions, the inhibition of precapillary vasoconstriction, the reduction of the peripheral edema formation and the ability to restore normal deformability of red blood cells (Vanhoutte, 1982; Van Nueten & De Clerck, 1984). Investigation of the antihypoxic effect of this type of drugs revealed that its calcium channel blocking activity, ability to increase red blood cell deformability and consequently lower whole blood viscosity apparently play a dominant role in cerebral protection (Van Nueten & Vanhoutte, 1984; Weir, 1984). But its interaction with arachidonic acid metabolism might be also significant (Higgs et al., 1985; Nikolov et al., 1984). Brain protective action during hypoxic conditions has been shown for flunarizine (Van Nueten & De Clerck, 1984; Van Nueten & Vanhoutte, 1984; Wauquier, 1982), while lidoflazine did not effect CBF in an animal model of total cerebral ischemia (Dean et al., 1984).

Nimodipine, another calcium entry blocker, induces an increase of CBF in forebrain regions without altering flow in hindbrain structures. A low drug dosage induced the greatest increase in local CBF suggesting that the effect of increased dosage is counteracted by the concomitant systemic hypotension (Mohamed et al., 1984). Other investigators found modest increase in basal CBF without significant alteration in cerebral metabolism or systemic blood pressure, keeping the autoregulation mechanism intact. Nimodipine appeared to block the cerebrovascular mechanism sensitive to CO_2 (McCalden et al., 1983). Infusion of the dose that produced maximal increase in flow, decreased the cerebral reactivity to changes in pCO_2, suggesting that nimodipine may be a relatively selective cerebrovascular dilator (McCalden et al., 1984b). An homogeneous increase in local cerebral glucose utilization was found in the rat brain after intravenous administration of the drug (d'Avella et al., 1984). Although theoretically useful in the treatment of cerebral ischemia, flunarizine and verapamil have been disappointing in some animal experiments (Berger et al., 1984; Newberg et al., 1984). Clinical applications of nimodipine are currently limited to the prevention of cerebral ischemia following arterial vasospasm (Auer, 1983) and as a possible antimigraine agent (Peroutka, 1983; Spierings, 1984). It may also have a beneficial effect in the treatment of patients with ischemic stroke (Gelmers, 1984). In a group of patients suffering from migraine and cluster headache, where CBF measurements were performed during oxygen inhalation, the normal vasoconstrictor response was reduced with high drug doses (Meyer &

Hardenberg, 1983). Following a single oral dose in cerebrovascular patients, a global increase in CBF was observed 1 hour after administration with the greatest regional increases in low flow areas (Gaab et al., 1982). Increased CBF was seen in patients with subarachnoid hemorrhage, where regional analysis revealed a more generalized rise in CBF compared with atherosclerotic stroke (Gaab et al., 1982). Measurement of CBF after nifedipine showed an increase in flow in four out of five patients where the drug was being used for acute antihypertensive treatment in contrast to clonidine which reduced blood flow in all patients by 28% (Bertel et al., 1983). Animal experiments and CBF assessments in humans give grounds for moderate optimism that this group of drugs may become useful in neurological practice. We await adequate clinical trials.

"Metabolic Activators" and Other Vasodilating Drugs

Vincamine, an indolic alkaloid isolated from Vinca minor is employed in the treatment of cerebrovascular disorders in some countries (Spagnoli & Tognoni, 1983). It possesses "anti-anoxic" properties (Gotti & Depoortere, 1980) similar to 1-eburnamonine (Lacroix et al., 1979). Vinpocetine and its metabolite apovincaminic acid cause an increase in CBF in anesthetized dogs (Imamoto et al., 1984). A new eburnamonine derivative appears to facilitate EEG recovery following experimental ischemia in the gerbil (Barzaghi et al., 1982). No effect was observed on CBF in humans when an infusion of 30 mg was administered but increased dosage resulted in significant increase in mean hemispheric flow (Heiss, 1980). In another study, increased CBF corresponded to the peak plasma concentration of vincamine in all except one patient where CBF did not change. The reason for that was due to decreased pCO_2 (Witzmann et al., 1977). In chronic, stable neurological disease, including hydrocephalus, dementia and old cerebral infarction, vincamine leads to an increase in CBF with more pronounced action seen in the ischemic regions (Depresseux, 1977; Heiss, 1980). Increases in CBF together with reductions in hemispheric asymmetry, were seen after 2 weeks of vincamine treatment (Risberg et al., 1982). Bromvincamine did not influence regional CBF following 2 weeks of treatment (Risberg et al., 1982) but after a longer period of therapy, increased CBF and improved psychometric performance in a group of mild to moderate mentally deteriorated patients has been reported (Kobayashi et al., 1984b). The CBF response to 1-eburnamonine varies greatly and inconclusive results have been reported after single infusion therapy (Gosetti et al., 1978).

Tinofedrine, a derivative of 1-norepinephrine possesses vasoactive properties and has been investigated with regard to its effect on CBF. Acute, single administration of this agent has no significant effect on CBF (Heiss, 1980; Heiss & Podreka, 1979). Significant increases in CBF were observed after the acute administration of tinofedrine in patients with multi-infarct dementia by another team, but higher doses were given (Merory et al., 1978). After long-term treatment with tinofedrine, improvement of brain-blood flow was observed in a group of cerebrovascular patients in a subacute stage of disease. Flow increases were reported both in infarcted and noninfarcted hemispheres (Ott & Lechner, 1980).

Bencyclan also belongs to the group of vasoactive substances allegedly useful in the treatment of cerebrovascular disease (Rossignol & Ebiqwei–Ibru, 1980). Acute parenteral administration of this drug does not alter CBF to any significant degree (Heiss, 1980; Herrschaft, 1976).

Piracetam belongs to the novel class of drugs called nootropics, sometimes used in the treatment of cerebral vascular disorders and other organic brain syndromes. A protective effect against hypoxia-induced brain damage has been reported (Giurgea et al., 1971) but not confirmed (Dirks et al., 1984). Experimental animal investigations suggest a beneficial effect in learning (Wolthuis, 1971), and learning impairment (Myslivečkova–Hassmanova et al., 1978). Therapeutic benefits have been reported in senile dementia (Macchione et al., 1976; Stegink, 1972), cerebrovascular disease (Kartin et al., 1979), acute alcohol withdrawal (Dencker et al., 1978), speech rehabilitation (Mubrin et al., 1983), but not all the studies are convincing. CBF is augmented in patients with acute stroke (Herrschaft, 1978). No effect was seen either on mental functions or on regional CBF after long-term treatment in patients with organic dementia (Gustafson et al., 1978). Acute administration of piracetam or its derivative etiracetam failed to show any effect on CBF in anesthetized patients (Van Aken & Rolly, 1980).

Pyrithioxine is marketed as a "metabolic activator" and is composed of two B_6 vitamine (pyridoxine) molecules. Experimental data show that it activates protein metabolism (Kanig, 1973), changes the EEG activation pattern (Zimmermann et al., 1982), activates the brain-stem reticular formation, causing an increase in CBF and metabolism (Stoica et al., 1973) and may be beneficial in dementia (Cooper & Magnus, 1980) and in cerebrovascular disorders (Tazaki et al., 1980). In the group of cerebrovascular patients, increased gray-matter flow was observed after infusion of pyrithioxine which was attributed to the activation of cerebral oxygen metabolism (Herrschaft, 1975; Herrschaft, 1976). But in another study, pyritinol failed to influence disturbed CBF or pathologically changed cerebral oxygen consumption in patients with organic brain disorders (Hoyer et al., 1977).

Hemodilutional Therapy

Glycerol is a polyhydric alcohol soluble in water. As a hyperosmolar solution, it is used to reduce brain edema. Experimental investigations have shown reduced perivascular spaces and improved EEG recovery after glycerol treatment in an animal model of ANOXIC brain injury (Gomerčić et al., 1983; Marković et al., 1983) as well as a temporary increase in CBF after subarachnoid hemorrhage (Hashi et al., 1972). On the other hand, deleterious effects of glycerol treatment, particularly in relation to CBF and metabolism were seen after glycerol treatment of cerebral microembolism in the rat (Bralet et al., 1983). A clinical trial with glycerol in patients with acute cerebral infarction has been reported and a significant improvement in neurological status compared with placebo (Mathew et al., 1972) or mannitol (Kalousek et al., 1978) was observed. In patients with acute stroke, IV glycerol leads to increased hemispheric flow and a reduction in cerebral oxygen consumption and carbon dioxide production (Meyer et al., 1972).

Mannitol is also a polyhydric alcohol and it is used in similar situations. Using an animal model of cerebral infarction, mannitol suppressed brain swelling during recirculation after 3 hours, but was ineffective after 6 hours of arterial occlusion (Suzuki et al., 1980). When a very high dose of mannitol (2gm/kg) was administered to the intact animal, small increases in CBF occurred, lasting less than 10 minutes and followed by a significant reduction of approximately 3 hours duration. These findings suggest that either the effect of mannitol on CBF is quantitatively different when flow is reduced or that the protective effect is based upon a different mechanism than the augmentation of flow in situations where it is compromised (Kassel et al., 1982). In acute head injury, mannitol increased CBF in nearly all patients but cerebral metabolic rate increased, together with the blood flow in only a few patients. Intracranial pressure was independent of the CBF changes and the relationship of these parameters was unpredictable (Bruce et al., 1973).

Dextran, an branched polysaccharide, is used as a plasma expander. The results of hemodilution therapy following acute cerebral infarction are encouraging (Gottstein, 1979). A critical trial where dextran has been administered to patients with acute focal ischemia revealed neurological improvement attributed to the augmentation of collateral perfusion secondary to reduced blood viscosity (Wood & Fleischer, 1982). In cerebrovascular patients, dextran has been reported to increase cerebral blood flow even in ischemic regions (Heiss, 1980; Heiss & Podreka, 1979; Heiss et al., 1972; Herrschaft, 1975).

Other Drugs Including Antihypertensives and Diuretics

Antihypertensives. It is known that hypertensive patients have altered autoregulation and baroreflex function which can make them sensitive to a reduction in blood pressure (Strangaard et al., 1973). Experimental data where chronic antihypertensive treatment was administered in hypertensive rats revealed a return to the normal values of previously impaired autoregulation (Barry et al., 1983; Vorstrup et al., 1984a). In acute stroke, increased systemic blood pressure will aggravate ischemic brain edema (Fenske et al., 1978). On the other hand, when systemic blood pressure is rapidly lowered and drops below the lower limit of cerebral autoregulation, impairment of brain tissue perfusion will result. Alpha-adrenergic blockers are able to protect the brain against consequences of hypotension induced low blood flow states (Gygax & Wiernsperger, 1983; MacKenzie et al., 1984).

Clinical studies of CBF during hypotensive treatment have shown that control of hypertension can be achieved without jeopardizing cerebral blood flow or inducing signs and symptoms of cerebral ischemia even in cerebrovascular patients. Furthermore, control of hypertension reduces both, the risk of stroke and the recurrence rate of repeated strokes (Gifford, 1983). Acute reduction of systemic blood pressure by intravenous injection of diazoxide in hypertensive patients showed preserved autoregulation after first administration of drug but repeated administration revealed some degree of dysautoregulation (Goldberg et al., 1977). Acute antihypertensive treatment with nifedipine induced an increase in CBF in the majority of patients examined, whereas clonidine reduced CBF in all patients (Bertel et al., 1983). Controlled hypotension with sodium nitroprusside in patients operated for cerebral aneurysms revealed only a minor change relating mainly to an increase in CBF after termination of the hypotensive period. Regional changes were not accentuated during hypotension nor were ischemic regions disclosed (Henriksen et al., 1983). Only in patients where autoregulation was impaired, were relatively severe flow disturbances noted postoperatively at the site of retraction and in some of these patients ischemic deficits ensued (Farrar et al., 1981).

Captopril is commonly used in the treatment of congestive heart failure because it lowers peripheral vascular resistance and blood pressure. A single-dose study, in control subjects and patients with congestive heart failure, was performed using single photon emission tomography. Despite the marked decrease in blood pressure CBF increased slightly in the patients with severe congestive heart failure, although after correction of pCO_2, CBF remained unchanged. In control subjects, different results were seen, namely little effect on systemic blood pressure with small, insignificant decrease in CBF (Paulson et al., 1984). Using the ^{133}Xenon intravenous technique, rCBF has been examined after captopril treatment in patients with congestive heart failure. CBF increased almost to the values of control subjects after 4–15 days treatment despite a fall in mean blood pressure. The reason for this effect remains obscure (Rajagopalan et al., 1984).

Diuretics represent a group of drugs frequently employed in everyday clinical practice. Carbonic anhydrase inhibitors are the most frequently studied in respect of their effect on CBF. When used in mildly demented geriatric patients, increased CBF was found and this persisted for at least 6 weeks, but no consistent improvement in mentation was observed (Wyper et al., 1976). Similar results were found after intravenous administration, while oral treatment had no significant effect on CBF (Heiss, 1980; Heiss & Podreka, 1979). A local vasodilatory effect on cerebral vessels was also suggested, based on the findings of increased CBF after intravenous treatment (Hauge et al., 1983). The acute effect of acetazolamide has also been investigated in patients where the regulation of cerebral circulation was considered normal. CBF significantly increased leaving $CMRO_2$ unchanged, which was explained by decrease in brain pH due to inhibition of oxygen unloading in the cerebral capillaries (Vorstrup et al., 1984b). Cardiac glycosides, such as digoxin and methylproscillaridin, do not affect CBF to any significant degree, but ouabain increases CBF. This change possibly reflects a direct influence on cerebral vessels (Heiss, 1980; Heiss & Podreka, 1979). Ouabain, like acetazolamide, is a specific inhibitor of carbonic anhydrase and the explanations for their effects on CBF may be similar (Vorstrup et al., 1984b).

Dexamethasone is frequently used for treatment of brain edema in certain clinical conditions, such as tumors, head injury, etc. (see Marshall, 1980; McGillicuddy, 1985). In children with severe closed head injury, dexamethasone appears beneficial (James et al., 1979) although an analysis of results from three different countries did not confirm better outcome in patients treated with steroids as opposed to other methods of treatment (Jannett et al., 1980). In experimental brain edema, dexamethasone reduces adjacent edema (Gaab et al., 1979) but in focal ischemia, and even in combination with mannitol it fails to modify the size of resulting cerebral infarction (Little, 1978). Following dexamethasone treatment in patients with brain tumors, hemispheric CBF was significantly improved and cerebral vasomotor response was markedly or completely restored. Improvement in brain function and neurological symptoms was also observed, suggesting that dexamethasone tends to counteract the factors responsible for alteration of cerebral vasomotor function and serves to remove edema fluid around brain tumors (Hadjidimos et al., 1973).

Concluding Remarks

The great advantages of inhalation and intravenous methodology are relative noninvasiveness, good reproducibility, and safety. Some resolution is sacrificed but this may not matter if it is used in appropriate situations. A major disadvantage, however, is that blood flow is the only parameter measured. Without a coincidental measurement of $CMRO_2$ we can never be certain that we have affected cerebral function and increased CBF is often equated with improved CBF. Coupling of CBF with metabolism has been demonstrated experimentally by Raichle et al. (1976) and confirmed with PET studies in normal humans (Lebrun–Grandié et al., 1983) and patients with dementia (Frackowiack et al., 1981). While it may be safe to assure coupling in many pathological states, it is clear that many procedures (e.g., Hct reduction) and perhaps many drugs affect the ratio of CBF to metabolism without affecting the latter per se. Considerable caution is therefore warranted when assessing the clinical significance of drugs which increase CBF. Numerous claims for the efficacy of cerebral "vasodilators" have emerged from CBF laboratories but their significance remains questionable without adequate clinical descriptions of patient outcome. CBF measurements may suggest that some drugs are efficacious and others deleterious, and so point the way to controlled clinical trials, but they are not in themselves a reliable clinical indicator.

REFERENCES

Albrecht, R. F., Miletich, D. J., & Madala, L. R. (1983). Normalization of cerebral blood flow during prolonged halothane anesthesia. *Anesthesiology, 58,* 26–31.

Alman, R. W., Rosenberg, M., & Fazekas, J. F. (1952). Effects of histamine on cerebral hemodynamics and metabolism. *Arch. Neurol. Psychiat., 67,* 354–356.

Altura, B. T., & Altura, B. M. (1984). Effects of barbiturates, phencyclidine, ketamine and analogs on cerebral circulation and cerebrovascular muscle. *Microcirc. Endoth. Lymphat., 1,* 169–184.

Aoyagi, M., Deshmukh, V. D., Meyer, J. S., Kawamura, Y., & Tagashira, Y. (1976). Effect of beta-adrenergic blockade with propranolol on cerebral blood flow, autoregulation and CO_2 responsiveness. *Stroke, 7,* 291–295.

Astrup, J., Nordström, C.–H., & Rechncrona, S. (1977). Rate of rise in extracellular potassium in the ischemic rat brain and the effect of preischemic metabolic rate: Evidence for a specific effect of phenobarbitone. *Acta Neurol. Scand., 56*(Suppl. 64), 148–149.

Astrup, J., Resenørn, J., Cold, G. E., Bendtsen, A., & Møller Sørensen, P. (1984). Minimum cerebral blood flow and metabolism during craniotomy. Effect of thiopental loading. *Acta Anaesthesiol. Scand., 28,* 478–481.

Auer, L. M. (1983). Cerebrovascular activity of the calcium antagonist nimodipine. In M. Reivich, & H. I. Hurtig (Eds.). *Cerebrovascular diseases* (pp. 375–384). New York: Raven Press.

Awad, I., Little, J. R., Lucas, F., Skrinska, V., Slugg, R., & Lesser, R. P. (1983). Modification of focal cerebral ischemia by prostacyclin and indomethacin. *J. Neurosurg., 58,* 714–719.

Barry, D. I., & Hemmingsen, R. (1984). Cerebral blood flow autoregulation during acute ethanol intoxication in the rat. *Acta Pharmacol. Toxicol., 54,* 227–232.

Barry, D. I., Svendsen, U. G., Vorstrup, S., Jarden, J. O., Braendstrup, O., Graham, D. I., & Strandgaard, S. (1983). The effect of chronic hypertension and antihypertensive drugs on the cerebral blood flow. *Acta Med. Scand.* (Suppl. 678), 37–42.

Barzaghi, F., Dragonetti, M., & Boissier, J. R. (1982). Effect of a new eburnamenine derivative (RU 24722) on EEG recovery in the conscious gerbil after cerebral ischemia. *Drug Dev. Res., 2,* 533–541.

Berger, J. R., Busto, R., & Ginsberg, M. D. (1984). Verapamil: Failure of metabolic amelioration following global forebrain ischemia in the rat. *Stroke, 15,* 1029–1032.

Berglund, M., & Ingvar, D. H. (1976). Cerebral blood flow and its regional distribution in alcoholism and in Korsakoff's psychosis. *J. Stud. Alco., 37,* 586–597.

Berglund, M., Nielzen, S., & Risberg, J. (1977). Regional cerebral blood flow in a case of bromide psychosis. *Arch. Psychiat. Nervenkr., 223,* 197–201.

Berglund, M., & Risberg, J. (1980). Regional cerebral blood flow in a case of amphetamine intoxication. *Psychopharmacology, 70,* 219–221.

———. (1981). Regional cerebral blood flow during alcohol withdrawal. *Arch. Gen. Psychiat., 38,* 351–355.

Berntman, L., Carlsson, C., Hägerdal, M., & Siesjö, B. K. (1978). Circulatory and metabolic effects in the brain induced by amphetamine sulphate. *Acta Physiol. Scand., 102,* 310–323.

Bertel, O., Conen, D., Radü, E. W., Müller, J., Lang, C., & Dubach, U. C. (1983). Nifedipine in hypertensive emergencies. *Brit. Med. J., 286,* 19–21.

Bidabe–Renou, A. M., Constant, P., Caille, J. M., & Vernet, J. (1978). Vasoreactivité des infarctus cerebraux aux barbituriques et autres anesthesiques intraveineux. *Ann. Anesthesiol. Fr., 19,* 821–826.

Black, K. L., Hoff, J. T., Radin, N. S., & Deshmukh, G. D. (1984). Eicosapentaenoic acid: Effects on brain prostaglandins, cerebral blood flow and edema in ischemic gerbils. *Stroke, 15,* 65–69.

Bleyaert, A. L., Nemoto, E. M., Safar, P., Stezoski, S. W., Moosy, J., Rao, G. R., & Mickell, J. (1977). Thiopental amelioration of post-ischemic encephalopathy in monkeys. *Acta Neurol. Scand., 56*(Suppl. 64), 144–145.

Bradbury, M. W. B. (1984). The structure and function of the blood-brain barrier. *Federation Proc., 43,* 186–190.

Bralet, J., Beley, P., Bralet, A.–M., & Beley, A. (1983). Comparison of the effects of hypertonic glycerol and urea on brain edema, energy metabolism and blood flow following cerebral microembolism in the rat. Deleterious effect of glycerol treatment. *Stroke, 14,* 597–604.

Brodersen, P., Gjerris, F., Hansen, A., Sørensen, P. M., & Nørholm, T. (1977). Cerebral blood flow and intracranial pressure during hypocapnic halothane anesthesia in brain tumor patients. *Acta Neurol. Scand., 56*(Suppl. 64), 500–501.

Brodie, J. D., Christman, D. R., Corona, J. F., Fowler, J. S., Gomez–Mont, F., Jaeger, J., Micheels, P. A., Rotrosen, J., Russell, J. A., Volkow, N. D., Wikler, A., Wolf, A. P., & Wolkin, A. (1984). Patterns of metabolic activity in the treatment of schizophrenia. *Ann. Neurol., 15*(Suppl.), S166–S169.

Bruce, D. A., Langfitt, T. W., Miller, J. D., Schutz, H., Vapalahti, M. P., Stanek, A., & Goldberg, H. I. (1973). Regional cerebral blood flow, intracranial pressure, and brain metabolism in comatose patients. *J. Neurosurg., 38,* 131–144.

Busija, D. W. (1983). Role of prostaglandins in the response of the cerebral circulation to carbon dioxide in conscious rabbits. *J. Cerebr. Blood Flow Metabol., 3,* 376–380.

Busija, D. W., & Heistad, D. D. (1983). Effects of indomethacin on cerebral blood flow during hypercapnia in cats. *Am. J. Physiol., 244,* H519–H524.

Calne, D. B. (1980). *Therapeutics in neurology* (2d ed.). Oxford, England: Blackwell Scientific Publications.

Capon, A., De Rood, M., Verbist, A., & Fruhling, J. (1977). Action of vasodilators on regional cerebral blood flow in subacute or chronic cerebral ischemia. *Stroke, 8,* 25–29.

Capraro, J. A., Reedy, D. P., Latchaw, J. P., Slugg, R. M., Stowe, N. T., Lesser, R. P., & Little, J. R. (1984). Treatment of acute focal cerebral ischemia with propranolol. *Stroke, 15,* 486–491.

Carpi, A. (1972). Classification of drugs acting on cerebral circulation. In A. Carpi (Ed.). Pharmacology of the cerebral circulation (Vol. 1, pp. 81–86). Oxford, England: Pergamon Press.

Chin, P.–W., Imai, S., Nakano, U., Takeda, K., Tamatsu, H., & Ushijima, T. (1983). Effects of drugs on the cerebral circulation of the dog in relation to the cerebral oxygen consumption. *Br. J. Pharmacol., 79,* 897–906.

Cook, P., & James, I. (1981a). Cerebral vasodilators (1st of 2 pts.). *N. Engl. J. Med., 305,* 1508–1513.

______. (1981b). Cerebral vasodilators (2d of 2 pts.). *N. Eng. J. Med., 305,* 1560–1564.

Cooper, A. J., & Magnus, R. V. (1980). A placebo-controlled study of pyritinol (''Encephabol'') in dementia. *Pharmatherapeutica, 2,* 317–322.

D'Avella, D., Cicciarello, R., La Torre, F., Princi, P., Greenberg, R. P., d'Aquino, S., & Caputi, A. P. (1984). The effect of the calcium antagonist nimodipine upon local cerebral glucose utilization in the rat brain. *Life Sci., 34,* 2583–2588.

Dean, M. J., Hoehner, P. J., Rogers, M. C., & Traystman, R. J. (1984). Effects of lidoflazine on cerebral blood flow following twelve minutes total cerebral ischemia. *Stroke, 15,* 531–535.

Dencker, S. J., Wilhelmson, G., Carlsson, F., & Bereen, F. J. (1978). Piracetam and chlormethiazole in acute alcohol withdrawal. A controlled clinical trial. *J. Int. Med. Res. 6,* 395–400.

Depreseux, J. C. (1977). The cerebral hemodynamic effect of vincamine. *Acta Neurol. Scand.*, *56*(Suppl. 64), 408–409.

Dirks, Von B., Seibert, A., Sperling, G., & Krieglstein, J. (1984). Vergleich der Wirkungen von Piracetam und Metohexital auf dem zerebralen Energiestoffwechsel. *Arzneim.-Forsch.*/Drug Res., 34 I, 258–266.

Eadie, M. J., & Tyrer, J. H. (1980). *Neurological clinical pharmacology. Lancaster:* MTP Press.

Escuret, E., Roquefeuil, B., Frerebeau, P., & Baldy–Moulinier, M. (1977). Effect of hyperventilation associated with administration of central nervous depressants in brain injuries. *Acta Neurol. Scand.*, *56*(Suppl. 64), 154–155.

Farrar, J. K., Gamache, F. W., Ferguson, G. G., Barker, J., Vorkey, G. P., & Drake, C. G. (1981). Effects of profound hypotension on cerebral blood flow during surgery for intracranial aneurysms. *J. Neurosurg.*, *55*, 857–864.

Fazekas, J. F., Thomas, A., Johnson, J. V. V., & Young, W. K. (1960a). Effect of arterenol (norepinephrine) and epinephrine on cerebral hemodynamics and metabolism. *Arch. Neurol. 2*, 435–438.

Fazekas, J. E., Thomas, A., Johnson, J. V. V., & Young, W. K. (1960b). Effect of norepinephrine on cerebral hemodynamics in severe hypotension. *Arch. Neurol.*, *2*, 305–308.

Fazekas, J. F., & Alman, R. W. (1964). Comparative effects of isoxsuprine and carbon dioxide on cerebral hemodynamics. *Amer. J. Med. Sci.*, *248*, 16–19.

Fenske, A., Kohl, J., Regli, F., & Reulen, H. J. (1978). The effect of arterial hypertension on focal ischemic edema. *J. Neurol.*, *219*, 241–251.

Forster, A., Juge, O., & Morel, D. (1982). Effects of midazolam on cerebral blood flow in human volunteers. *Anesthesiology*, *56*, 453–455.

Forster, A., Juge, P., & Model, D. (1983). Effects of midazolam on cerebral hemodynamics and cerebral vasomotor responsiveness to carbon dioxide. *J. Cerebr. Blood Flow Metabol.*, *3*, 246–249.

Frackowiak, S. J., Pozzilli, C., Legg, N. J., Du Boulay, G. H., Marshall, J., Lenzi, G. L., & Jones, T. (1981). Regional cerebral oxygen supply and utilization in dementia. A clinical and physiological study with oxygen-15 and positron tomography. *Brain*, *104*, 753–778.

Frost, E. A. M. (1984). Some inquiries in neuroanesthesia and neurological supportive care. *J. Neurosurg.*, *60*, 673–686.

Gaab, M. R., Brawanski, A., Bockhorn, J., Haubitz, I., Rode, C. P., & Maximilian, V. A. (1982). Calcium antagonism: A new therapeutic principle in stroke and cerebral vasospasm? *rCBF Bull.*, 3, 47–51.

Gaab, M., Herrmann, F., Kerscher, J., Rausch, K., Lochner, J., & Pflughaupt, K. W. (1979). Comparison of the effects of dexamethasone, barbiturate, and THAM on experimental brain edema. *Acta Neurochir.*, (Suppl. 28), 493–497.

Gelman, S., Fowler, K. C., & Smith, L. R. (1984). Regional blood flow during isoflurane and halothane anesthesia. *Anesth. Analg.*, *63*, 557–565.

Gelmers, H. J. (1984). The effects of nimodipine on the clinical course of patients with acute ischemic stroke. *Acta Neurol. Scand.*, *69*, 232–239.

Gifford, R. W. (1983). Effect of reducing elevated blood pressure on cerebral circulation. Hypertension, *5* (Suppl. 3), 3–17–3–20.

Giurgea, C., Lefevre, D., Lescrenier, C., & David–Remacle, M. (1971). Pharmacological protection against hypoxia-induced amnesia in rats. *Psychopharmacologia*, *20*, 160–168.

Globus, M., Keren, A., Eldad, M., Granot, C., Tzivoni, D., Lavy, S., & Stern, S. (1983). The effect of chronic propranolol therapy on regional cerebral blood flow in hypertensive patients. *Stroke*, *14*, 964–967.

Goldberg, H. I., Codario, R. A., Banka, R. S., & Reivich, M. (1977). Patterns of cerebral dysautoregulation in severe hypertension to blood pressure reduction with diazoxide. *Acta Neurol. Scand.*, *56*(Suppl. 64), 64–65.

Gomerčić, V., Mubrin, Z., Marković, Z., & Davila, D. (1983). Histological assessment of osmotherapy of anoxic brain edema. *Iugoslav. Physiol. Pharmacol. Acta,* (Suppl. 2), 74–77.

Gosetti, B., Ventura, M., Damiano, M., Bait, C., & Zaccaria, A. (1978). CBF changes after eburnamonine infusion in patients with cerebrovascular insufficiency. *Eur. Neurol., 17*(Suppl. 1), 171–172.

Gotti, B., & Depoortere, H. (1980). Anti-anoxic action of vincamine. In A. Bès & G. Géraud (Eds.). *Circulation cérébrale* (pp. 105–107). Toulouse, France: Fournié.

Gottstein, U. (1965). Pharmacological studies of total cerebral blood flow in man with comments on the possibility of improving regional cerebral blood flow by drugs. Acta Neurol. Scand., *41*(Suppl. 14), 136–141.

———. (1979). Haemodilution therapy in arterial circulatory disorders. *Terapiewoche, 29,* 44.

Gottstein, U., & Paulson, O. B. (1972). The effect of intracarotid aminophylline infusion on the cerebral circulation. *Stroke, 3,* 560–565.

Grome, J. J., & Stefanovich, V. (1984). The effects of caffeine and theophylline administration on local cerebral glucose utilization in a rat brain. *Arch. Pharmacol., 325*(Suppl. 7), R79.

Gross, P. M., Harper, A. M., & Teasdale, G. M. (1981). Cerebral circulation and histamine; 1. Participation of vascular H_1- and H_2-receptors in vasodilatatory responses to carotid arterial infusion. *J. Cereb. Blood Flow Metabol., 1,* 97–108.

Gustafson, L., Risberg, J., Johanson, M., Fransson, M., & Maximilian, V. A. (1978). Effects of piracetam on regional cerebral blood flow and mental function in patients with organic dementia. *Psychopharmacology, 56,* 115–117.

Gygax, P., & Wiernsperger, N. (1983). Hypotension induced changes in cerebral microflow and EEG and EEG and their pharmacological alterations, Acta Med. Scand., Suppl. 678, 29–36.

Hachinski, V., Norris, J. W., Edmeads, J., & Cooper, P. W. (1978). Ergotamine and cerebral blood flow. Stroke, *9,* 594–596.

Hadjidimos, A., Steingass, U., Fischer, F., Reulen, H. J., & Schürmann, K. (1973). The effects of dexamethasone on rCBF and cerebral vasomotor response in brain tumors. Eur. Neurol., *10,* 25–30.

Hammer, R. P., Jr., & Herkenham, M. (1983). Altered metabolic activity in the cerebral cortex of rats exposed to ketamine. J. Comp. Neurol., *220,* 396–404.

Hartmann, A. (1981). Effect of pentoxifylline on regional cerebral blood flow in patients with cerebrovascular disease. Pharmatherapeutica, *2,* 528.

———. (1983). Effect of pentoxifylline on regional cerebral blood flow in patients with cerebral vascular disorders. Eur. Neurol., *22,* 108–115.

Hashi, K., Meyer, J. S., Shinmaru, S., Welch, K. M. A., & Teraura, T. (1972). Effect of glycerol and intracarotid phenoxybenazamine on cerebral hemodynamics and metabolism after experimental subarachnoid hemorrhage. J. Neurol. Sci., *17,* 23–28.

Hauge, A., Nicolayse, G., & Thoresen, M. (1983). Acute effects of acetazolamide on cerebral blood flow in man. Acta Physiol. Scand., *117,* 233–239.

Heiss, W.-D. (1973). Drug effects on regional cerebral blood flow in focal cerebrovascular disease. *J. Neurol. Sci., 19,* 461–482.

———. (1979). Effect of drugs on cerebral blood flow in man. In M. Goldstein, L. Bolis, C. Fieschi, S. Gorini, & C. H. Millikan (Eds.). *Cerebrovascular disorders and stroke* (pp. 95–114). New York: Raven Press.

———. (1980). Pharmakologische Beeinflussung der Zirkulation im Gehirn. *Bull. Schweiz. Akad. Med. Wiss., 36,* 183–207.

Heiss, W.-D., & Podreka, I. (1979). Assessment of pharmacological effects on cerebral blood flow. *Eur. Neurol., 17*(Suppl. 1), 135–143.

Heiss, W.-D., Prosenz, P., Tschabitscher, H., Lasek, C., & Herles, H. J. (1972). Effect of low molecular dextran on total cerebral blood flow and regional flow within ischemic lesions. *Eur. Neurol., 8,* 129–133.

Heiss, W.-D., & Zeiler, K. (1978). The influence of drugs on cerebral blood flow. *Pharmakotherapie, 1,* 137–144.

Henriksen, L., Thorshauge, C., Harmsen, A., Christensen, P., Søronsen, M. B., Lester, J., & Paulson, O. B. (1983). Controlled hypotension with sodium nitroprusside: Effects on cerebral venous blood gases in patients operated for cerebral aneurysms. *Acta Anaesthesiol. Scand., 27,* 62–67.

Herrschaft, H. (1975). The efficacy and course of action of vaso- and metabolic-active substances on regional cerebral blood flow in patients with cerebrovascular insufficiency. In M. Harper, B. Jennett, D. Miller, & J. Rowan (Eds.). *Blood flow and metabolism in the brain* (pp. 11.24–11.28). Edinburgh: Churchill Livingstone.

_______. (1976). The efficacy and course of action of vaso- and metabolic-active substances on regional cerebral blood flow in patients with cerebral ischemia. *Arzneim.-Forsch./Drug Res., 26,* 1240–1241.

_______. (1978). Diewirkung von Piracetam auf die Gehirndurchblutung des Menschen. Quantitative regionale Hirndurchblutungsmessungen bei der akuten zerebralen Ischämie. *Med. Klin., 73,* 195–202.

Herrschaft, H., Gleim, F., Schmidt, H., & Duus, P. (1975). Das Verhalten der regionalem Gehirndurchblutung unter dem Einfluss von Bencyclan. *Med. Klin., 70,* 896–903.

Herrschaft, H., & Schmidt, H. (1973). Das Verhalten der globalen und regionalen Hirndurchblutung unter dem Einfluss von Propanidid, Ketamine and Thiopental-Natrium. *Anaesthesist, 22,* 486–495.

_______. (1974). Der Einfluss von Methohexital-Natrium auf die globale und regionale Hirndurchblutung des Menschen. *Anaesthesist, 45,* 340–344.

Herrschaft, H., Schmidt, H., & Duus, P. (1971–1972). Cerebral blood flow in man under general anesthesia with regard to several narcotics. *Eur. Neurol., 6,* 373–382.

Hertz, M. M., & Paulson, O. B. (1983). Glucose transfer across the blood-brain barrier. In A. J. Szabo (Ed.). *CNS regulation of carbohydrate metabolism* (pp. 177–192). Orlando, Fla.: Academic Press.

Higgs, C. A., Mugridge, K. G., & Moncada, S. (1985). Arachidonic acid metabolism and calcium flux. In T. Godfraind, P. M. Vanhoutte, S. Govoni, & R. Paoletti (Eds.). *Calcium entry blockers and tissue protection* (pp. 51–58). New York: Raven Press.

Hillbom, M., & Kaste, M. (1983). Ethanol intoxication: A risk factor for ischemic brain infarction.ı Stroke, 14, 694–699.

Hougaard, K., Hansen, A., & Brodersen, P. (1974). The effect of ketamine on regional cerebral blood flow in man. *Anesthesiology, 41,* 562–567.

Hougaard, K., Nilsson, B., & Wieloch, T. (1983). Fatty acid cyclo-oxygenase inhibitors and the regulation of cerebral blood flow. *Acta Physiol. Scand., 117,* 585–587.

Hoyer, S., Oesterreich, K., & Stoll, K.–D. (1977). Effects of pyritinol-HCL on blood flow and oxidative metabolism of the brain in patients with dementia. *Arzneim.–Forsch./Drug Res., 27,* 671–674.

Hughes, R. J. D., James, I. M., & Dijane, A. (1981). The effect of beta-histine methanesulphonate upon cerebral blood flow. *Br. J. Clin. Pharmacol., 11,* 308–310.

Imamoto, T., Tanabe, M., Shimamoto, N., Kawazoe, K., & Hirata, M. (1984). Cerebral circulatory and cardiac effects of vinpocetine and its metabolite, apovincaminic acid, in anesthetized dogs. *Arzneim.–Forsch./Drug Res., 34,* 161–169.

James, I. M., Newbury, P. & Woollard, M. L. (1978). The effect of naftidrofuryl oxalate on cerebral blood flow in elderly patients. *Br. J. Clin. Pharmacol., 6,* 545–546.

James, H. E., Madauss, W. C., Tibbs, P. A., McCloskey, J. J., & Bean, J. R. (1979). The effect of high dose dexamethasone in children with severe closed head injury. *Acta Neurochir., 45,* 225–236.

Jennett, B., Teasdale, G., Fry, J., Braakman, R., Minderhound, J., Heiden, J., & Kurze, T. (1980). Treatment for severe head injury. *J. Neurol. Neurosurg. Psychiat., 43,* 289–295.

Kågström, E., Smith, M.–L., Wallstedt, L., & Siesjö, B. K. (1983). Cyclo-oxygenase inhibition by indomethacin and recirculation following cerebral ischemia. *Acta Physiol. Scand., 118,* 193–201.

Kalousek, M., Hudolin, V., Mubrin, Z., & Marković, Z. (1978). Terapija moždanog edema infuzijskom otopinom glicerola. *Lij. Vjes., 100,* 654–658.
Kanig, K. (1973). Encephalotropic drugs and cerebral RNA metabolism. In H. P. Zippel (Ed.). *Memory and transfer of information* (pp. 571–582). New York: Plenum.
Kartin, P., Povše, M., & Skondia, V. (1979). Clinical study of piracetam in patients with subacute cerebrovascular accidents. *Acta Therap., 5,* 235–243.
Kassel, N. F., Baumann, K. W., Hitchon, P. W., Gerk, M. K., Hill, T. R., & Sokoll, M. D. (1982). The effects of high dose mannitol on cerebral blood flow in dogs with normal intracranial pressure. *Stroke, 13,* 59–61.
Kety, S. S. (1974). Physiological and physical factors governing the initial stages of drug distribution. In T. Teorell, R. L. Dedrick, P. G. Condliffe (Eds.). *Pharmacology and pharmacokinetics* (pp. 233–240). New York: Plenum Press.
Kety, S. S., & Schmidt, C. F. (1948). The nitrous oxide method for the quantitative determination of cerebral blood flow in man: Theory, procedure and normal values. *J. Clin. Invest., 27,* 476–483.
Kobayashi, S., Yamaguchi, S., Katsube, T., Okada, K., Kitani, M., Murao, M. & Tsunematsu, T. (1984a). Effects of naftidrofuryl on the time course of the regional cerebral blood flow in acute ischemic stroke. *Arzneim.–Forsch./Drug Res., 34,* 1580–1583.
Kobayashi, S., Yamaguchi, S., Katsube, T., Kitani, M., Okada, K., Tsunematsu, T., & Murao, M. (1984b). Effect of long-term administration of BV26–723 (Brovincamine) on cerebral blood flow. *rCBF Bull., 7,* 144–148.
Krabbe, A. A., & Olesen, J. (1982). Effect of histamine on regional cerebral blood flow in man. *Cephalalgia, 2,* 15–18.
Kubota, K., Yamaguchi, T., Abe, Y., Fujiwara, T., Hatazawa, J., & Matsuzawa, T. (1983). Effects of smoking on regional cerebral blood flow in neurologically normal subjects. *Stroke, 14,* 720–724.
Kuschinsky, W., Suda, S., Bünger, R., Yaffe, S., & Sokoloff, L. (1983). The effects of intravenous norepinephrine on the local coupling between glucose utilization and blood flow in the rat brain. *Pflügers Arch., 398,* 134–138.
Lacroix, P., Quinion, M. J., Linee, P., & Le Polles, J. B. (1979). Cerebral metabolic and hemodynamic activities of l-eburnamonine in the anesthetized dog. *Arzneim.–Forsch. Drug. Res., 29,* 1029–1101.
Lavyne, M. H., Koltun, W. A., Clement, J. A., Rosene, D. L., Pickren, K. S., Zarvas, N. T., & Wurtman R. L. (1977). Decrease in neostriatal blood flow after d-amphetamine administration or electrical stimulation of the substantia nigra. *Brain Res., 135,* 77–86.
Lebrun–Grandié, P., Baron, J.–C., Soussaline, F., Loc'h, C., Sastre, J., & Bousser, M.–G. (1983). Coupling between regional blood flow and oxygen utilization in the normal human brain. A study with positron tomography and oxygen 15. *Arch. Neurol., 40,* 230–236.
Lenzi, G. L., Jones, T., Reid, J. L., & Moss, S. (1979). Regional impairment of cerebral oxydative metabolism in Parkinson's disease. *J. Neurol. Neurosurg. Psychiat., 42,* 59–62.
Le Poncin–Lafitte, M., Grosdemouge, C., Duterte, D., & Rapin, J. R. (1984). Simultaneous study of haemodynamic, metabolic and behavioural sequelae in a model of cerebral ischemia in aged rats: Effects of nicergoline. *Gerontology, 30,* 109–119.
Little, J. R. (1978). Modification of acute focal ischemia by treatment with mannitol and high-dose dexamethasone. *J. Neurosurg., 49,* 517–524.
Little, J. R., Latchaw, J. P., Slugg, R. M., Lesser, R. P., & Stowe, N. P. (1982). Treatment of acute focal cerebral ischemia with propranolol. *Stroke, 13,* 302–307.
Lognecker, D. E. (1984). Effects of general anesthetics on the microcirculation. *Microcirc. Endothel. Lymph., 1,* 129–150.
Macchione, C., Molaschi, M., Fabris, F., & Feruglio, F. S. (1976). Results with piracetam in the management of senile psycho organic syndromes. *Acta Therap., 2,* 261–269.

MacKenzie, E. T., Gotti, B., Nowicki, J.–P., & Young, A. R. (1984). Adrenergic blockers as cerebral antiischemic agents. In E. T. MacKenzie, J. Seylaz, & A. Bes (Eds.). *Neurotransmitters and the cerebral circulation* (pp. 219–243). New York: Raven Press.

Magnussen, I., Jakobsen, P., & Høedt–Rasmussen, K. (1977). Aminophylline and stroke. *Acta Neurol. Scand., 56*(Suppl. 64), 168–169.

Mankovsky, N. B., Mints, A. Ya., Lizogub, V. G., & Bo, K. (1979). Regional cerebral blood flow and its regulation in patients with the initial stage of cerebral atherosclerosis. *Kliniceskaya Med., 57,* 35–39.

Marcel, G. A., & George, C. (1983). Pentoxifylline and cerebrovascular diseases. *Eur. Neurol., 22*(Suppl. 1), 89–97.

Marković, Z., Mubrin, Z., & Gomerčić, V. (1983). Effects of osmotherapy on EEG changes during and after anoxic brain injury. *Iugoslav. Physiol. Pharmacol. Acta,* (Suppl. 2), 132–135.

Marshall, L. F. (1980). Treatment of brain swelling and brain edema in man. In J. Cervós–Navarro & R. Ferszt (Eds.). *Brain edema, pathology, diagnosis, and therapy* (pp. 459–469). New York: Raven Press.

Mathew, N. T., Meyer, J. S., Rivera, V. M., Charney, J., & Hartmann, A. (1972). Double-blind evaluation of glycerol therapy in acute cerebral infarction. *Lancet, 2,* 1327–1329.

Mathew, R. J., Barr, D. L., & Weinman, M. L. (1983). Caffeine and cerebral blood flow. *Brit. J. Psychiat., 143,* 604–608.

McCalden, T. A., Nath, R. G., & Thiele, K. (1983). The effects of nimodipine (Baye 9736) on the cerebral circulation in baboons. *Proc. West. Pharmacol. Soc., 26,* 127–129.

———. (1984a). The role of prostacyclin in the hypercapnic and hypoxic cerebrovascular dilatations. *Life Sci., 34,* 1801–1807.

———. (1984b). The effects of calcium antagonist /nimodipine/ on basal cerebral blood flow and reactivity to various agonists. *Stroke, 15,* 527–530.

McGillicuddy, J. E. (1985). Cerebral protection: Pathophysiology and treatment of increased intracranial pressure. *Chest, 87,* 85–93.

McHenry, L. C. Jr., Jaffe, M. E., Kawamura, J. & Goldberg, I. (1971). Hydergine effect on cerebral circulation in cerebrovascular disease. *J. Neurol. Sci., 13,* 475–481.

McHenry, L. C., Jaffe, M. E., West, J. W., Cooper, E. S., Kenton III, U. J., Kawamura, J., Oshiro, T., & Goldberg, H. I. (1972). Regional cerebral blood flow and cardiovascular effects of hexobendine in stroke patients. *Neurology, 22,* 217–223.

McHenry, L. C. Jr., Stump, D. A., Howard, G., Novack, T. T., Bivins, D. H., & Nelson, A. O. (1983). Comparison of the effects of intravenous papaverine hydrochloride and oral pavabid HP capsulets on regional cerebral blood flow in normal individuals. *J. Cerebr. Blood Flow Metabol., 3,* 442–447.

Melamed, E., & Lavy, S. (1979). Effect of papaverine on regional cerebral blood flow of the contralateral hemisphere in patients with acute cerebral infarction. Appl. Neurophysiol., *42,* 217–223.

Melamed, E., Lavy, S., Cooper, G., & Bentin, S. (1978). Regional cerebral blood flow in Parkinsonism; measurement before and after levodopa. J. Neurol. Sci., *38,* 391–397.

Merory, J., Du Boulay, G. H., Marshall, J., Morris, J., Ross Russell, R. W., Symon, L., & Thomas, D. J. (1978). Effect of tinofedrine /Homburg D8955/ on cerebral blood flow in multi-infarct dementia. J. Neurol. Neurosurg. Psychiat., *41,* 900–902.

Meyer, J. S., Fukuuchi, Y., Shimazu, K., Ohuchi, T., & Ericsson, A. D. (1972). Effect of intravenous infusion of glycerol on hemispheric blood flow and metabolism in patients with acute cerebral infarction. *Stroke, 3,* 168–180.

Meyer, J. S., & Hardenberg, J. (1983). Clinical effectiveness of calcium entry blockers in prophylactic treatment of migraine and cluster headaches. *Headache, 23,* 266–277.

Meyer, J. S., Kanda, T., Shinohara, Y., Fukuuchi, Y., Shimazu, K., Ericsson, A. D., & Gordon, W. H. Jr. (1971). Effect of hexobendine on cerebral hemispheric blood flow and metabolism.

Preliminary clinical observations concerning its use in ischemic cerebrovascular disease. *Neurology, 21,* 691–702.

Meyer, J. S., Okamoto, S., Sari, A., Koto, A., Itoh, Y., & Ericsson, A. D. (1974a). Effects of beta-adrenergic blockade on cerebral autoregulation and chemical vasomotor control in patients with stroke. *Stroke, 5,* 167–179.

Meyer, J. S., Okamoto, S., Shimazu, K., Koto, A., Ohuchi, T., Sari, A., & Ericsson, A. D. (1974b). Cerebral metabolic changes during treatment of subacute cerebral infarction by alpha and beta adrenergic blockade with phenoxybenzamine and propranolol. *Stroke, 5,* 180–195.

Meyer, J. S., Mathew, N. T., Hartmann, A., & Rivera, V. M. (1974c). Orally administered betahistine and regional cerebral blood flow in cerebrovascular disease. *J. Clin. Pharmacol., 14,* 280–289.

Miller, V. T., Coull, B. M., Yatsu, F. M., Shah, A. B., & Beamer, N. B. (1984). Prostacyclin infusion in acute cerebral infarction. *Neurology* (Cleveland) *34,* 1431–1435.

Mohamed, A. A., McCulloch, J., Mendelow, A. D., Teasdale, G. M., & Harper, A. M. (1984). Effect of the calcium antagonist nimodipine on local cerebral blood flow: Relationship to arterial blood pressure. *J. Cerebr. Blood Flow Metabol., 4,* 206–211.

Moncada, S. (1983). Biology and therapeutic potential of prostacyclin. *Stroke, 14,* 157–168.

Montgomery, E. B., Jr., Grubb, R. L., Jr. & Raichle, M. E. (1981). Cerebral hemodynamics and metabolism in postoperative cerebral vasospasm and treatment with hypertensive therapy. *Ann. Neurol., 9,* 502–506.

Moskowitz, M. A., & Coughlin, S. R. (1981). Basic properties of the prostaglandins. *Stroke, 12,* 696–701.

Mubrin, Z., Marković, Z., Šikić, N., Desnica–Ivičević, J., & Košiček, T. (1983). Piracetam facilitates the speech rehabilitation of children with minor brain damage. *Iugoslav. Physiol. Pharmacol. Acta,* (Suppl. 2), 143–145.

Myslivečkova–Hassmanova, J., Mysliveček, J., & Janda, F. (1978). Learning and memory under the influence of emotional stress and nootropic drug action. *Activ. Nerv. Sup., 20,* 246–266.

Nemoto, E. M., Kofke, W. A., Kessler, P., Hossman, K.–A., Stezoski, S. W., & Safar, P. (1977). Studies of the pathogenesis of ischemic brain damage and the mechanism of its amelioration by thipental. *Acta Neurol. Scand., 56* (Suppl. 64), 142–143.

Newberg, L. A., Steen, P. A., Milde, J. H., & Michenfelder, J. D. (1984). Failure of flunarizine to improve cerebral blood flow or neurologic recovery in a canine model of complete cerebral ischemia. *Stroke, 15,* 666–671.

Newlin, D. B., Golden, C. J., Quaife, M., & Graber, B. (1982). Effect of alcohol ingestion on regional cerebral blood flow. *Int. J. Neurosci., 17,* 145–150.

Nikolov, R., Nikolova, M., & Milanova, D. (1984). Study of the antihypoxic effect of cinnarizine and its interaction with prostacyclin. *Meth. Find. Exptl. Clin. Pharmacol., 6,* 135–138.

Nilsson, A., Risberg, J., Johanson, M., & Gustafson, L. (1977). Regional changes of cerebral blood flow during haloperidol therapy in patients with paranoid symptoms. *Acta Neurol. Scand., 56*(Suppl. 64), 478–479.

Nordström, C. H., Calderini, G., Rechncrona, S., & Siesjö, B. K. (1977). Effects of phenobarbital anesthesia on postischemic cerebral blood flow and oxygen consumption in the rat. *Acta Neurol. Scand., 56*(Suppl. 64), 146–147.

Norris, J. W., Hachinski, V. C., & Cooper, P. W. (1975). Changes in cerebral blood flow during migraine attack. *Br. Med. J., 3,* 676–684.

O'Brien, M. D., & Veall, N. (1966). Effect of cyclandelate on cerebral cortex perfusion-rates in cerebrovascular disease. *Lancet, 2,* 729–730.

Oiwa, K., Shimazu, K., Tamura, N., Hienuki, M., Kim, H.–T., Yamamoto, T., & Hamaguchi, K. (1984). Effect of aging on cerebral blood flow autoregulation—with special reference to the role of prostaglandins. *Monograph Neural Sciences, 11,* 210–215.

Okayashu, H., Meyer, J. S., Mathew, N. T., Amano, T., & Hardenberg, J. (1984). Lithium carbonate has no measurable effect on cerebral hemodynamics in cluster headaches. *Headache, 24,* 1–4.

Okuda, C., Miyazaki, M. & Kuriyama, K. (1984). Alterations in cerebral β-adrenergic receptor-adenylate cyclase system induced by halothane, ketamine and ethanol. Neurochem. Int., *6,* 237–244.

Olesen, J., & Paulson, O. B. (1971). The effect of intra-arterial papaverine on the regional cerebral blood flow in patients with stroke or intracranial tumor. *Stroke, 2,* 148–159.

Olesen, J. (1972). The effect of intracarotid epinephrine, norepinephrine and angiotensin on the regional cerebral blood flow in man. *Neurology, 22,* 978–987.

Olesen, J., & Skinhøj, E. (1972). Effects of ergot alkaloids (Hydergine®) on cerebral haemodynamics in man. *Acta Pharmacol. Toxicol., 31,* 75–85.

Olesen, J. (1976). Effect of intracarotid prostaglandin E_1 on regional cerebral blood flow in man. *Stroke, 7,* 566–569.

Olesen, J., Hougaard, K., & Hertz, M. (1978). Isoproterenol and propranolol: Ability to cross the blood-brain barrier and effects on cerebral circulation in man. *Stroke, 9,* 344–349.

Ott, E., & Lechner, H. (1980). Increase of cerebral blood flow in patients with subacute cerebral infarction following long term treatment with tinofedrine. In A. Bès & G. Géraud (Eds.). *Circulation cérébrale* (pp. 143–144). Toulouse, France: Fournié.

Pappius, H. M., & Wolfe, L. S. (1983). Effects of indomethacin and ibuprofen on cerebral metabolism and blood flow in traumatized brain. *J. Cerebr. Blood Flow Metabol. 3,* 448–459.

Passero, S., Nardini, M., & Battistini, N. (1981). Effect of pentoxifylline on cerebral blood flow in patients with chronic cerebrovascular disease. *J. Int. Med. Res., 9,* 211–214.

Paulson, O. B., Jarden, J. O., Godtfresden, J., & Vorstrup, S. (1984). Cerebral blood flow in patients with congestive heart failure treated with captopril. *Amer. J. Med., 76,* 91–98.

Peeke, S. C., & Peeke, H. V. S. (1984). Attention, memory, and cigarette smoking. *Psychopharmacology, 84,* 205–216.

Peroutka, S. J. (1983). The pharmacology of calcium channel antagonists: A novel class of anti-mirgaine agents? *Headache, 23,* 278–283.

Philippon, B. L., Thivolle, P., & Berger, M. (1982). Nicergoline et hemodetournement en faveur des zones d'hypodebit dans les accidents ischemiques cerebraux. *Rev. Electroencephalogr. Neurophysiol. Clin., 12,* 361–366.

Pickard, J. D., Rose, J. E., Cooke, M. B. D., Blair, I., & Strathdee, A. (1977). The effect of salicylates on cerebral blood flow in man. *Acta Neurol. Scand., 56*(Suppl. 64), 422–423.

Pickard, J. D., & Walker, V. (1984). Current concepts of the role of prostaglandins and other eicosanoids in acute cerebrovascular disease. In E. T. MacKenzie, J. Seylaz, & A. Bès (Eds.). *Neurotransmitters and the cerebral circulation* (pp. 191–218). New York: Raven Press.

Pizzolato, G., Soncrant, T. T., & Rapoport, S. I. (1984). Haloperidol and cerebral metabolism in the conscious rat: Relation to pharmacokinetics. *J. Neurochem., 43,* 724–732.

Preskorn, S. H., Simpson, G. H., Friesen, D., Rinne, J., & Jerkovich, G. (1981). Medical therapies for mood disorders alter the blood-brain barrier. *Science, 213,* 469–471.

Purves, M. J. (1972). *The physiology of the cerebral circulation* (Ch. 12, Some aspects of the pharmacology of cerebral vascular smooth muscle; pp. 334–351). Cambridge,: University Press UK.

Raichle, M. E., Grubb, R. L., Gado, M. H., Eichling, J. O., & Ter–Pogossian, M. M. (1976). Correlation between regional cerebral blood flow and oxidative metabolism. *Arch. Neurol., 33,* 523–526.

Rajagopalan, B., Raine, A. E. G., Cooper, R., & Ledingham, J. G. G. (1984). Changes in cerebral blood flow in patients with severe congestive cardiac failure before and after captopril treatment. *Amer. J. Med., 76,* 86–90.

Rapoport, S. I., Hori, M., & Klatzo, I. (1971). Reversible osmotic opening of the blood-brain barrier. *Science, 173,* 1026–1028.

Rapoport, S. I., & Thompson, H. K. (1973). Osmotic opening of the blood-brain barrier in the moneky without associated neurological deficit. *Science, 180,* 971.

Renou, A. M., Orgogozo, J. M., Vernhiet, J., Constant, P., & Caille, J. M. (1977). Vascular reactivity with althesin /R/ in focal cerebral ischemia. *Acta Neurol. Scand., 56*(Suppl. 64), 172–173.

Risberg, J., Gustafson, L., & Prohovnik, I. (1981). rCBF measurements by ^{133}Xe inhalation: Applications in neuropsychology and psychiatry. *Prog. Nucl. Med., 7,* 82–94.

Risberg, J., Hagstadius, S., & Gustafson, L. (1982). rCBF-measurements in the study of drug effects. *rCBF Bull., 3,* 56–57.

Rogers, R. L., Meyer, J. S., Shaw, T. G., Mortel, K. F., Hardenberg, J. P., & Zaid, R. R. (1983). Cigarette smoking decreases cerebral blood flow suggesting increased risk for stroke. *JAMA, 250,* 2796–2800.

Rogers, R. L., Meyer, J. S., Shaw, T. G., Mortel, K. F. & Thornby, J. (1984). The effects of chronic cigarette smoking on cerebrovascular responsiveness to 5 per cent CO_2 and 100 per cent O_2 inhalation. *J. Amer. Geriat. Soc., 32,* 415–420.

Rolly, G., & Van Aken, J. (1979). Influence of enflurane on cerebral blood flow in man. *Acta Anaesth. Scand.,* (Suppl. 71), 59–63.

Rossignol, R., & Ebiqwei–Ibru, M. (1980). Drugs against brain hypoxia. *Trend Pharmacol. Sci., 1,* 287–289.

Rovere, A. A., Raynald, A. C., & Scremin, O. U. (1977). On the mechanisms of the amphetamine induced vasodilation at the rat's cerebral cortex. *Experientia, 33,* 1461–1463.

Sakabe, T., Maekawa, T., Fujii, S., Ishikawa, T., Tateishi, A., & Takeshita, H. (1983). Cerebral circulation and metabolism during enflurane anesthesia in humans. *Anesthesiology, 59,* 532–536.

Shaw, T. G., & Meyer, J. S. (1978). Double-blind trial of oral papaverine in chronic cerebrovascular ischemia. *Angiology, 29,* 839–851.

Shenkin, H. A. (1951). Effects of various drugs upon cerebral circulation and metabolism of man. *J. Appl. Physiol., 3,* 465–471.

Siesjö, B. K., & Wieloch, T. (1983). Prostaglandins and the cerebral circulation. In B. Samuelsson, R. Paoletti, & P. Ramwell (Eds.). *Advances in prostaglandin, thromboxane, and leukotriene research* (pp. 339–344). New York: Raven Press.

Simard, D., & Paulson, O. B. (1973). Cerebral vasomotor paralysis during migraine attack. *Arch. Neurol., 29,* 207–209.

Simeone, F.A., Frazer, G., & Lawner, P. (1979). Ischemic brain edema: Comparative effects of barbiturates and hypothermia. *Stroke, 10,* 8–12.

Skinhøj, E., & Paulson, O. B. (1970). The mechanism of action of aminophylline upon cerebral vascular disorders. *Acta Neurol. Scand., 46,* 129–140.

Smith, A. L. (1975). Mechanisms for cerebral vasodilation by halothane. In T. W. Langfitt, L. C. McHenry, M. Reivich, & H. Wollman (Eds.). *Cerebral circulation and metabolism* (pp. 353–354). Berlin: Springer–Verlag.

Smith, A. L., Hoff, J. T., Nielsen, S. L., & Larson, C. P. (1975). Barbiturate protection against cerebral infarction. In T. W. Langfitt, L. C. McHenry, M. Reivich, & H. Wollman (Eds.). *Cerebral circulation and metabolism* (pp. 347–348). Berlin: Springer–Verlag.

Spagnoli, A., & Tognoni, G. (1983). ''Cerebroactive'' drugs. Clinical pharmacology and therapeutic role in cerebrovascular disorders. *Drugs, 26,* 44–69.

Spierings, E. L. H. (1984). Clinical evaluation of calcium entry blockers in migraine. In T. Godfraind, A. G. Herman, & D. Wellens (Ed.). *Calcium entry blockers in cardiovascular and cerebral dysfunctions* (pp. 271–281). Boston: Martinus Nijhoff.

Stegink, K. J. (1972). The clinical use of piracetam a new nootropic drug. The treatment of senile involution. *Arzneim.–Forsch./Drug Res., 22,* 957–977.

Steiner, L., Forster, M. C., Bergvall, U., & Carlsson, L. A. (1972). Effect of prostaglandin E_1 on cerebral circulatory disturbances. *Eur. Neurol., 8,* 23–31.

Stoica, E., Meyer, J. S., Kawamura, Y., Hiromoto, H., Hashi, K., Aoyagi, M., & Pascu, I. (1973). Central neurogenic control of cerebral circulation. Effects of intravertebral injection of pyrithioxin on cerebral blood flow and metabolism. *Neurology, 23,* 687–698.

Strangaard, S., Olesen, J., Skinhøj, E., & Lassen, N. A. (1973). Autoregulation of brain circulation in severe arterial hypertension. *Br. Med. J., 1,* 507–510.

Suzuki, J., Tanaka, S., & Yashimoto, T. (1980). Recirculation in the acute period of cerebral infarction: Brain swelling and its suppression using mannitol. *Surg. Neurol., 14,* 467–472.

Tazaki, Y., Omae, T., Kuromaru, S., Ohtomo, E., Hasegawa, K., Mori, A., Kurihara, M., Kutsusawa, N., & Okada, T. (1980). Clinical effect of encephabol (pyritinol) in the treatment of cerebrovascular disorders. *J. Int. Med. Res., 8,* 118–126.

Toda, N. (1983). Dopamine vasodilates human cerebral artery. *Experientia, 39,* 1131–1132.

Todd, M. M., & Drummond, J. C. (1984). A comparison of the cerebrovascular and metabolic effects of halothane and isoflurane in the cat. *Anesthesiology, 60,* 276–282.

Tsuda, Y., Kimura, K., Yoneda, S., Asai, T., Handa, N., Tanouchi, J., Inoue, M., & Abe, H. (1983). Hemodynamics in Shy–Drager syndrome and treatment with indomethacin. *Eur. Neurol., 22,* 421–427.

Uyama, O., Nagatsuka, K., Fukunega, R., Kusunoki, M., Takano, T., Yoneda, S., Kimura, K., & Abe, H. (1983). Role of prostacyclin in the response of cerebral blood flow to CO_2. *Brain Res., 259,* 344–347.

Van Aken, J., & Rolly, G. (1980). Influence of piracetam and etiracetam compared to placebo, on rCBF and parameters of brain metabolism. *Acta Anesthesiol. Belg., 31*(Suppl.), 21–28.

Van den Kerchkoff, W., Hossmann, K.–A., & Hossmann, V. (1983). No effect of prostacyclin on blood flow, regulation of blood flow and blood coagulation following global cerebral ischemia. *Stroke, 14,* 724–730.

Vanhoutte, P. M. (1982). Effects of calcium entry blockers on tissue hypoxia. *J. Cerebr. Blood Flow Metabol., 2*(Suppl. 1), S42–S44.

Van Nueten, J. M., & De Clerck, F. (1984). Vascular reactivity and calcium entry blockers. In P. Greengard (Ed.). *Advances in cyclic nucleotide and protein phosphorilation research* (pp. 575–583). New York: Raven Press.

Van Nueten, J. M., & Vanhoutte, P. M. (1984). Flunarizine. In A. Scriabine (Ed.). *New drugs annual: Cardiovascular drugs* (pp. 245–266). New York: Raven Press.

Vasileva, T. (1981). The effect on brain hemodynamics exerted by papaverine hydrochloride in conjunction with smoking and alcohol consumption. *Folia Medica, 23,* 26–31.

Vorstrup, S., Barry, D. I., Jarden, J. O., Svendsen, U. G., Braendstrup, O., Graham, D. I., & Strandgaard, S. (1984a). Chronic antihypertensive treatment in the rat reverses hypertension-induced changes in cerebral blood flow autoregulation. *Stroke, 15,* 312–318.

Vorstrup, S., Hendriksen, L., & Paulson, O. B. (1984b). Effect of acetazolamide on cerebral blood flow and cerebral metabolic rate for oxygen. *J. Clin. Invest., 74,* 1634–1639.

Wauquier, A. (1982). Brain protective properties of etomidate and flunarizine. *J. Cerebr. Blood Flow Metabol., 2*(Suppl. 1), S53–S56.

Weber, G., Kreisel, T., Peter, S., & Künzel, J. (1980). A double-blind placebo controlled cross-over study in patients with peripheral vascular diseases, using a new capillary viscometer. *Angiology, 31,* 1–5.

Weindl, A. (1983). The blood-brain barrier and its role in the control of circulating hormone effects on the brain. In D. Ganten & D. Pfaff (Eds.). *Central cardiovascular control. Basic and clinical aspects* (pp. 151–186). Berlin: Springer–Verlag.

Weir, B. (1984). Calcium antagonists, cerebral ischemia and vasospasm. *Can. J. Neurol. Sci., 11,* 239–246.

Wennmalm, Å. (1982). Effect of cigarette smoking on basal and carbon dioxide stimulated cerebral blood flow in man. *Clin. Physiol., 2,* 529–535.

Wennmalm, Å., Eriksson, S., Hagenfeldt, L., Law, D., Patrono, C., & Pinca, E. (1983). Effect of prostaglandin synthesis inhibitors on basal and carbon dioxide-stimulated cerebral blood flow in man. In B. Samuelsson, R. Paoletti, & P. Ramwell (Eds.). *Advances in prostaglandin, thromboxane, and leukotriene research* (pp. 351–355). New York: Raven Press.

Wesnes, K., & Warburton, D. M. (1983). Effects of smoking on rapid information processing performance. *Neuropsychobiology, 9,* 223–229.

White, R. P., & Hagen, A. A. (1982). Cerebrovascular actions of prostaglandins. *Pharm. Ther., 18,* 313–331.

Whittle, B. J. R., & Moncada, S. (1983). Pharmacological interactions between prostacyclin and thromboxanes. *Br. Med. Bull., 39,* 232–238.

Witzmann, H. K., Siegers, C. P., Heiss, W. D., & Kohlmeyer, K. (1977). Effect of vincamine on CBF under pharmacokinetic aspects. *Acta Neurol. Scand., 56*(Suppl. 64), 410–411.

Wollman, H., Smith, A. L., & Alexander, S. C. (1969a). Effects of general anesthetics in man on the ratio of cerebral blood flow to cerebral oxygen consumption. In M. Brock, C. Fieschi, D. H. Ingvar, N. A. Lassen, & K. Schürmann (Eds.), *Cerebral blood flow. Clinical and experimental results* (pp. 242–243). Berlin: Springer-Verlag.

Wollman, H., Smith, A. L., Neigh, J. L., & Hoffman, J. C. (1969). Cerebral blood flow and oxygen consumption in man during electroencephalographic seizure patterns associated with ethrane anesthesia. In M. Brock, C. Fieschi, D. H. Ingvar, N. A. Lassen, & K. Schürmann (Eds.). *Cerebral blood flow. Clinical and experimental results* (pp. 246–248). Berlin: Springer–Verlag.

Wolthuis, O. L. (1971). Experiments with UCB 6215, a drug which enhances acquisition in rats: Its effects compared with those of methampethamine. *Eur. J. Pharmacol., 16,* 283–297.

Wood, J. H., & Fleischer, A. S. (1982). Observations during hypervolemic hemodilution of patients with acute focal cerebral ischemia. *JAMA, 248,* 2999–3004.

Wyper, D. J., McAlpine, C. J., Jawad, K., & Jennett, B. (1976). Effects of a carbonic anhydrase inhibitor on cerebral blood flow in geriatric patients. *J. Neurol. Neurosurg. Psychiat., 39,* 885–889.

Zimmermann, P., Fünfgeld, E. W., Seidel, R., & Nischwitz, W. (1982). Electrophysiological profile of neurotropics (hydergine, piracetam, pyritinol) in organic brain disease in the aged. *Drug Dev. Res., 2,* 481–488.

Ziylan, Y. Z. (1984). Pathophysiology of the opening of the blood-brain and blood-cerebrospinal fluid barriers in acute hypertension. Exp. Neurol., *84,* 18–28.

7 Measurement of Cerebral Blood Flow in Cerebrovascular Diseases (Neurology, Part I)

Alexander Hartmann
H. Lagrète
University Hospital of Neurology, Bonn, Federal Republic of Germany

Despite introduction of the principle to measure regional cerebral blood flow (rCBF) more than twenty years ago (Lassen et al., 1963; Hoedt-Rasmussen et al., 1966) only a few neurological centers do use it in clinical practice. In the decade before that the radioactive tracer was administered by injection into one internal carotid artery (Heiss et al., 1979; Hartmann et al., 1977; Herrschaft, 1975; Kohlmeyer, 1985). This limited the applicability to a few procedures and repeated estimations could be done only with considerable risk to the individual patient. However, with the modification of the atraumatic technique as first described by Veall and Mallett (1967) and later by Obrist et al. (1975), it became possible to measure rCBF over both hemispheres repeatedly on a day-to-day basis even in outpatients. The reason that most of the neurologists do not use blood flow data for the clinical practice is based on the fact that neurophysiologists and other colleagues who are working in the field of cerebral blood flow, have failed to underline the importance of the actual CBF value for the neurological condition.

The concept of flow thresholds, which is explained in detail in the chapter by Symon, supports the view that any drastic flow reduction might be harmful to the functional integrity of the brain. This leads to the fact that any doctor who is involved in therapy of patients with diseases which go along with reduced blood flow should know the blood-flow value as well as those of the blood pressure and heart rate. Therapy of factors complicating intracerebral tumors depend primarily on the knowledge of intracranial pressure and visualization of the tumor size and brain edema as provided by cranial computerized tomography. In patients with cerebrovascular diseases (CVD), however, the dominant factor is cerebral blood

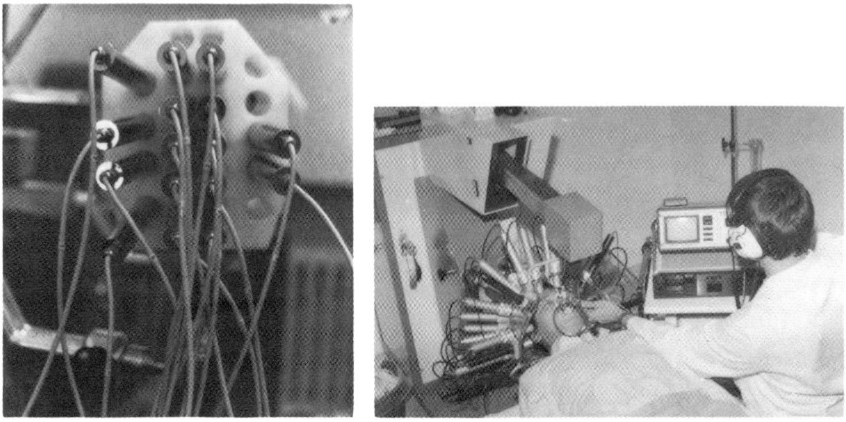

FIGURE 7.1. (a) Device of detector arrangement with slightly angeled detectors over the superior, inferior, frontal and occipital part of the skull. (b) New helmet arrangement of all 32 detectors, which allow high accurate re-positioning of the detectors in successive measurements.

flow. Therefore, it seems carelessness to us, not to be aware of the circulatory condition of the brain in these conditions.

This chapter will describe certain aspects of cerebrovascular disease where measurement of rCBF appears appropriate for diagnostic and therapeutic purposes in individual patients. In our laboratory, rCBF is measured with a 32 detector Novo instrument.

METHOD

For measurement of rCBF a 32 detector setup, as manufactured by Novo, is used. From 1979 to 1980 a detector holder with parallel arrangements of 16 detectors over both sides of the skull was used. However, due to the fact that the most vertical and most basical detectors showed more artifacts than all others, we constructed our own detector holder, in which the detectors of the upper and lowest row are slightly angled inward (Fig. 7.1). From 1983 up to now we are using a helmet as provided by the company. In patients with stable regular breathing it does not matter whether the ^{133}Xenon is administered by intravenous injection or by inhalation (Fig. 7.2). However, it is of utmost importance that any leakage from the nose and mouth is avoided. In our experience, a rubber tube, positioned in front of the teeth and behind the lips is of advantage, compared with a face mask (Fig. 7.3). The nose must be closed by a plastic-clamp.

In our laboratory data are stored on-line to a computer and then processed for calculation of CBF data by the initial slope index, the modified stochastic analy-

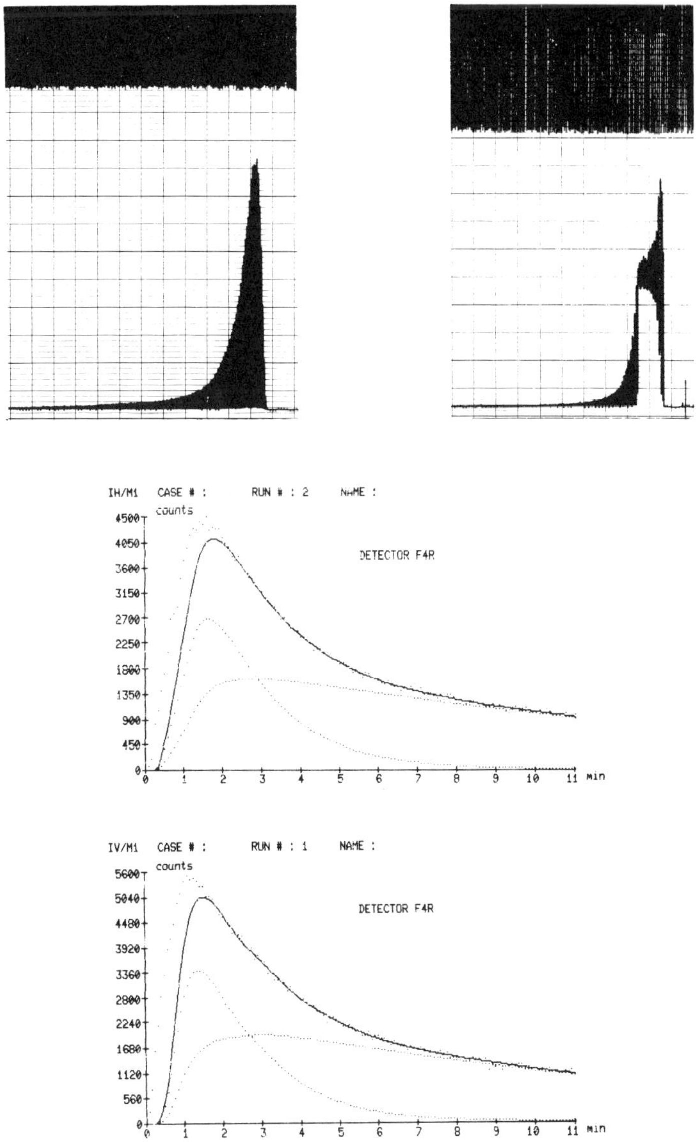

FIGURE 7.2. Intravenous (left) and inhalation technique. Two measurements were performed, immediate successive. The upper part of each recording indicates the CO_2 in volume percentage, the lower part, the concentration of the endexpiratory ^{133}Xenon. Two examples of calculated clearance curves are given, both from identical locations. Despite different administration of ^{133}Xenon, both curves have similar shapes and give identical CBF-values.

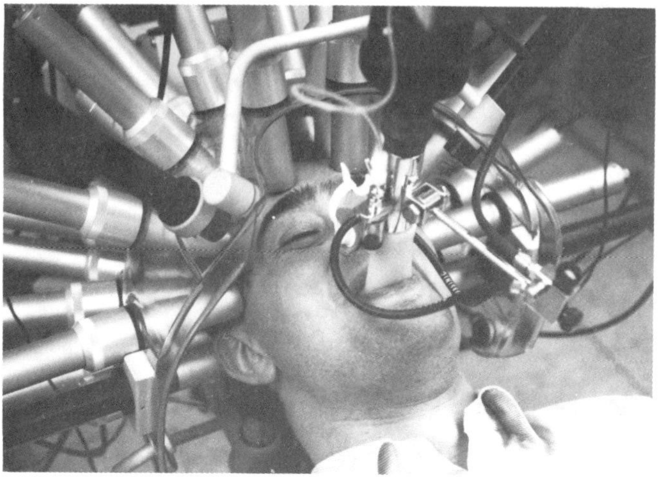

FIGURE 7.3. Rubber mouth piece for $Xenon^{133}$ intoxication study.

sis and the bicompartmental technique (Fig. 7.4). Partition coefficient (lambda) for Xe between blood brain tissue is estimated from the hemoglobin concentration, end-tidal CO_2 (Vol. %) is recorded continuously on a plotter (Fig. 7.5).

We feel it important that the environment of the laboratory is under constant condition. Therefore, each measurement is performed in darkness, except for a small light for the computer. The noise level of the laboratory is reduced as much as possible. The patient is asked to keep his or her eyes closed during the measurement. About every other minute the physician performing the measurement assures the patient that everything is going alright. This procedure has proven to promote the most stable results in respect to breathing rhythm, end-tidal CO_2, blood pressure, heart rate and—as tracked in several measurements—electroencephalographic activity.

SUPERFICIAL TEMPORAL ARTERY: MIDDLE CEREBRAL ARTERY-ANASTOMOSIS

Superficial temporal artery to middle cerebral artery anastomosis (STA-MCAA) has been developed by Yasargil (1969) and has been used for the prevention of recurrent strokes with some success (Gratzl et al., 1976; Chater, 1976; Yasargil and Yonekawa, 1977). However, the only clinical controlled long-term study, which was started several years ago, finished in 1985, shows in selected patients that surgical treatment, in general, is no better than conservative management. STA-MCAA has the following theoretical rationale:

1. Improvement of marginal perfusion (penumbra) (Astrup et al., 1981) in tissue where viable tissue is still present.

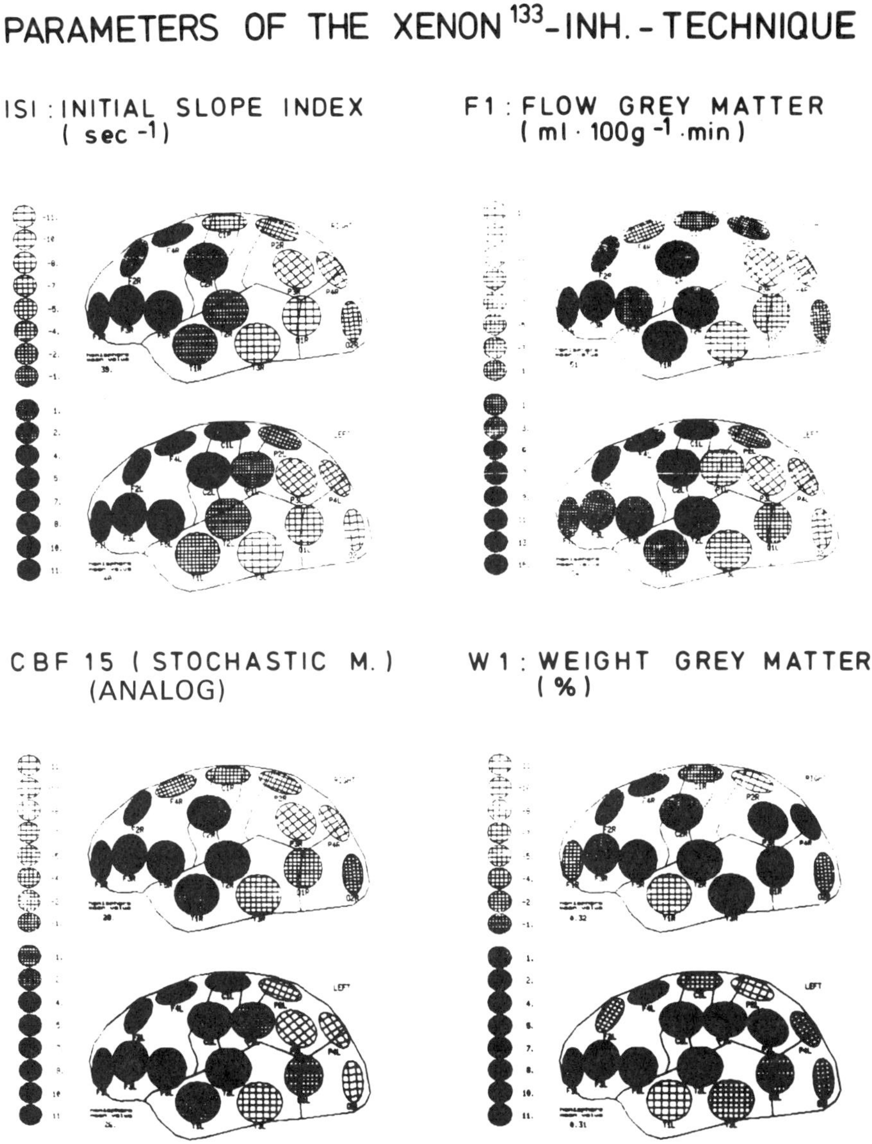

FIGURE 7.4. ISI, F1, CBF 15 and percentage weight of gray matter in a normal patient. All data expressed as percentage deviation from total mean. The relative flow map indicates similar distribution of flow for all calculation procedures with typical hyperfrontality. Only relative distribution of gray-matter weight is more homogeneously.

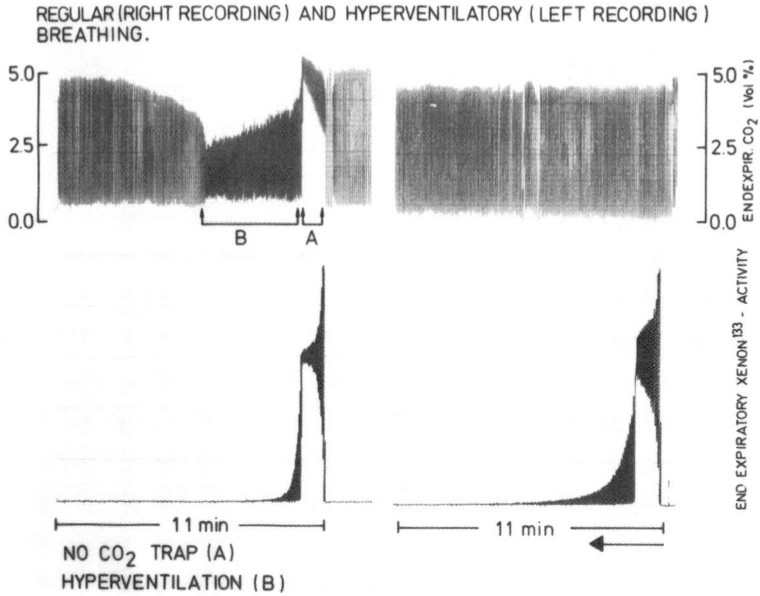

FIGURE 7.5. Regular and hyperventilatory breathing during inhalation method. The recording reads from right to left. The upper part of each tracing indicates end-expiratory CO_2 in volume percentage, the lower part the end-expiratory ^{133}Xenon concentration. The right side indicates normocapnic conditions, the left side recording during hyperventilation. Hyperventilation was performed during "A" and "B" (upper tracing, left). During the "A" the CO_2 trap was bypassed to indicate the change of CO_2 during the time of breathing from the air bag (saturation phase). The figure indicates that: (a) hyperventilation can be studied easily with this technique thus permitting activation tests; (b) the CO_2 trap is of high importance to allow constant CO_2 values.

2. Bypassing a local stenosis with hemodynamic relevants.
3. Preservation of autoregulation for situation of transient perfusion pressure drop.

The selection of appropriate candidates and the assessment of postoperative results has been performed mainly on clinical grounds. Since STA-MCAA intends improvement of rCBF it seems appropriate to measure the possible effect by rCBF measurement and to try to identify subgroups of patients in whom surgery might prove beneficial. Several reports have appeared in the literature. As yet there is no consensus of opinion as to whether STA-MCAA improves blood flow in only one or both hemispheres and whether metabolism is influenced also.

Unilateral occlusion of the internal carotid artery is the most commonly reported vascular alteration for which STA-MCAA has been performed (Chater and Popp, 1976; Gratzl et al., 1976; Popp and Chater, 1977; Reichman, 1975; Sundt et al., 1976; Yasargil and Yonekawa, 1977). Since only one sort of patient with internal carotid artery occlusion will continue to have further ischemic attacks (Dyken et al., 1874; Fields and Lemak, 1976; Grilla and Patterson, 1975; Hardy et al., 1962; McDowell et al., 1961), the results of the STA-MCAA must be compared with these experiences (Fig. 7.6).

Most of the CBF studies in patients with STA-MCAA did not report on a control group. Tolonen et al. (1985) did not find any change of CBF in the first 3 months following unilateral ischemia, treated conservatively. This is in contrast to our experience (see chapter 3), which indicates that CBF in acute cerebral infarction changes over the time.

Meyer et al. (1970) found bilateral CBF-changes in patients with unilateral ischemia who did not receive a STA-MCAA. The parallel increase of flow in both hemispheres in patients being operated on might be explained by this fact. A therapeutic benefit in respect to CBF in patients with STA-MCAA can only be suggested if CBF changes differ from that in the control group.

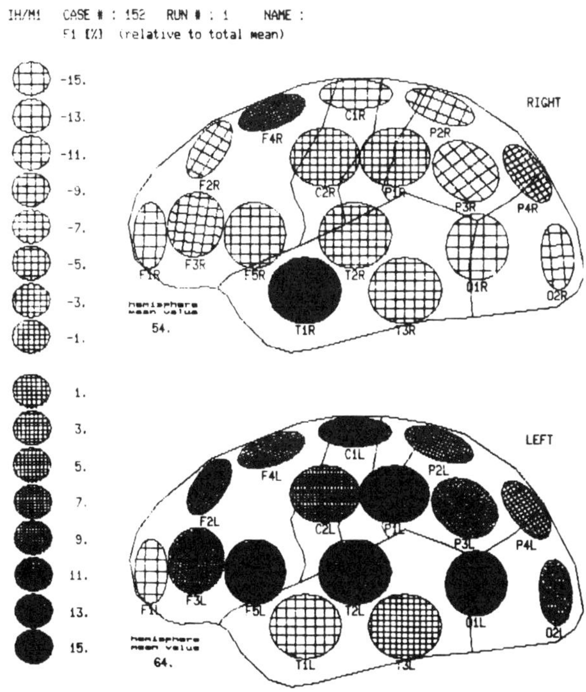

FIGURE 7.6. Regional cerebral blood flow in acute occlusion of the internal carotid artery. F1 is expressed as relative deviation from the total mean value of the brain. Light areas indicate low flow, dark ones high flow. Over the right hemisphere F1 flow is significantly lower than over the contralateral side.

The first report on CBF in patients with STA-MCAA appeared from Roberts et al. (1975). The authors concluded that flow in the target tissue was supplied primarily from the connected bypass (indicated by monoexponential curves) as well as from the internal carotid artery (biexponential curves). The study involved intra-arterial Xenon injections into either the contralateral ICA or the superficial temporal artery, making interpretation of data difficult. CBF was not measured prior to the bypass, so this study could not give any guidelines on patient selection for the procedure.

Schmiedeck et al. (1976) and Gratzl et al. from Munich (1976) also used the intra-arterial ^{133}Xe technique and the multidetector setup to study 110 patients with cerebrovascular diseases (CVD), of which 53 received a STA-MCAA. In 40 patients CBF measurements were repeated after bypass operation, usually within 1 week after surgery. In patients with occlusion of the internal carotid artery the contralateral side was used for the injection of the tracer. However, the authors did not mention whether the amount of tracer which reached the involved hemisphere was sufficient for reliable count rates. Postoperative measurements were performed with tracer injection into either the external or internal carotid artery on the involved side. In all patients a postoperative basic study was followed by CO_2 inhalation test which was able to delineate the ischemic focal sharply from the environmental tissue. The authors recommended to operate only on those patients in whom preoperative rCBF was not generally reduced (which in the opinion of the authors indicated a generalized small vessel disease). Only patients with focal reduction of cerebral blood flow were considered for STA-MCAA by the authors. In patients with a normal flow, the authors did not consider bypass because "it seems superfluous to add additional collateral blood supply to normal perfused cortex." In our experience we do not agree on these points since patients with normal flow and a history of hemodynamic cause of transient ischemia might suffer from disturbed autoregulation which then could be compensated for by the bypass duing critical situation of perfusion pressures. Alternative conclusions could be derived from the data presented. Patients with severe occlusive intracranial disease may have normal resting flow but fail to respond to CO_2, suggesting maximal dilation even under resting conditions (Norrving et al., 1982). They may suffer delayed ischemic episodes whenever systemic blood pressure falls because of the reduced vascular reserve and could perhaps benefit from a bypass. In patients with generalized reduction of blood flow, STA-MCAA could be considered if the territory of the middle cerebral artery presents with maximal reduction of flow compared to the other tissue.

Little et al. (1979) used the intra-arterial ^{133}Xe design as well as fluorescence angiography during surgery for STA-MCAA. They observed improvement of flow immediately after connection of the anastomosis. However, the design of the study did not allow measurements after surgery, therefore, it was not able to make any suggestment in respect to significant flow by the anastomosis.

The varying results in regard to CBF changes using hemispheric blood flow data in different studies may be due to local flow resdistribution following surgery. Only regional measurements are able to answer this question. The only study which deals with regional data was presented by Laurent et al. (1982). The study was retrospective and not controlled. However, with the inhalation design it was possible to observe a postoperative increase of flow in the anterior cerebral artery of 46%, in the middle cerebral artery of 15%, and in the watershed area of 85%.

Like others, the authors noted an improvement of CBF on both the operated and the contralateral side. Contrary to Schmiedek et al. (1976) and Chater (1976), the authors believed that in patients with generalized reduction of cerebral blood flow STA-MCAA is not indicated.

It may be important to observe not only the resting flow but also the capacity of the vascular system to react to changes of pCO_2. Halsey et al. (1982) reported on hemispheric flow in 19 patients before and after STA-MCAA. There was a progressive increase of flow over the months up to the 26th week, more in the operated than in the contralateral side. In all instances, CBF was retested under hypercapnia and a negative correlation emerged between preoperative and postoperative reactivity, i.e., the postoperative changes of vascular reactivity were greater in those patients who showed a reduced preoperative reactivity.

The authors believe that the postoperative resting cerebral blood flow changes are primarily due to the natural cause of recovery of brain function in patients with minor infarction and patients with transient ischemic attacks. However, they did not substantiate their hypothesis by following a control group and secondly in patients with transient ischemic attacks one would not expect spontaneous significant increase in flow several months after the attack. In our laboratory, we have never seen a patient with a transient ischemic attack who initially presented with contralateral cerebral blood-flow reduction. Only this would explain the improvement in CBF postoperatively if it is independent of the bypass. It seems important to note, however, that the increase in CO_2 reactivity was greatest in those patients who had a poor reactivity prior to surgery. This suggests that a functioning bypass might improve the vascular reserve in those patients in whom it was compromised prior to surgery. No explanation was given in the study as to why CO_2 reactivity also improved after surgery on the contralateral side.

The improvement of CO_2 reactivity was also described by Tsuda et al. (1984) using the intra-arterial ^{133}Xe injection technique before and after STA-MCAA in ten patients. In some patients a gamma camera was positioned over the vertical aspect of the skull and in other patients over the lateral aspect. CO_2 reactivity was tested by hyperventilation. Reduced CO_2 reactivity was noted primarily in patients with watershed infarction plus TIA. CBF increased mostly in those patients in whom pre-operative flow was low. This underlines the importance of STA-MCAA also in patients with low preoperative resting flow. CO_2 reactivity in this study improved more in those cases with high preoperative CO_2 reactivity.

The authors raise the question whether postoperative CBF increase (more than 30% in some subgroups) is due to the spontaneous course or the increased offer of blood. Because CBF increase of 30% was never observed in patients with transient ischemic attack in the chronic phase, one could assume that this increase does not reflect the natural course. CBF changes in the chronic phase of complete infarction might be observed within the first 6 weeks of recovery but rather mild thereafter (Tolonen et al., 1981; Demeurisse et al., 1983, Meyer et al., 1982).

However, there is some truth in the statement of Halsey et al., that resting flow level is not affected in many patients with STA-MCAA. The goal of the anastomosis is improvement of flow in areas with critical perfusion, in whom moderate additional drop of perfusion pressure might then cause functional impairment. Furthermore, the improvement of CO_2 reactivity was observed by Tsuda et al. (1984), Halsey et al. (1982), and suggested by Vorstrup et al. (1984) and points to the important role of the anastomosis in the local regulation of flow. Since the natural course of CBF following minor or complete infarction of the brain may vary, the results of STA-MCAA on CBF may be best evaluated by long-term studies.

Yonekura et al. (1982) have used the intravenous technique to follow blood flow in 107 patients with STA-MCAA for two years following surgery. From the clinical point of view, it was stated, that over a period of 25 months, 82% of patients with transient ischemic attacks, 77% of those with transient ischemic attacks plus mild stroke, and in those patients who suffered from mild stroke only 70% recovered well. However the criteria of judgement were not fully explained. The mean blood-flow changes in the total group increased by 10% within one week following anastomosis and then slowly fell down over two years to 86% compared with the preoperative resting flow. By separating patients with internal carotid artery lesions from those with middle cerebral artery diseases, there was a stronger increase of flow in the latter group in the first week but not thereafter. No differences could be detected between young and older patients with TIA and those with completed strokes. The trend of bilateral identical percentage change of CBF was explained by the reduction of intracerebral steal. This is surprising since it would anticipate a loss of autoregulation in the side contralateral to the STA-MCAA.

It was not mentioned whether all patients with a postoperative contralateral CBF increase had suffered from arterial lesions or ischemic attacks in that side. Only this could explain the loss of autoregulation as a prerequisite to the increase of flow after STA-MCAA. Since the ipsilateral and contralateral flow increase—matched for all patients—was less than 10% in the first week, the CBF changes could be due to the statistical error of the technique.

Two controlled studies have been published so far. Twenty patients with similar lesions who underwent STA-MCAA were studied by de Weerd et al. (1982). The patients were divided into two groups, one receiving a STA-MCAA.

CBF was measured using the inhalation technique and calculations of flow were done by the initial flow index. Unfortunately, patients with a recent stroke (2 days) and those with ischemic attacks months back were grouped together. In 5 out of 10 operated patients CBF increased in both sides and in the other 5 CBF decreased on both sides. Five out of 10 patients in the control group showed a CBF reduction over a period of 3 months. The asymmetry of CBF decreased after surgery but there were no significant differences in rCBF between patients who underwent surgery and those who did not. The study indicated that there is no general trend of CBF behavior after STA-MCAA.

The other control study was performed by Tanahashi et al. from the group in Houston (1985). Regional data in this study which was done for up to 4 years in individual patients, were not reported. Two weeks after surgery, there was a significant increase of cerebral blood flow which began to decrease 2 years postoperatively. From the third year on there was no significant difference between the treated and the nontreated group. There was no difference between both ipsilateral and the contralateral hemisphere at any time. The authors state that the final answer in respect to the benefit of STA-MCAA could not be given by the CBF studies but only by clinical evaluation.

One disadvantage of the two-dimensional studies is the inability to record flow changes in the depth of the brain. A new development, the ^{133}Xe-SPECT-tomography, as described by Lassen et al. (1985), may be able to record flow changes even in distance of the cortical surface of the brain. Vorstrup et al. (1984) have used this new system to measure the local flow before and STA-MCAA in 22 patients. Only those patients were operated on who presented with a flow deficit more extensive than hypodense alteration in the cranial computerized tomography. The postoperative evaluation of the patients showed a significant increase of CBF in only 2 out of 22 cases. A control group was not performed and regional variations were not described.

Not only blood-flow measurements may be important for selection of patients for STA-MCAA, apart from clinical and angiographic evaluation but measurement of metabolism as well. Grubb et al. (1979) studied rCBF and regional cerebral metabolic rate of oxygen with intra-arterial injection of $H_2{}^{15}O$ (CBF) and ^{15}O-oxyhemoglobin ($CMRO_2$) in nine patients before and after STA-MCAA. In five patients in whom anastomosis contributed significantly to the perfusion of the MCA both rCBF and $rCMRO_2$ were reduced prior to the surgery. After installation of the STA-MCAA both values increased. In four patients with patent but functionally nonimportant anastomosis both rCBF and $rCMRO_2$ showed a parallel trend of behavior either in increase or no change. The important observation in this study was that all those patients benefited from the STA-MCAA in whom CBF prior to surgery was decreased independently on the observation of $rCMRO_2$ and "marked neurological deficits." Even if not drawn by the authors, it may be concluded that CBF measurements apart from clinical and angiographical evaluation may be sufficient to select patient for STA-

MCAA. Because a technique as described in this report is expensive and requests arterial puncture, it seems less appropriate for pre- and postoperative evaluation of patients with STA-MCAA.

Another metabolic study was reported by Baron et al. (1981) on one patient with a left-sided intracarotid artery occlusion who suffered from several attacks of transient neurological deficits assumed to be due to hemodynamic origin. CBF was measured by the $C^{15}O_2$-technique. Forty-five days before surgery cerebral blood flow was decreased and oxygen extraction rate increased in the territory of the middle cerebral artery in the affected hemisphere. Thirty-two days after surgery both values had returned to normal. In the opinion of the author, STA-MCAA improved the "misery perfusion syndrome," characterized by reduced CBF and increased oxygen extraction. These data, albeit from a single patient, support the observations by Grubb et al. (1979) on three patients in whom there were increases in both CBF and $CMRO_2$ after surgery in areas which prior to surgery had low flow and high metabolism. However, these reports of all together four cases do not prove that one needs both, CBF- and O_2 metabolism measurements to select patients for bypass surgery.

Powers et al. (1984) used positron emission tomography with intraarterial time activity recording to measure interhemispheric ratio of CBF, $CMRO_2$, cerebral blood volume (CBV) and fractional extraction of oxygen (OEG) in 17 patients 1 day to 7 weeks before STA-MCAA and 7 days to 4 weeks post surgery. Data were compared to 14 normal volunteers who were measured once. Before surgery, hemispheric cerebral blood flow of the symptomatic side was reduced in 13 out of 17 cases, in 12 out of these 13 cases $CMRO_2$ was depressed as well. In 7 out of 17 patients cerebral blood volume was increased. Interhemispheric CBF-ratio increased post STA-MCAA in the symptomatic hemisphere in 6 patients. Cerebral blood volume in 6 cases in whom CBF increased postsurgically was decreased or increased prior to operation. Postsurgery $CMRO_2$ or CBF did not change but oxygen extraction fraction did decrease. The following may be concluded from this study:

1. Selection of patients for STA-MCAA does not require measurement of oxygen metabolism since CBF was only increased in those patients who had reduced CBF preoperatively.

2. Since cerebral blood volume did not change after STA-MCAA it is not necessary to measure it as a tool for selection of patients for surgery.

3. Since oxygen extraction fraction did decrease after STA-MCAA parallel to an increase of cerebral blood flow it may be assumed that in patients with no clinical deficit at the time of surgery reduction of blood flow was compensated for by increase of OEF. After surgery cerebral blood flow increased and, therefore, OEF could decrease to a normal value.

To the best of our knowledge no controlled long-term study exists in the literature with reports on *regional* blood-flow measurements over both hemispheres in patients before and after STA-MCAA. To evaluate the question, whether (a) blood flow does change by STA-MCAA and, (b) blood flow measurements might be used as a diagnostic tool in selection of patients for STA-MCAA we have performed a prospective controlled study on patients with unilateral cerebral ischemia in the territory of the middle cerebral artery, transient ischemic attacks, prolonged reversible ischemic neurological deficits or permanent strokes with complete recovery or only mild neurological deficits at the time of the surgery. All patients agreed in the operation. The blood-flow data, which were collected till the end of the first year after surgery were compared with 16 patients with identical diagnosis and similar treatment except for not getting the STA-MCAA. In the operated group, blood flow was estimated before surgery once and after surgery three times, whereas in the control group blood-flow data were collected three times over a period of several months.

From the angiographical diagnosis patients had complete occlusion of one internal carotid artery, inaccessible high stenosis of the internal carotid artery, and stenosis or complete occlusion of one middle cerebral artery.

Prior to STA-MCAA installation blood flow was measured a few days before time of operation; after surgery 2 to 9 days (CBF2), 4 to 8 weeks (CBF3) and 8 to 12 months (CBF4).

Clinical symptomatology was not altered by surgery. At CBF1 (blood-flow

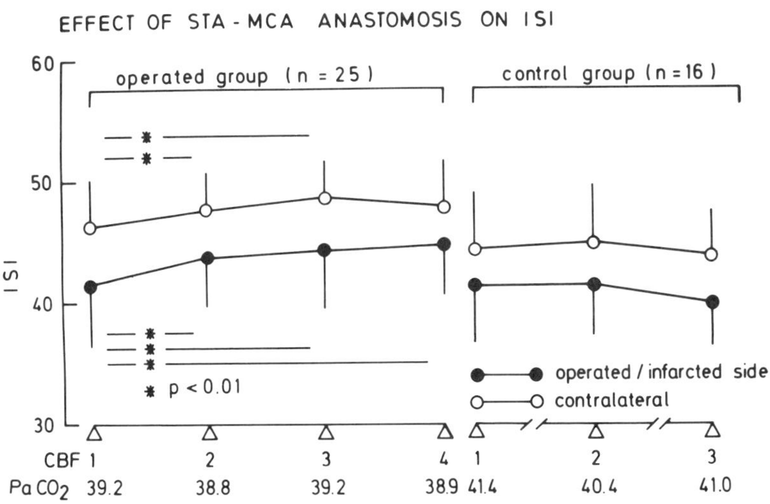

FIGURE 7.7. Effect of superficial temporal artery-middle cerebral artery anastomosis on initial slow index (ISI), compared with 16 patients with identical diagnosis and clinical presentation but no surgical therapy. CBF1: prior to surgery (see text); CBF2: short time after bypass-surgery; CBF3: weeks after surgery; CBF4: months after surgery.

measurement before surgery in the operated group) there was no significant difference between the infarcted sides and between the contralateral sides of both groups. At CBF2 and CBF3 mean initial slope index of both the ipsi- and the contralateral side of the operated groups was significantly higher than that of the control group (Fig. 7.7). In contrast to Meyer's observation (1982) but in agreement with Halsey et al. (1982) we did not observe a flow reduction parallel to that of the control group in the operated hemispheres.

Furtheron we observed a significant increase of flow in the contralateral side in only three cases from CBF1 to CBF3 and in one case from CBF1 to CBF4. We, therefore, believe that neutralization of intracerebral steal phenomenon is not a major benefit of STA-MCAA. The mild increase of mean hemispheric flow for the whole group indicates that in patients with focal cerebral ischemia mean blood flow does not change significantly after installation of STA-MCAA. However, compared with the control group, mean flow of the operated side increases significantly within a few weeks and thereafter remains unchanged for months.

The main advantage of the multidetector inhalation system is the repeated measurements of regional flow course. Due to our experience from test–retest maneuvers in normal volunteers, we consider any regional flow value which is more than 15% below or above mean hemispheric value as being relatively hypoemic or hyperemic. Fig. 7.8 indicates the percentage of classified areas with relative hyperemia, normoemia, and hyperemia at all four measurements in the operated and the contralateral side. In the contralateral side there was no change

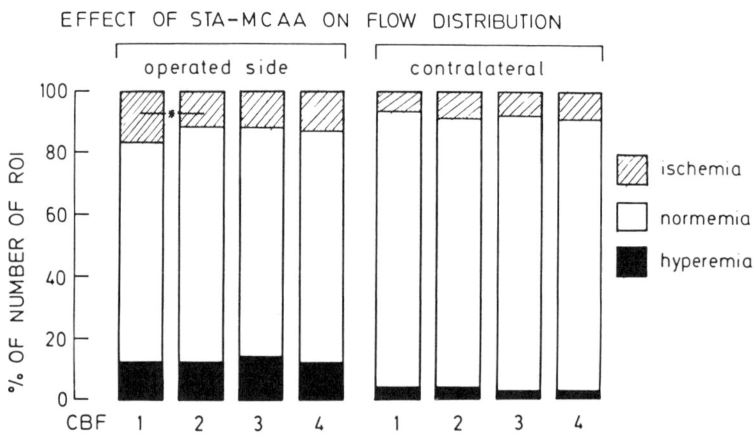

FIGURE 7.8. Effect of superficial temporal artery-middle cerebral artery anastomosis on number of areas with ischemia, normoemia, and hyperemia at CBF1–CBF4 in the operated and the contralateral side. From CBF1 to CBF2 there was a significant reduction of areas with focal ischemia. At CBF4 there were still areas with ischemia and hyperemia, indicating that the bypass did not normalize flow maps.

of distribution of the classified areas. However, in the operated side there was a significant reduction of regions of interest with relative hypoemia from CBF1 to CBF2. In the same time the number of regions of interest with flow within the normal relative distribution increased. However, since even at CBF4 there was still a significant number of areas with relative hyperemia and areas with relative hypoemia, the STA-MCAA did not achieve a normalization of flow distribution which was observed in only 3 out of 25 cases.

Because some authors believe that STA-MCAA improves flow also in territories which are not directly connected to the operated arteries, we have counted the number of areas in each territory, which benefitted significantly from STA-MCAA, i.e., increased flow by at least 15%. Fig. 7.9 indicates that mostly the territory of the middle cerebral artery benefited from the anastomosis. Since areas with a significant reduction of flow were distributed all over the hemisphere, a direct steal between neighboring areas was not observed.

In contrast to Schmiedek et al. (1976), we have also observed rCBF increases in areas with major reductions in flow. Our belief is that, in addition to the prophylactic goal of STA-MCAA, the connection of an extracranial artery to major intracerebral arteries may improve local flow to an extent which brings it

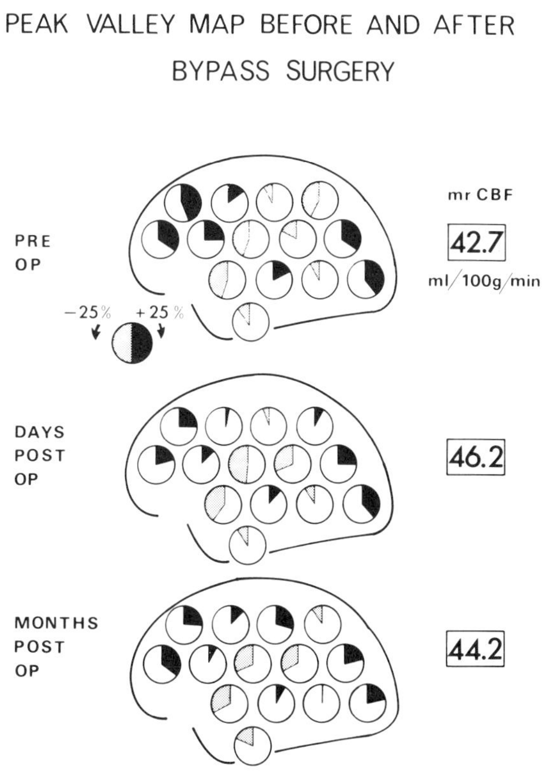

FIGURE 7.9. Peak valley map before and after bypass operation in one patient. Flow expressed as a percentage of deviation from mean 90° value of the operated hemisphere. Mean flow given on the right side. CBF-measurement before surgery (upper map, pre-op), six days after surgery (middle map) and 8 months after surgery. Six days after surgery there was no significant improvement of CBF, even in the ischemic tissue of the territory supplied by the middle cerebral artery. Months after surgery rCBF increased significantly in one area (most upper row of detectors, third from the left).

above a certain critical threshold. In no case CBF measurements did predict the clinical outcome of the patient. However, since blood flow rose more in tissue with low than in tissue with normal flow, the procedure may have some therapeutic role. Due to selection of patients included into the protocol the multicenter study is inconclusive (see "Special Reports" in *New England Journal of Medicine,* 809–810 and 814–824 (1987)).

REGIONAL CBF IN TRANSIENT ISCHEMIC ATTACKS

Transient ischemic attacks (TIA) consist of sudden onset of neurological symptoms due to cerebral ischemia of the brain or the retina (amaurosis fugax) which by definition resolve within 24 hours, usually within 5 to 30 minutes. TIAs are an important warning sign of stroke: About half of these patients experience a stroke and report on preceding warning signs. TIAs are due to emboly from extracranial or intracranial arteries or from the heart, to alterations of hemodynamic conditions, platelet function, or state of coagulation, to vasculopathies and to compression of arteries in their extra- or intracranial course. Work-up of patients with one or several TIAs include Doppler sonography, transcranial Doppler sonogaphy, DSA, cranial computerized tomography (CCT), a careful examination of the heart and evaluation of the neurological conditions. Formerly it was believed that TIAs were not associated with frank alteration of tissue in cranial computerized tomography but publications from Perone et al. (1979) and Ladurner et al. (1985) have indicated hypodensic areas on CCT. However, sequential examinations have not been done. Nowadays it is believed but not proven that TIA might often be associated with permanent alteration of cerebral tissue. TIA is a rather arbitrary description and does not define the length and course of the ischemia itself. It defines only the duration of clinical symptoms.

Studies of regional cerebral blood flow in patients with TIA are rare. Since most of the patients suffering from such a disease enter the hospital after the neurological symptoms have disappeared, clinical and neuroradiological workup is performed—if at all—with some delay. Fartheron, the intra-arterial technique did not allow repeated measurements in patients without any neurological signs. Because TIA may precede a completed stroke, it is of interest to know for how long and to what extent CBF might be reduced.

Three intra-arterial studies on patients with TIA have been published: Rees et al. (1970) reported on 11 patients with history of TIA and observed alteration of blood flow (reduction and increase) in 7 cases 8–90 days after the last TIA. Bicompartmental analysis suggested that fast clearing tissue was predominantly involved by the ischemic process. In the majority of cases rCBF disturbances correlated with the tissue localization of ischemia, as judged by clinical manifestations.

This observation is in contrast to the report from Skinhoj et al. (1970) who studied 12 cases with transient ischemic attacks, 40 minutes to 4 years after the last attack. In most of the cases focal abnormalities were not observed, one patient—who was studied 30 minutes after TIA—presented with focal hyper-mia, but another patient showed disturbed autoregulation to blood pressure in-crease. The authors concluded that abnormalities of cerebral autoregulation could be noted only in the phase immediately following the ischemic attack. Six of the 12 patients studied were evaluated in the first 4 days following the TIA. The authors concluded that alteration of blood flow might be observed primarily within this period. Wong et al. (1973), however, found focal CBF abnormalities in about 80% of the 22 patients with TIA, who were studied 1 to 90 days after the ischemic attacks. In this study there was a high level of correlation between the localization of the lesion as judged by clinical examination and the area of rCBF disturbances. This is of interest, since in the first days after an ischemic attack in the majority of CCT no tissue alteration might be observed. The study again indicated that in addition to symptomatic lesions rCBF measurement might de-tect so-called silent areas, which do not present with clinical symptoms at the time of the examination but may indicate region which might be endangered by further hemodynamic attacks.

Tsuda et al. (1983) have used the intra-arterial technique to test CO_2-respon-siveness in patients with TIA and obstructive disease of the internal carotid artery. In patients with complete occlusion of the internal carotid artery the detectors were placed over the vertical aspect of the skull. Diminished CO_2-responsiveness was noted primarily in patients with internal carotid artery occlu-sion but not internal carotid artery stenosis.

In none of these four publications CBF data could be correlated to the con-tralateral hemisphere and to repeated measurements.

Four studies have been detected in the literature which employed the ^{133}Xe inhalation technique. However, these studies again did not perform repeated measurements to follow the CBF course. These studies are:

1. Ackerman (1979) reported on 32 patients with TIA, 23 of them having symptoms from the hemispheres. It was reported that mean rCBF was reduced compared with a normal control group and that only 1 out of 7 patients who underwent endarterectomy had a CBF increase after surgery. No difference was observed between the symptomatic and the asymptomatic side. This led to the suggestion that TIA as a warning sign with bilateral reduction of flow might be a precedent of diaschisis observed during a completed stroke. Since repeated stud-ies were not done this question remained unanswered.

2. Naritomi et al. (1977) reported on 15 patients with TIA and mentioned a normal autoregulation in all cases. It was not stated, whether focal abnormalities were observed. However, the authors reported on bilateral focal flow reduction persisting for about 3 weeks after the onset of symptoms in TIAs due to carotid diseases. These statements in respect to alteration of flow following an ischemic

attack were done by single measurements in different patients at different time after the attack.

3. Yonekua et al. (1980) investigated 87 patients with TIA but did not mention the time distance from the last attack to the CBF measurement. With the intravenous technique they found the highest hemispheric blood flow in the contralateral side of patients with unilateral middle cerebral artery stenosis and the lowest hemispheric flow in the ipsilateral side of patients with intracarotid artery occlusion and stenosis. There was a significant difference in hemispheric rCBF between the symptomatic and the contralateral hemisphere. However, there was no significant difference between groups with TIA, TIA plus minor stroke, and minor stroke only. In respect to focal flow disturbances, there was a significant reduction of flow over the ipsilateral temporal lobe in patients with focal TIA plus bilateral lesion, whereas in patients with focal TIA flow abnormalities were noted over the occipital, frontal, and parietal lobe but not over the temporal aspect of the hemispheres.

4. Meyer et al. (1979) studied 19 patients with unilateral carotid transient ischemic attacks about 75 days after the onset of symptoms. Again, the authors described bilateral reduction of regional blood flow in patients with unilateral TIA which resolved within 3 weeks after the last TIA. These observations were not done with repeated measurements. There was a significant difference of flow over the tissue area responsible for the clinical symptoms in patients who were measured within 3 weeks after the onset of symptoms when compared with those who were measured later on.

Vorstrup et al. (1983) have employed the ^{133}Xenon inhalation single photon emission computer tomography (SPECT) to study rCBF in 14 cases with TIA days to weeks after the ischemic attack. Four of the 14 patients showed reduction of flow which roughly correlated to hypodense areas on CCT and was interpreted as being due to incomplete infarctions. Other patients showed a flow reduction with no abnormality in the CCT. The reconstructive vascular surgery did not change the flow pattern thus suggesting "irreversible ischemic tissue damage without cross embolition."

Lenzi et al. (1978) have measured both regional cerebral blood flow and oxygen metabolism in 11 patients with TIA. The time distance between onset of symptoms and measurements of CBF and metabolism was not mentioned. It was noted that blood-flow disturbances were more prominent than metabolic alterations. Repeated measurements have not been done.

It is still uncertain whether TIAs might be associated with *prolonged* alterations of cerebral tissue appearance as judged by computerized tomography or by early and successive measurements in the regional cerebral blood flow. Between 1979 and 1983 we studied 20 patients with transient ischemic attacks, during the attack or within 6 hours after clinical recovery. The application of the non-traumatic inhalation technique made it possible to study blood flow as soon as a patient entered the hospital. All patients had TIAs in the territory of the internal carotid artery and did not have any symptoms of vertebro-basilar insufficiency. Thirteen of 20 patients experienced their first attack; 7 patients had a history of several similar attacks. In most of the cases CBF was measured during the attack. CBF measurement number 2 (CBF2) was undertaken on the day following admission at a time when all clinical signs had vanished. CBF3 was done between the sixth and the eighth day after the transient ischemic attack. rCBF-measurements were compared with 20 patients in our CBF laboratory who had no history of acute cerebral ischemic attacks but suffered from at least 2 risk factors for cerebral vascular disease. The data in these 20 patients were collected over a period of 3 years independently of the TIA protocol. However, in all patients at least 3 CBF-measurements were performed within two weeks.

Compared with the control group, mean rCBF in the TIA group was significantly reduced in both hemispheres on Day 1 (Fig. 7.10). Between both sides of the TIA group there was a significant difference on Day 1 with a reduced mean rCBF over the involved side. From Day 1 to Day 2 mean rCBF in the involved side increased significantly and remained unchanged from Day 2 to Day 7. Seven days after onset of symptoms mean rCBF of both the involved and the contralateral hemisphere was significantly lower compared with that of the control group. However, looking at the individual cases we observed 10 patients in whom mean rCBF increased significantly from CBF2 to CBF3.

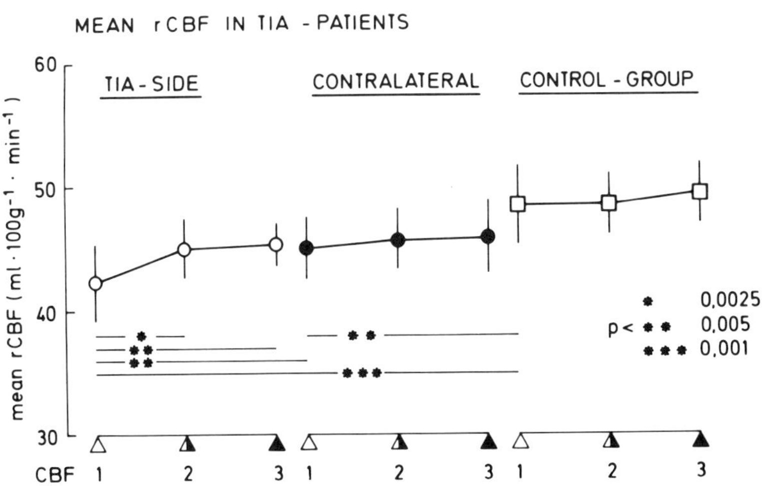

FIGURE 7.10. Mean rCBF in patients with TIA and control patients. CBF1: day of transicent ischemic attack (TIA); CBF2: the following day, when clinical symptoms had disappeared; CBF3: seven days after TIA. CBF data were separated for the involved and the contralateral side in TIA patients but matched for the control group which did not suffer from clinical signs of ischemia but had risk factors for cerebrovascular disease.

The data indicate, that during CBF1 blood flow is significantly reduced in the affected side, compared with the contralateral hemisphere and to a control group with a similar risk profile but no history of TIA. From Day 1 to Day 2 there is a significant increase of cerebral blood flow only in the hemisphere suffering from transient ischemia but not in the conteralateral side.

Mean hemispherical data do not give any impression about focal abnormalities and even might mask focal hypo- and hyperemic zones. In our experiences one should calculate always the relative flow distribution of each hemisphere to receive impressions on regional flow behavior. Measurements in 10 normals for F1, initial slope index and mean flow have indicated that any percentage of deviation of regional flow from mean regional cerebral blood flow of more than 15% may be considered statistically significant. We consider areas with a significantly reduced flow compared with mean rCBF as being relatively hypoemic and those with the significant higher flow compared to mean rCBF as being relatively hyperemic. Fig. 7.11 gives an impression of relative flow distribution (F1) in 10 normals, measured with parallel arrangement of detectors. Hyperfrontality and occipital increase of flow during steady state ($paCO_2$ = 40 mm Hg, dark room, low noise, and closed eyes) are indicated. The only significant difference between corresponding areas of the right and left hemispheres were observed in the lower part of the frontal lobe, where in the right side rCBF was higher than mean rCBF and over the left side rCBF was lower than mean rCBF.

Repeated measurements of flow in our patients with TIA have revealed that

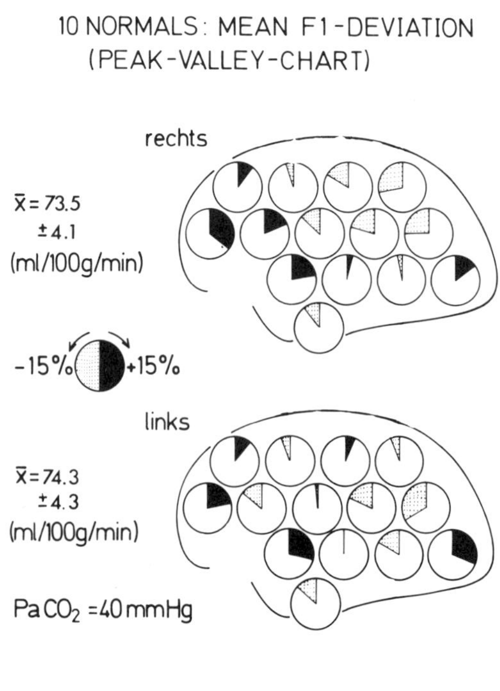

FIGURE 7.11. Regional deviation of F1 flow from mean CBF in 10 young normal patients (volunteers). Black segments to the right indicate a regional flow above mean rCBF, dotted areas to the left indicate regional flow below mean rCBF. The only significant difference between corresponding right and left areas was observed in the second area from the left in the second row, where rCBF in the right side was above mean rCBF and rCBF in the left side below mean rCBF.

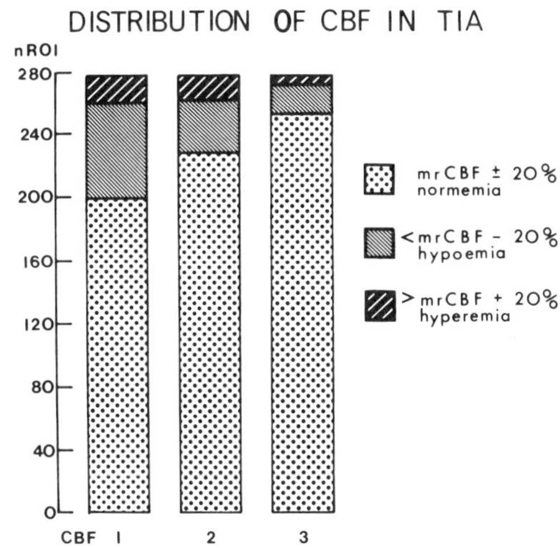

FIGURE 7.12. Number of areas with normemia 90° (dotted), hypoemia (striped with fine lines) and hyperemia (striped with big lines) at CBF1, 2, and 3 in patients with TIA. There is a reduction of areas with hypoemia from CBF1 to 2 and from CBF2 to 3.

even on the seventh day after onset of symptoms regional distribution of flow is not normal. On Day 1, about 60 out of 280 regions of interest in the involved hemisphere showed relative hypemia, whereas 20 regions of interest presented with relatively hyperemia. The following day the total amount of hypoemic regions was significantly reduced but still present (Fig. 7.12). The trend to normalization of relative flow distribution was still going on to Day 7 and at this time the flow map may represent a stable flow distribution no more influenced by the ischemic attack. However, the change of flow from Day 2 to Day 7 was

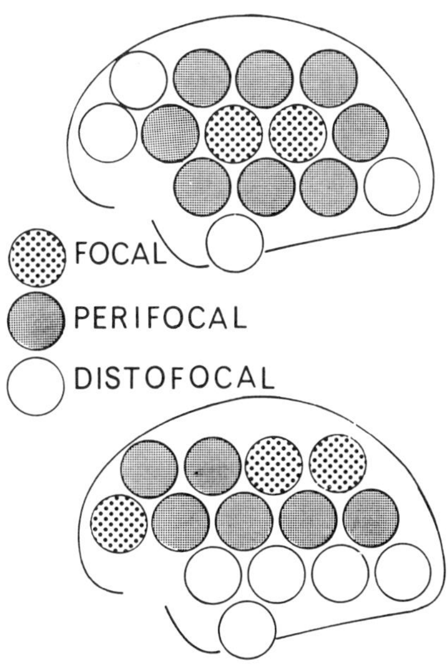

FIGURE 7.13. Classification of areas into focal, perifocal, and distofocal areas (detectors), according to the anatomical localization suggested from clinical presentation.

believed to be due only to the transient ischemic attack since there was a significant deviation of flow behavior in comparison to the control group.

If one tries to correlate the localization of the ischemic attack as judged by clinical examination and EEG-findings to observation in rCBF measurements, one is able to classify the external detectors as focal, perifocal, and distal detectors. The detectors over the ischemic focus are so-called focal detectors, all the surrounding detectors are called the perifocal detectors and the rest of the detectors in the respective hemisphere are classified as being distal detectors (Fig. 7.13). Looking at the individual cases we have observed different types of behavior in the focal detectors, which are partly indicated in Fig. 7.14. In some cases a normalization of focal flow were observed over the perifocal and distal focal tissue and over the contralateral side. In other cases we have observed an unchanged flow from Day 1 to Day 2 over the focal detectors without any involvement of the perifocal, distal or contralateral tissue. However, in other patients an increased flow (luxury perfusion) was observed on Day 1 or Day 2. In those patients, in whom hyperemic flows over the focal detectors were observed on Day 2 but not on Day 1 and Day 7, reduction of flow was noted in the perifocal and distal tissue. Again the contralateral side was not involved. In some cases focal blood flow was reduced on Day 1 compared with the contralateral side and did not change until Day 7. This persistent focus might be due not to the acute ischemic attack but to persistent chronic alteration of blood flow on the basis of generalized cerebrovascular disease.

Our data indicate that in respect to regional blood-flow behavior there is a varying course between individual patients suffering from acute onset of transient cerebral ischemica. Early normalization, late normalization, early or delayed luxury perfusion and persistent ischemic flow may be observed and might be correlated with reduction of flow in the perifocal tissue. Contralateral flow reduction as observed in completed infarction as observed in completed infarction (diaschisis) is not an important finding in patient with transient ischemic attacks. However, since flow abnormalities could be observed on Day 1 and Day 2 at a time when cranial computerized tomography is not able to detect any tissue alteration in the majority of patients with TIA and completed stroke, measurement of regional cerebral blood flow might be important to indicate flow reduction and the exact side of ischemia. Ready availability of the method enables the doctor to start these measurements at a time when the patient enters the hospital.

Because blood-flow reduction in patients with TIA might be observed on Day 2 the cerebral tissue might be at a state where any additional hemodynamic crisis might harm again the tissue and convert a second transient ischemic attack into a completed stroke. In our opinion patients with transient ischemic attack and reduced blood flow (compared with a control group or to the contralateral hemisphere) should be treated like patients with completed ischemic stroke. Since our present regimen of treating ischemic stroke involves hemorrheological maneuver, we treat patients with transient ischemic attacks with either isovolemic or hypervolemic hemodilution for at least three days.

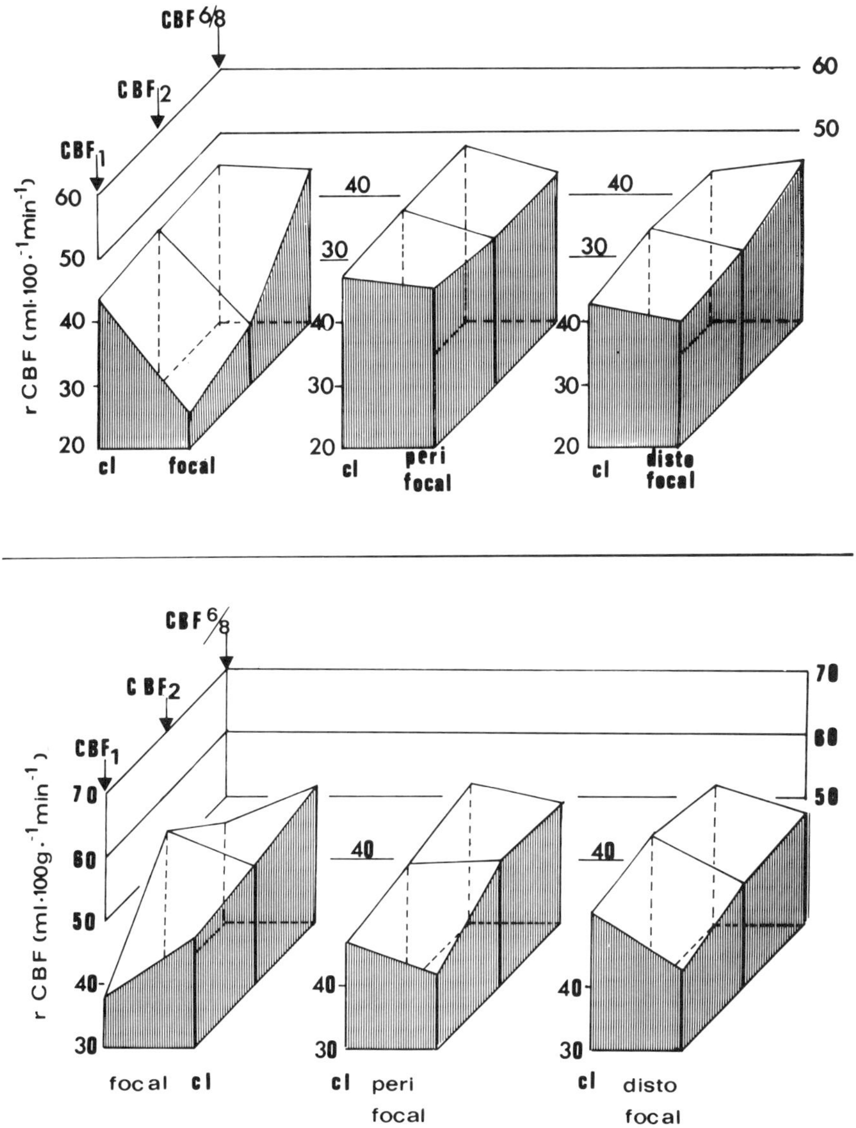

FIGURE 7.14. Change of rCBF in focal, perifocal, and distofocal areas at CBF1, 2, and, 3 in patients with TIA. The upper picture represents patients with prolonged hypoemia in the focal areas at CBF2. Flow in perifocal and distofocal detectors and flow in the contralateral hemisphere (cl) is not affected. The lower picture represents selected cases with delayed hyperemia. At CBF2 (1 day after TIA) rCBF in the focal area, which at CBF1 was hypoemic, is now hyperemic and normalizes till CBF3. The perifocal detector indicates ischemia at CBF1, but normal flow at CBF2. Flow in the contralateral side (cl) is not affected.

rCBF IN ACUTE CEREBRALINFARCTION

Most of the studies measuring rCBF in acute cerebral infarction have not included repeated bilateral measurements. Single estimation of CBF may not be able to separate acute flow alterations due to the ischemic stroke from chronic changes due to the underlying chronic cerebrovascular process. In the following paragraphs we will review the literature on measurement of regional cerebral blood flow in the acute state of infarction and after that report on our own experiences. Hemispheric blood flow studies, as done in the time before regional flow techniques, have already documented the reduction of hemispheric flow in acute and chronic cerebrovascular disease (Heymas et al., 1953; Shenkin et al., 1953; Novack et al., 1953; Scheinberg et al., 1976; Fazekas et al., 1955; Kempinski et al., 1961; Ekberg et al., 1965). Most of the reports on regional blood flow measurements have used the intraarterial injection technique, which limits the usefulness of the desaturation technique.

Hoedt–Rasmussen and Skinhoj (1964) noted a reduction of flow in the contralateral side in patients, who presented with signs and symptoms of unilateral hemispheric vascular disease. The authors did not exclude the possibility that contralateral blood flow was reduced prior to the stroke. They state that mean tissue flow (gray and white matter) was as low as 23 to 35 ml/100 g/min and that at flow levels below this limit clinical symptoms such as dementia did appear. However, in our own experience, mean rCBF in this range might be measured even without any clinical symptoms.

Fieschi et al. (1966) using the krypton 85 technique compared their data on stroke patients with 10 control subjects without cerebrovascular disease. The importance of this study is that CBF was estimated within 5 days after onset in 23 patients, whereas in 27 other patients the measurement was performed at a later state. Hemispheric flow of the stroke patients was reduced by more than 30% in the fast clearing compartment but less than 25% in the slow compartment. These values appeared to be independent of the time interval between ictus and measurement. Like Rasmussen and Skinhoj, the authors observed in 4 patients a reduction of flow in the contralateral side of the stroke.

Fujishima et al. (1974) have employed the intravenous RISA dilution technique in 29 patients with unilateral infarction. Flow was expressed as ml/min and was observed to be reduced in more than 50% of all patients in the involved side and in 45% bilaterally. Contralateral flows tended to normalize with longer intervals since the stroke. Only in patients with a persistent impairment of consciousness bilateral CBF reduction was noted more than 2 months after the stroke. In contradiction to Meyer et al. (1970; 1971), who supplied data for their hypothesis that contralateral flow reduction was primarily due to metabolic depression, Fujishima et al. (65) believe that primarily a bilateral increase of cerebrovascular resistance causes the flow reduction.

Levy et al. (1975) and Melamed et al. (1971) have used the intra-arterial technique to measure rCBF in the contralateral side in patients with acute infarction in the territory of the internal carotid artery. Measurement of CBF was done within 72 hours after onset of stroke. Despite the fact that in the normal healthy control group of 60 years and older mean rCBF was remarkably low (less than 40 ml/100 g/min) the stroke patients had a significantly lower CBF. These data support the observation of Hoedt-Rasmussen and Skinjoh (1964), Fieschi et al. (1966), and McHenry (1966), who observed a reduction of both CBF and $CMRO_2$.

Paulson et al. (1970) reported on a group of patients with acute occlusion of the middle cerebral artery and observed a reduction of mean flow in 8 out of 10 cases. In some patients focal hyperemia was found in tissue neighboring the ischemic focus, in others focal hyperemia was accompanied by ischemia in the perifocal tissue. Repeated studies were done in 3 instances and confirmed a persistence of the ischemic focus with loss of autoregulation. In these cases an occlusion of the middle cerebral artery was of permanent nature.

In a further paper Paulson (1970) reported on 31 patients with ischemic stroke and without arterial occlusion. In these areas CBF was studied only once and at different times (1 day to 11 years) after onset of symptoms. Hyperemic focuses during resting condition were found only in the first few days after onset of stroke. Focal vasoparalysis as measured with hyper- or hypocapnia was seen also in the acute phase of stroke. Ischemic focal disturbances, however, were observed throughout all stages after onset of stroke. It was not proven that focal ischemia changes in nature or intensity since repeated measurements have not been done. In this study ischemic and hyperemic areas were never found in the same hemisphere.

One of the most extensive studies on rCBF in infarction was performed by Meyer et al. with the atraumatic ^{133}Xe inhalation technique (1970, 1971). They estimated CBF once in 32 patients with unilateral infarction but did not perform repeated CBF studies. However, in 10 cases autoregulation was tested by tilting the supine patient by 30 degrees. It was stated that a reduction of blood pressure by about 12 mm Hg did not change flow significantly for the total group except for the territory of the middle cerebral artery. In patients with acute cerebral infarction CBF was reduced over both sides whereas in patients in whom stroke had occurred more than 4 weeks before, CBF was reduced only within the affected hemisphere. In contrast to our own experiences, CBF was also bilaterally reduced in patients with TIA for 1 to 3 weeks after the attack. Since consecutive measurements were not performed, the observed results in TIA patients could reflect the chronic state of cerebrovascular disease and must not be the consequence of the acute ischemic attack.

An attempt was made to correlate the degree of focal ischemia in the affected side and corresponding areas of the contralateral side with the time duration from the onset of the stroke. In the first 3 weeks after infarction there was a rather symmetrical reduction of focal flow in the territory of the middle cerebral artery over both sides. After that time focal flow was better in the contralateral side. Comparing the rCBF values for both F1 and mean flow, it was estimated that the clinical prognosis of the patient was good when F1 was above 37 ml/100 g/min and mean flow above 23 ml/100 g/min. This observation may fit into the concept of flow thresholds as described by Astrup et al. (1977).

The authors concluded from the observation that diaschisis plays an important part in acute cerebral infarction. Meyer et al. (1979) suggested that contralateral flow reduction (diaschisis) as a mirror focus of the affected hemisphere is provoked by neuronal depression via brain stem connections or the corpus callosum.

As noted, the majority of previous studies lacked longitudinal observations. We have attempted to supply such observations by following 38 patients with unilateral MCA ischemic infarction during the acute phase of their illness. All patients were admitted and evaluated within 48 hours after onset of symptoms. Blood-flow measurements were done on the day of admission (CBF1) subsequently on Day 6 to 8 (CBF2), 13 to 16 (CBF3), and 22 to 27 (CBF4). All patients reported here were treated with hemodiluting agents.

Mean rCBF in the infarcted hemisphere was significantly lower than that in the contralateral side at CBF1–CBF3. At CBF4 there was no significant difference between both sides but there were more patients in whom CBF of the contralateral side was higher than that of the infarcted side. In the contralateral side mean rCBF dropped from CBF1 to CBF2, probably due to development of increased intracranial pressure accompanying brain edema. However, this was not accompanied by a drop of mean rCBF in the infarcted side. We cannot exclude that the decrease of CBF in the contralateral side is due to unknown processes, such as late diaschisis. From CBF2 to CBF3 both sides presented with a significant increase of CBF. The infarcted hemispheres, but not the contralateral ones, further increased flow from CBF3 to CBF4. Table 7.1 lists the number of patients in whom CBF of the infarcted side was higher than contralaterally. At CBF1 to CBF3 only a few cases presented with this sign, proba-

TABLE 7.1
Differences of Mean rCBF Between Infarcted and Contralateral Hemispheres at CBF 1–4

	CBF1	*CBF2*	*CBF3*	*CBF4*
mCBF inf. lower than mCBF cl.	21	19	15	13
mCBF inf. same as mCBF cl.	14	12	19	22
mCBF inf. higher than mCBF cl.	3	6	2	0
n	38	37	36	35

inf. = infarcted side
cl. = contralateral side

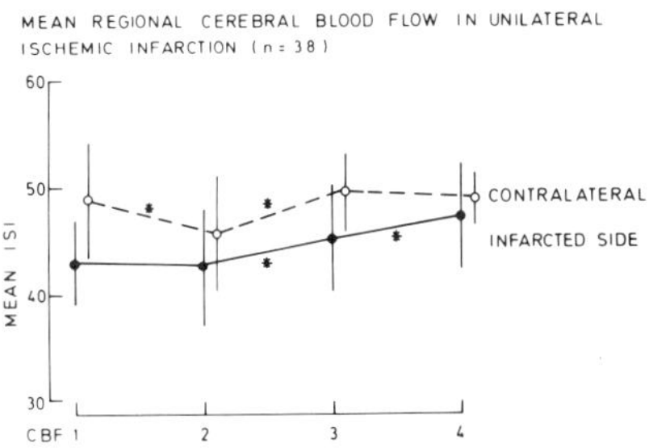

FIGURE 7.15a. Mean rCBF in unilateral ischemic infarction. CBF was measured on Day 1 (CBF1), Day 7 (CBF2), Day 14 (CBF3) and Day 21 (CBF4). ISI (initial slope index) decreased over the contralateral side from CBF1 to CBF2 and normalized again to CBF3. In the symptomatic side mean CBF increased significantly from CBF2 (Day 7) to CBF4 (Day 21).

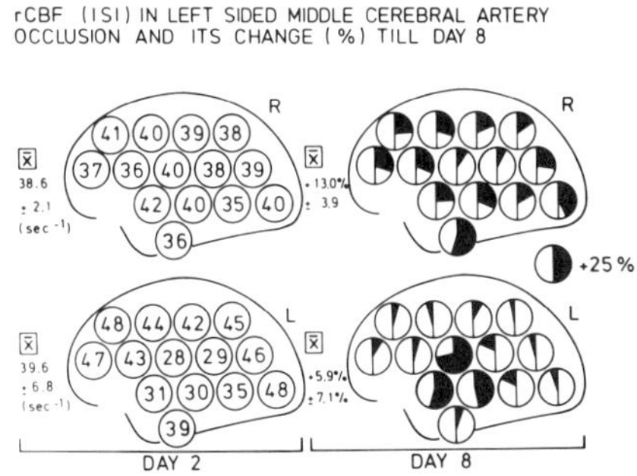

FIGURE 7.15b. Indicates the actual flow (ISI·sec^{-1}) in the right and in the left hemisphere in a patient with leftsided occlusion of the middle cerebral artery. The increase of CBF from day 2 to day 8, given as regional percentage changes in both right brain drawings, was bigger in the right (the "normal") than in the left hemisphere. Furthermore it may be recognized that the increase of flow in the left side concerned primarily the territory of the middle cerebral artery but in the right side the total surface of the hemisphere.

bly reflecting luxury perfusion. At CBF4 (3–4 weeks after infarction) none of our cases had a mean flow in the infarcted hemisphere which was above that of the other side.

In 8 out of 38 cases mean rCBF of the contralateral hemisphere increased significantly from CBF1 to CBF2, thus indicating an early flow depression (diaschisis). All of these patients suffered from either emboli to the middle cerebral artery or complete occlusion of the internal carotid artery, none from stenosis to both arteries. The size of infarction did not predict the possible occurrence of diaschisis. Classifying the hypodense area in the CCT, which was done in the first 6 days, as representing a big infarct if more than 50% of the area supplied by the middle cerebral artery was involved, 5 out of 8 cases with early diaschisis had a big infarct and 3 had a small one.

To exclude the possibility of a look-through phenomenon as simulating diaschisis the regional flow distribution was calculated for each case. In the majority of patients ischemia in the contralateral side was not confined to the territory of the middle cerebral artery but rather distributed over the total hemisphere. This was also observed in cases where ischemia in the involved side was observed exclusively in the area of the middle cerebral artery. Fig. 7.15b represents one of those cases where initial CBF on Day 2 indicated bilateral reduction of flow which then increased subsequently on both sides. It is obvious from the initial appearance of flow distribution and from its change over the time to Day 8 (CBF2) that ischemia in the side contralateral to the infarct involved the total hemisphere.

Our observations do not explain the nature of diaschisis. Meyer et al. (1982) believe that loss of metabolic control—indicated by reduced oxygen consumption and glucose utilization—leads to contralateral flow reduction. On the other side, Lavy et al. (1975) state that transneural depression is responsible for the CBF alterations. Both mechanisms do not explain our observation of focal decrease in the infarcted and homogenous flow reduction in the contralateral side. In contrast to Slater et al. ( ), we did not observe CBF decreases over the contralateral sides in all patients who presented with ipsilateral ischemia nor did we observe a prolonged contralateral ischemia. Contralateral flow reduction is rather limited in time (1 to 2 weeks) but extensive in topography involving the total hemisphere.

Luxury perfusion means tissue perfusion in excess of metabolic requirements. According to this notion, one needs both measurements of flow and metabolism to identify the phenomenon. However, we tried to bypass the problem by defining relative luxury perfusion, which indicates a regional flow, being 15% above mean hemispheric flow *and* decreasing to the next measurement without change of neurological condition. This was observed in four patients: Focal relative hyperemia was noted on Days 1–2 but not on Days 6–8. In all four instances it was accompanied by perifocal ischemia, which persisted for 21 days at least. In six other cases absolute focal hyperemia with flow levels above that of normal volunteers was noted again, accompanied by perifocal ischemia. The close topographical correlation of both relative and absolute hyperemia with transient but prolonged ischemia in the neighborhood supports the theory of vasoparalysis during the acute phase of cerebral infarction. However, the therapeutic consequences are rather unknown except that vasodilators are contraindicated.

REFERENCES

Ackerman, R. H., Gouluiamons, A. D., Grotta, J. C., Correira, J. A., Chang, J. T. (1979). Extracranial vascular disease and cerebral blood flow in patients with transient ischemic attacks. *Acta Neurol. Scand.*, Suppl. 60:442–443.

Astrup, J., Siesjo, B. K., Symon, 1. (1981). Thresholds in cerebral ischemia—the ischemic penumbra. *Stroke,* 12:723–725.

Astrup, J., Symon, L., Branston, N. M., et al. (1977). Cortical evoked potential and extracellular K^{++} and H^{+} at critical levels of brain ischemia. *Stroke,* 8:51–57.

Baron, J. C., Bousser, M. G., Rey, A., Guillard, A., Comar, D., Castaigne, P. (1981). Reversal of focal misery perfusion syndrome by extra-intracranial bypass in hemodynamic cerebral ischemia: A case study with 15 O positron emission tomography. *Stroke,* 12:454–459.

Chater, N. (1976). Patient selection and results of extra- to intra-cranial anastomosis in selected cases of cerebrovascular disease. IN: Keener, E. B., Carmel, P., Friedman, H., et al. (eds): *Clinical Neurosurgery*. Baltimore, Williams & Wilkins, Vol. 23, 287–309.

Chater, N., Popp, J. (1976). Microsurgical vascular bypass for occlusive cerebrovascular disease. Review of 100 cases. *Surg. Neurol.* 6:115–118.

Demeurisse, G., Verhas, M., Capon, A., Paternot, J. (1983). Lack of evolution of the cerebral blood flow during clinical recovery of a stroke. *Stroke,* 14:77–81.

De Weerd, A. W., Veering, M. M., Mosmans, P. C. M., van Huffelen, A. C., Tulleken, C. A. F., Jonkman, E. J. (1982). Effect of extra-intracranial (STA-MCA) arterial anastomosis on EEG and cerebral blood flow. *Stroke,* 13:674–679.

Dyken, M. L., Klatte, E., Kolar, O. J., et al. (1974). Complete occlusion of common or internal carotid arteries. Clinical significance. *Arch. Neurol.,* 30:343–346.

Ekberg, R., Cronquist, S., Ingvar, D. H. (1965). Regional cerebral blood flow in cerebrovascular disease. *Acta Neurol. Scand.,* 41 (Suppl. 14):164–168.

Fazekas, J. F., Klen, J., Finnerty, F. A. (1955). Influence of age and vascular disease on cerebral hemodynamics and metabolism. *Amer. J. Med.,* 18:477.

Fields, W. S., Lemak, N. A. (1976). Joint study of extracranial arterial occlusion. X. Internal carotid artery occlusion. *JAMA,* 235:2734–2738.

Fieschi, C., Agnoli, A., Battistini, N., et al. (1966). Regional cerebral blood flow in patients with brain infarct—a study with 85 Kr clearance technique. *Arch. Neurol.,* 15:653–663.

Fujishima, M., et al. (1974). Bilateral reduction of hemispheric blood flow in patients with unilateral cerebral infarction. *Stroke,* 5:648–653.

Gratzl, O., Schmiedeck, P., Spetzler, R., et al. (1976). Clinical experience with extra-intracranial arterial anastomosis in 65 cases. *J. Neurosurg.,* 44:313–324.

Grilla, P., Patterson, R. G., Jr. (1975). Occlusion of the carotid artery: Prognosis (natural history) and the possibilities of surgical revascularization. *Stroke,* 6:17–20.

Grubb, R. L., Ratcheson, R. A., Raichle, M. E., Kliefoth, A. B., Gado, M. H. (1979). Regional cerebral blood flow and oxygen utilization in superficial temporal-middle cerebral artery anastomosis patients. *J. Neurosurg.,* 50:733–741.

Halsey, J. H., Morawetz, R. B., Blauenstein, U. W. (1982). The hemodynamic effect of STA-MCA bypass. *Stroke,* 13:163–167.

Hardy, W. G., Lindner, D. W., Thomas, L. M., et al. (1962). Anticipated clinical course in carotid artery occlusion. *Arch. Neurol.,* 6:138–150.

Hartmann, A., Lange, D., Alberti, E., Dorndorf, W. (1977). Die Bestimmung der regionalen Gehirndurchblutung mit der Gamma-Kamera. *Forschr. Roentgenstr.* 126:52–60.

Heiss, W. D., Podreka, I., Roszucky, A. (1979). Regional cerebral blood flow measurement with scintillation camera after intra-carotid and intravenous Xenon application. IN: Meyer, J. S., Lechner, H., Reivich, M: *Cerebral Vascular Diseases 2,* Excerpta Medica, Amsterdam, 25–33.

Herrschaft, H. F. (1975). Die regionale Gehirndurchblutung. Berlin, Heidelberg, New York: Springer.

Heymas, A., Patterson, J. F., Duke, T. W., Hattey, L. L. (1953). The cerebral circulation and metabolism in arteriosclerotic and hypertensive cerebrovascular disease. *New Engl. J. Med.,* 249:223.

Hoedt-Rasmussen, K., Sveinsdottir, E., Lassen, N. A. (1966). Regional cerebral blood flow in man determined by intra-arterial injection of radioactive inert gas. *Circ. Res.,* 18:237–247.

Kempinski, W. H., Boniface, W. H., Keating, J. B. A., Morgan, P. P. (1961). Serial hemodynamic study of cerebral infarction in man. *Circulat. Res.,* 9:1051.

Kohlmeyer, K. (1985). The intraarterial $Xenon^{133}$ method: Principles and clinical application. IN: *Cerebral Blood Flow and Metabolism Measurement.* Eds. Hartmann, A., Hoyer, S., Springer Verlag, Heidelberg-New York-Berlin, 1–18.

Ladurner, G., Sager, E. D., Lechner, H. (1980). Morphologisch faBbare Veranderungen bei transitorish ischamichen attacken im computertomogramm. *Fortschr. Neurol. Psychiat.,* 48:220–223.

Lassen, N. A. (1985). Cerebral blood flow tomography using Xenon[133] inhalation-methodological consideration. IN: Hartmann, A., Hoyer, S. (Eds.), *Cerebral Blood Flow and Metabolism* Measurement. Heidelberg-New York-Berlin, Springer Verlag, 224–233.

Lassen, N. A., Hoedt-Rasmussen, K., Sorensen, S. C., Skinhoj, E., Cronquist, S., Bodforss, B., Ingvar, D.H. (1963). Regional cerebral blood flow in man determined by krypton[85]. *Neurology,* 13(9):719–727.

Laurent, P., Lawner, P. M., O'Connor, M. (1982). Reversal of intracerebral steal by STA-MCA anastomosis. *J. Neurosurg.,* 57:629–632.

Lavy, S., Melamed, E., Portnoy, Z. (1975). The effect of cerebral infarction on the regional cerebral blood flow of the contralateral hemisphere. *Stroke,* 6:160–163.

Lenzi, G. L., Jones, T., Mc Kenzie, G. G., Moss, S. (1978). Noninvasive regional study of chronic cerebrovascular disorders using the oxygen 15 inhalation technique. *J. Neurol. Neurosurg. Psychiat.,* 41:11–17.

Little, J. R., Yamamoto, Y. L., Feindel, W., Meyer, E., Hodhe, C. P. (1979). Superficial temporal artery to middle cerebral artery anastomosis. *J. Neurosurg.,* 50:560–569.

McDowell, F. H., Potes, J., Groch, S. (1961). The natural history of internal carotid and vertebral-vasilar artery occlusion. *Neurology,* 11 (4, Part 2):153–157.

Mc Henry, L. C., Jr. (1966). Cerebral blood flow studies in middle cerebral and internal carotid artery occlusion. *Neurology (Minneap),* 16:1145–1151.

Melamed, E., Lavy, S., Portnoy, Z., Sadan, S., Carmon, A. (1971). Correlation between regional cerebral blood flow and EEG frequency in the contralateral hemisphere in acute cerebral infarction. *J. Neurol. Science,* 26:21–27.

Meyer, J. S., Nakajima, S., Okabe, T., Amano, T., Centeno, R., Lee, Y. Y., Levine, J., Levinthal, R., Rose, J. (1982). Redistribution of cerebral blood flow following STA-MCAA bypass in patients with hemispheric ischemia. *Stroke,* 13:774–784.

Meyer, J. S., Naritomi, H., Sakai, F., Ishihara, N., Grant, P. (1979). Regional cerebral blood flow, diaschisis and steal after stroke. *Neur. Res.,* 1:101–119.

Meyer, J. S., Shinohara, Y., Kanda, T., Fukuuchi, Y., Ericsson, A. D., Kok, N. K. (1970). Diaschisis resulting from acute unilateral cerebral infarction. Quantitative evidence for man. *Arch. Neurol.,* 23:241–147.

Meyer, J. S., Shinohara, Y., Kanda, T., et al. (1970). Diaschisis resulting from acute unilateral cerebral infarction. *Arch. Neurol.,* 23:241–247.

Meyer, J. S., et al. (1971). Clinical prognosis correlated with hemispheric blood flow in cerebral infarction. *Stroke,* 2:383–394.

Naritomi, H., Meyer, J. S., Deshmikh, V. D., Pollack, P. (1977). Noninvasive measurement of rCBF in TIA's and stroke due to carotid and vertebrobasilar disease. *Acta Neurol. Scand.,* 65 (Suppl. 64):474–475.

Norrving, B., Nilsson, B., Risberg, J.: (1982). rCBF in patients with carotid occlusion. *Stroke,* 13:155–162.

Novack, P., Shenkin, H. A., Bortin, L., Goluboff, B., Soffe, A. M. (1953). The effects of carbon dioxide inhalation upon the cerebral blood flow and cerebral oxygen consumption in vascular disease. *J. Clin. Invest.,* 32:696.

Obrist, W. D., Thompson, H. K., Wang, H. S., Wilkinson, W. F. (1975). Regional cerebral blood flow estimated by Xenon[133] inhalation. *Stroke,* 6:245–256.

Paulson, O. B. (1970). Regional cerebral blood flow in apoplexy due to occlusion of the middle cerebral artery. *Neurology,* 20:63–77.

Paulson, O. B., Lassen, N. A., Skinhoj, E. (1970). Regional cerebral blood flow in apoplexy without arterial occlusion. *Neurology,* 20:125–138.

Perrone, P., Candelise, G., De Grandi, C., Scalfia, G. (1979). CT evaluation in patients with transient ischemic attacks. *Eur. Neurol.* 18:217–221.

Popp, A. J., Chater, N. (1977). Extracranial-to-intracranial vascular anastomosis for occlusive cerebrovascular disease: Experience in 110 patients. *Surgery*, 82:648–654.

Powers, W. J., Martin, W., Herscovitch, P., Raichle, M. E., Grubb, R. L. (1984). Extracranial-intracranial bypass surgery—hemodynamic and metabolic effects. *Neurology*, 34:1168–1174.

Rasmussen, K. H., Skinhoj, E. (1964). Transneural depression of the cerebral hemispheric metabolism in man. *Acta Neurol. Scand.* 40:41–46.

Rees, J. E., Bull, J. W. D., Ross Russell, R. W., Du Boulay, G. H., Marshall, J., Symon, L. (1970). Regional cerebral blood flow in transient ischemic attacks. *Lancet*, II:1210–1213.

Reichman, O. H. (1975). Extracranial-intracranial arterial anastomosis. IN: Whisnant, P. J., Sandok, B. A. (Eds.): *Cerebral Vascular Disease. Ninth conference* New York: Grune & Stratton, 175–185.

Roberts, T., Heilbrun, M., Reichman, O., Anderson, R. (1975). Regional cerebral blood flow studies following superficial temporal-middle cerebral artery anastomosis. *J. Neurosurg.*, 43:706–716.

Scheinberg, P., et al. (1976). Cerebral circulation and metabolism. *Stroke*, 7:213–234.

Schmiedek, P., Gratzl, O., Spetzler, R., Steinhoff, H., Enzenbach, R., Brendel, W., Marguth (1976). Selection of patients for extra-intracranial arterial bypass surgery based on rCBF measurements. *J. Neurosurg.*, 44:303–312.

Shenkin, H. A., Novack, P., Goluboff, B., Soffe, A. M., Mortin, L. (1953). The effects of aging, arteriosclerosis and hypertension upon the cerebral circulation. *J. Clin. Invest.*, 32:459.

Skinhoj, E., Hoedt-Rasmussen, K., Paulson, O. B., Lassen, N. A., (1970). Regional cerebral blood flow and its autoregulation in patients with transient focal cerebral ischemic attacks, 485–493.

Slater R. et al. (1977). Diaschisis with cerebral infarction. *Stroke*, 8:684–690.

Sundt, T. M., Jr., Siekart, R. G., Piepgras, D. G., et al. (1976). Bypasssurgery for vascular disease of the carotid system. *Mayo Clin. Proc.* 51:667–692.

Tanahashi, N., Meyer, J. S., Rogers, R. L., Kitagawa, Y., Mortel, K. F., Kandula, P., Levinthal, R., Rose, J. (1985). Long-term assessment of cerebral perfusion following STA-MCA bypass in patients. *Stroke*, 16:85–91.

Tolonen, U., Ahonen, A., Sulg, A., Kuikka, J., Kallanranta, T., Koskinen, M., Hokkanen, E. (1981). Serial measurements of quantitative EEG and cerebral blood flow and circulation time after brain infarction. *Acta Neurol. Scandinav.*, 63:145–155.

Tsuda, Y., Kimura, K., Iwata, Y., Hayakawa, T., Etani, H., Fukunaga, R., Yoneda, S., Abe, H. (1984). Improvement of cerebral blood flow and/or CO_2 reactivity after superficial temporal artery in patients with transient ischemic attacks and watershed-zone infarctions. *Surg. Neurol.*, 22:595–604.

Tsuda, Y., Kimura, K., Yoneda, S., Etani, H., Asai, T., Nakamura, M., Abe, H. (1983). Cerebral blood flow and CO_2-reactivity in transient ischemic attacks: Comparison between TIA's due to ICA occlusion and ICA mild stenosis. *Neurological Res.*, 5(No.3):17–37.

Veall, N., Mallett, B. L. (1967). The Xe^{133}-inhalation technique for regional cerebral blood flow studies. IN: Fellinger, K., Hofer, R. (Eds.): *Radioactive Isotope in Klinik und Forschung, Vol. III*. Munich, Urban & Schwarzenberg, 166–171.

Vorstrup, S., Hemmingsen, R., Henriksen, L., Lindewald, H., Engel, H. C., Lassen, N. A. (1983). Regional cerebral blood flow in patients with transient ischemic attacks studied by $Xenon^{133}$ inhalation and emission tomography. *Stroke*, 14:903–910.

Vorstrup, S., Paulson, O. B., Boysen, G., Engell, H. C., Lassen, N. A. (1984). The effect of extracranial-intracerebral bypass on cerebral blood flow. *Acta Neurol. Scand.*, Suppl. 98:303–304.

Wong, E., Bull, J. W. D., Du Boulay, G. H., Marshall, J., Ross Russel, R. W., Symon, L.

(1973). Regional cerebral blood flow in completed strokes and transient ischemic attacks. *Neurology,* 23:949–953.

Yasargil, M. G. (1969). Microsurgery applied to neurosurgery. Stuttgart, Georg-Thieme.

Yasargil, M. G., Yonekawa, Y. (1977). Results of microsurgical extra- intra-cranial arterial bypass in the treatment of cerebral ischemia. *Neurosurgery,* 1:22–24.

Yonekura, M., Austin, G., Hayward, W. (1982). Long-term evaluation of cerebral blood flow, transient ischemic attacks and stroke after STA-MCA anastomosis. *Surg. Neurol.,* 18:123–130.

Yonekura, M., Austin, G., Poll, N., Hayward, W. (1980). Evaluation of cerebral blood flow in patients with transient ischemic attacks and minor stroke. *Surg. Neurol.* 15:58–65.

8 Neurology II: Other Applications

J. Wade
Senior Registrar in Neurology,
St. Bartholomew's Hospital, London

S. Knezevic
Consultant Neurologist,
University Hospital, Zagreb

rCBF AND HYPERTENSION

Fog (1938) was the first to demonstrate that the diameter of the pial arterioles in the cat varies inversely with the intravascular pressure and he suggested that these vasomotor responses tend to keep the blood pressure constant under various physiological conditions. Lassen (1959), in a comprehensive review of the cerebral circulation in man, tabulated the results of a large number of studies performed during controlled hypertension and developed the concept of a lower limit of autoregulation. When mean blood pressure falls below this threshold, the resistance vessels are maximally dilated and flow diminishes progressively with further reductions on mean pressure (Harper, 1966).

The notion of an upper limit to autoregulation was suggested by Haggendal, Nilsson, and Nordback (1969) and then demonstrated in dogs by Ekstrom–Jodal et al. (1971). In 1973, Skinhoj, and Strangaard, using the intracarotid ^{133}Xenon method, reported increases in CBF in the region of 60% when acute severe hypertension was induced by angiotensin infusion in three subjects. Subsequent publications by McHenry et al. (1974), Strangaard et al. (1973), and Strangaard (1976) served to confirm these observations and established that the upper limit to autoregulation was set at higher levels of mean arterial blood pressure in chronically hypertensive subjects. It became clear that the plateau of constant CBF was shifted to the right along the axis of increasing blood pressure and the therapeutic implications of this were reviewed by Strangaard (1978).

The hypothesis that abrupt "therapeutic" reductions of blood pressure to "normal" values in patients with severe hypertension might be dangerous received support in a pathological study by Graham (1975). Watershed infarcts led to the deaths of two subjects treated for hypertension in whom the blood pressure was rapidly reduced to normal. Ledingham and Rajagopalan (1979) documented 10 further cases of neurological deterioration following the abrupt treatment of accelerated hypertension and found areas of ischemic damage in the brains of the three cases who were examined pathologically. Measurements using the noninvasive ^{133}Xenon inhalation technique in patients with accelerated hypertension have shown that readaptation of autoregulation can occur within days of treatment although it may take much longer (Gulliksen et al., 1982). Thus sequential measurements of rCBF may alert the clinician to dangerous falls in blood flow during the treatment of this rare but extremely dangerous condition.

HYPERTENSIVE ENCEPHALOPATHY

Measurements of rCBF have transformed our understanding of the pathophysiology of hypertensive encephalopathy. The pathological hallmark of this condition is cerebral oedema which Byrom (1954) attributed to intense focal arteriolar constriction in response to the severe pressure rise, causing decreased flow, ischemia and increased permeability of the blood-brain barrier. Byrom thought that the regions of focal narrowing were at fault but the converse in now more probable. With acutely induced hypertension, breakthrough may occur with a consequent rise in CBF (Strangaard et al., 1975). Regions of arteriolar constriction are thus regarded as the normal homeostatic response to elevated blood pressure and pathological significance is attached to the other regions where smooth muscle contractility is overcome by the intravascular pressure. This may be associated with blood-brain barrier dysfunction and extravasation of plasma into the brain tissue (Johansson, 1982).

HYPERTENSION IN PATIENTS WITH ACUTE STROKE

Patients with acute strokes are often hypertensive, either because they have longstanding hypertension or because the blood pressure has risen acutely as a consequence of the stroke. The risk of further neurological decline precipitated by overenthusiastic therapy of hypertension is very real (Britton, de Faire, & Helmers, 1980) as might be predicted from Strangaard's work since the autoregulatory plateau may be shifted toward higher blood pressure values and CBF may fall to ischemic levels when the blood pressure is rapidly returned to normal. Again, this is an area where sequential CBF measurements may lead to more rational and safer therapy.

rCBF IN MIGRAINE RESEARCH

The pathophysiology of migraine is not well understood and the dispute of whether migraine is primarily a phenomenon related to epilepsy (thus neuronal in origin) or a vascular disorder continues from the last century. It has been widely believed in the last 50 years that migraine is closely connected to a disturbance in cerebral blood vessels (Lance, 1982). The current view suggests that during the prodromal phase vasospasm causes cerebral ischemia and focal symptoms, whereas vasodilatation appears later during the headache phase of migraine (Wolff, 1963).

Several CBF studies have been reported in the last 15 years but due to the episodic nature of the disease and due to methodological difficulties many studies have provided inconclusive results. The results of several studies supported the vascular concept in that reduction of rCBF was demonstrated during the prodromal phase and a hyperemia was usually shown to accompany the headache later (Edmeads 1977; Hachinski et al., 1977; Mathew, Hrastnik, & Meyer 1976; Norris, Hachinski, & Cooper 1975; O'Brien 1971; Sakai & Meyer, 1978; Simard & Paulson, 1973; Skinhoj 1973; Skinhoj & Paulson, 1969).

This concept was questioned in 1981 when Olesen, Larsen, and Lauritzen studied six patients with provoked classical migraine attacks. They used the intra-arterial technique with 254 detectors to monitor rCBF changes. The attacks were initiated by focal hyperemia in three patients, and during the prodromes all patients had occipitoparietal rCBF reduction (oligemia). Oligemia gradually spread anteriorly, and in four patients severe headache was present during the oligemic phase.

This concept of spreading oligemia was similar to the spreading depression (SD) of Leao (Leao, 1944). This connection inspired a study in rats which showed that the rise of cortical blood flow during SD was followed by 20–25% reduction of flow below normal after SD. Spreading oligemia lasted at least for an hour. The authors speculated that the spreading oligemia of migraine may be a phenomenon physiologically related to the finding of an oligemia after SD in rats (Lauritzen et al. 1982).

The initial clinical study by Olesen was extended and Lauritzen et al. (1983) published results on nine patients who developed a characteristic attack following arteriography. rCBF was studied with 254 detectors at 5–10 min intervals. In eight patients the wave of oligemia originated in the posterior parts of the brain and spread anteriorly at a speed of 2 mm/min. It never crossed the Rolandic or Sylvian sulcus and it typically reached the primary sensorimotor area after symptoms from that area had begun and persisted there long after the focal symptoms disappeared. This time sequence suggests that focal symptoms in classical migraine are not secondary to oligemia, and the headache usually appears at a time of hypoperfusion. The way in which spreading oligemia progresses is similar to spreading depression of Leao and if so it may be an epiphenomenon of prolonged inhibition of cortical neurons after SD. The focal neurological signs may also be its result but the connection to pain remains unknown.

This study differed from the previously published ones. One of the reasons why the increase of flow was reported earlier may be due to larger detectors (in 32 detectors systems) detecting the flow changes in larger areas including the hyperemic state which spreads before the wave of spreading oligemia. When reduced blood flows were reported the results also suffered from the same criticism. The major criticism of Lauritzen's work was that all migrainous attacks were provoked, and it was also not clear whether all of the changes described were the result of cortical changes (as the method integrates the flow in the cortical and deeper areas), or some deeper areas of the brain were also involved.

Lauritzen and Olesen (1984) extended their work recently and using the SPECT method they reported rCBF studies in 12 patients with common migraine and 11 patients with classical migraine occurring spontaneously. All the patients with common migraine had normal results of rCBF investigation. Eight patients with classical migraine displayed unilateral regions of hypoperfusion while 3 had normal rCBF patterns. The low-flow regions were always at the side opposite to the focal neurological symptoms and the hypoperfusion remained through the headache period for 4 to 6 hours. While the previous studies have shown the progression of spreading oligemia, this study provided the exact localization of this vasomotor dysfunction. The hypoperfusion was always confined to the cortical regions and in 7 of the 8 patients only on the lateral aspect of the hemisphere. Subcortical structures were always normally perfused. The cortical changes appeared unrelated to the distribution of major cerebral arteries and they probably represent a manifestation of disturbed cerebral metabolism, in close connection to the SD of Leao. In 1 of the patients hypoperfusion was also found in the frontal lobes simultaneously with the low flow of the temporal and parietal lobes. As the spreading oligemia does not cross primary sulci this suggests that the insula may be the pathway of the spreading oligemia to the frontal lobe.

The studies which we have briefly described suggest that the primary disturbance in patients with classical migraine is probably neuronal, and that the spreading depression and spreading oligemia follow an unknown disturbance in the cortical function. They also show that the pathophysiology of classical and common migraine are different, at least as reflected by accompanying CBF changes.

rCBF INVESTIGATIONS IN EPILEPSY

Electrophysiological investigations have greatly influenced the study of epilepsy and related disorders in the last 50 years. EEG has been valuable in the diagnosis and treatment of many patients and our concepts and understanding of paroxysmal disorders have been based on various more or less sophisticated electrophysiological techniques. X-ray methods have been much less useful and even the CT scanning has not proved to be very instructive except for detecting macroscopic abnormalities which are relatively rare. The investigation of regional changes of cerebral circulation and metabolism have offered a completely new view on epileptic phenomena and they will be briefly reviewed here. Besides showing the different neurophysiological aspect, the rCBF studies can also offer a better spatial resolution than EEG recordings but they are still much slower and thus the results have a worse temporal resolution than EEG.

Although the cerebral circulation was studied as long as 45 years ago (Penfield, von Santha, & Cipriani 1939), the clinical application using new techniques is possible in the last 15 years. Ingvar (1973) found a fourfold increase in CBF in the epileptic focus during continuous paroxysmal focal EEG activity. In several other investigations (Brodersen et al., 1973) ictal hyperemia has been confirmed and it supports Jackson's idea of increased metabolism in the epileptic focus. Investigations in the interictal state have shown inconclusive results. Hougaard et al. (1976) were the first to demonstrate focal flow increase in areas presumed to comprise the epileptic focus. In contrast to their results, several studies showed hypoperfusion of the epileptic focuses in the interictal period (Baldy–Moulinier et al., 1985; Lavy et al., 1976; Rosadini et al., 1983). These differences may have resulted from different patient populations or different methods for rCBF investigations but it seems well established now that a decrease in CBF is constantly seen in epileptic focuses of patients with temporal lobe epilepsy and especially so when the focus is in the left temporal lobe and when it is fixed and unilateral. It is interesting to note that the zones of hypoperfusion do not obligatorily correspond to a lesional focus. However, some patients with temporal lobe epilepsy have multiple hypoactive areas, as well as the patients with secondary generalized epilepsies. In the patients with primary generalized epilepsies neither hypo- nor hyperperfused areas were found during interictal studies (Baldy–Moulinier, 1983; Baldy–Moulinier et al., 1985)

In the last several years PET studies have been widely used in the investigations of epilepsy and using fluorine 18 labeled fluorodeoxyglucose (Engel, 1984) and oxygen 15 (Bernardi et al., 1983) they have measured directly regional cerebral metabolism and blood flow in vivo. The results essentially confirm those mentioned herein but due to a three-dimensional reconstruction and good spatial resolution they have also helped in the surgical therapy of temporal lobe epilepsy. From the pathophysiological point of view these results are also important because the involvement of deeper structures of the brain and cerebellum has been recorded. The investigation of rCBF and metabolism in epilepsy has been very important as they have offered a new view at an old problem and it is quite clear that some of our concepts will have to be changed in respect of the new information obtained. It is to be hoped that the new classification of epileptic phenomena will be possible and that it will result in our better understanding of the epileptic manifestations, more efficient therapy and improved prognosis in our patients.

REFERENCES

Baldy–Moulinier, M. (1983). Concluding remarks. In M. Baldy–Moulinier, D. H. Ingvar, & B. S. Meldrum (Eds.). *Cerebral blood flow, metabolism and epilepsy* (Current problems in epilepsy) (pp. 393–395). London: John Libbey, Eurotext.

Baldy–Moulinier, M., Valmier, J., Touchon, J., Billiard, M., Besset, A., & Cadilhac, J. (1985). Debits cerebraux diminués en periode intercritique dans l'epilepsie du lobe temporal. *Rev. Neurol.* (Paris), *141*, 18–27.

Bernardi, S., Trimble, M. R., Frackowiak, R. S. J., Wise, R. J. S., & Jones, T. (1983). An interictal study of partial epilepsy using positron emission tomography and the oxygen-15 inhalation technique. *Journal of Neurology, Neurosurgery and Psychiatry, 46*, 473–477.

Britton, M., de Faire, U., & Helmers, C. (1980). Hazards of therapy for excessive hypertension in acute stroke. *Acta Medica Scandinavica, 207*, 253–257.

Brodersen, P., Paulson, O. B., Bolwig, T. G., Rogon, Z. E., Rafaelsen, O. J., & Laseen, N. A. (1973). Cerebral hyperemia in electrically induced epileptic seizures. *Arch. Neurol., 28*, 334–338.

Byrom, F. B. (1954). The pathogenesis of hypertensive encephalopathy and its relation to the malignant phase of hypertension. *Lancet ii*, 201–211.

Edmeads, J. (1977). Cerebral blood flow in migraine. *'gadache, 17*, 148–152.

Ekstrom–Jodal, B., Haggendal, E., Linder, L. E., & Nilsson, N. J. (1971). Cerebral blood flow autoregulation at high arterial pressures and different levels of carbon dioxide tension in dogs. *European Neurology, 6*, 6–10.

Engel, J. (1984). The use of positron emission tomographic scanning in epilepsy. *Ann. Neurol., 15* (Suppl.), S180–S191.

Fog, M. (1938). The relationship between the blood pressure and the tonic regulation of the pial arteries. *Journal of Neurology and Psychiatry, 1*(new series), 187–197.

Graham, D. I. (1975). Ischaemic brain damage of cerebral perfusion failure type after treatment of severe hypertension. *British Medical Journal, 2*, 739.

Gulliksen, G., Hojer–Pedersen, E., Moller, M., Harvald, B., & Enevoldsen, E. (1982). Autoregulation of cerebral blood flow in patients with malignant hypertension and hypertensive encephalopathy. In S. Strandgaard & D. I. Barry (Eds.). *Cerebral blood flow, hypertension and antihypertensive treatment. Acta Medica Scandinavica* (Suppl. *678*) 43–49.

Hachinski, V. C., Olesen, J., Norris, J. W., Larsen, B., Enevoldsen, E., & Lassen, N. A. (1977). Cerebral hemodynamics in migraine. *Can. J. Neurol. Sci., 4*, 245–249.

Haggendal, E., Nilsson, N. J., & Nordback, B. (1969). Aspects of the autoregulation of cerebral blood flow. In J. B. Loftstrem (Ed.). *Peripheral circulation and anaesthesia. International Anaesthesiology Clinics, 7*, 353–367.

Harper, A. M. (1966). Autoregulation of cerebral blood flow: Influence of the arterial blood pressure on the blood flow through the cerebral cortex. *Journal of Neurology, Neurosurgery and Psychiatry, 29*, 398–403.

Hougaard, K., Oikawa, T., Sveinsdottir, E., Skinhoj, E., Ingvar, D. H., & Lassen, N. A. (1976). Regional cerebral blood flow in focal cortical epilepsy. *Arch. Neurol., 33*, 527–535.

Ingvar, D. H. (1973). Regional cerebral blood flow in focal cortical epilepsy. *Stroke, 4*, 359–360.

Johansson, B. B. (1982). The blood-brain barrier and cerebral blood flow in acute hypertension. In S. Strangaard & D. I. Barry (Eds.). *Cerebral blood flow hypertension and antihypertensive treatment. Acta Medica Scandinavica*, Suppl. *678*, 107–112.

Lance, J. W. (1982). Mechanism and management of headache (4th ed.). London: Butterworth.
Lassen, N. A. (1959). Cerebral blood flow and oxygen consumption in man. *Physiological Reviews, 39,* 183–238.
Lauritzen, M., Jorgensen, M. B., Dimer, D. H., Gjedde, A., & Hansen, A. J. (1982). Persistent oligemia of rat cerebral cortex in the wave of spreading depression. *Ann. Neurol., 12,* 469–474.
Lauritzen, M., & Olesen, J. (1984). Regional cerebral blood flow during migraine attacks by Xe-133 inhalation and emission tomography. *Brain, 107,* 447–461.
Lauritzen, M., Skihoj Olsen, T., Lassen, N. A., & Paulson, O. B. (1983). Changes in regional cerebral blood flow during the course of classic migraine attacks. *Ann. Neurol., 13,* 633–641.
Lavy, S., Melamed, E., Portnoy, Z., & Carmon, A. (1976). Interictal regional cerebral blood flow in patients with partial seizures. *Neurology, 26,* 418–422.
Leao, A. P. P. (1944). Spreading depression of activity in cerebral cortex. *J. Neurophysiol., 7,* 359–390.
Ledingham, J. G. G., & Rajagopalan, B. (1979). Cerebral complications in the treatment of accelerated hypertension. *Quarterly Journal of Medicine, 48,* 25–41.
Mathew, N. T., Hrastnik, F., & Meyer, J. S. (1976). Regional cerebral blood flow in the diagnosis of vascular headache. *Headache, 15,* 252–260.
McHenry, L. C., West, J. W., Cooper, E. S., Goldberg, H. I., & Jaffe, M. E. (1974). Cerebral autoregulation in man. *Stroke, 5,* 695–706.
Norris, J. W., Hachinski, V. C., & Cooper, P. W. (1975). Changes in cerebral blood flow during a migraine attack. *Br. Med. J., 3,* 676–677.
O'Brien, M. D. (1971). Cerebral blood changes in migraine. *Headache, 10,* 139–143.
Olesen, J., Larsen, B., & Lauritzen, M. (1981). Focal hyperemia followed by spreading oligemia and impaired activation of rCBF in classic migraine. *Ann. Neurol., 9,* 344–352.
Penfield, W., von Santha, K., & Cipriani, A. (1939). Cerebral blood flow during induced epileptiform seizures in animal and man. *J. Neurophysiol., 2,* 257–267.
Rosadini, G., Ferillo, F., Rodriguez, G., Sannita, W. G., & Arvigo, F. (1983). In M. Baldy–Moulinier, D. H. Ingvar, & B. S. Meldrum (Eds.). *Cerebral blood flow, metabolism and epilepsy* (Current problems in epilepsy, pp. 26–32). London: John Libbey, Eurotext.
Sakai, F., & Meyer, J. S. (1978). Regional cerebral hemodynamics during migraine and cluster headache measured by the Xe133 inhalation method. *Headache, 18,* 122–132.
Simard, D., & Paulson, O. B. (1973). Cerebral vasomotor paralysis during migraine attack. *Arch. Neurol., 29,* 207–209.
Skinhoj, E., & Paulson, O. B. (1969). Regional blood flow in internal carotid distribution during migraine attack. *Br. Med. J., 3,* 569–570.
Skinhoj, E. (1973). Hemodynamic studies within the brain during migraine. *Arch. Neurol., 29,* 95–98.
Skinhoj, E., & Strangaard, S. (1973). Pathogenesis of hypertensive encephalopathy. *Lancet, i,* 461–462.
Strangaard, S. (1976). Autoregulation of cerebral blood flow in hypertensive patients. The modifying influence of prolonged antihypertensive treatment on the tolerance to acute, drug-induced hypotension. *Circulation, 53,* 720–727.
———. (1978). Autoregulation of cerebral circulation in hypertension. *Acta Neurologica Scandinavica,* Suppl. *66.*
Strangaard, S., Jones, J. V., MacKenzie, E. T., & Harper, A. M. (1975). The upper limit of cerebral blood flow autoregulation in experimental renovascular hypertension in the baboon. *Circulation Research, 37,* 164–167.
Strangaard, S., Olesen, J., Skinhoj, E., & Lassen, N. A. (1973). Autoregulation of brain circulation in severe arterial hypertension. *Br. Med. J., i,* 507–510.
Wolff, H. G. (1963). *Headache and other head pain* (2d ed.). New York: Oxford University Press.

9 The Use of Cerebral Blood-Flow Measurements in Clinical Neurosurgery

Lindsay Symon
Gough Cooper Department of Neurological Surgery, Institute of Neurology, London

Practical clinical measurement of cerebral blood flow has been with us since the development of inert gas clearance techniques in the mid-1960s (Høedt–Rasmussen, Sveinsdottir, & Lassen, 1966; Lassen et al., 1963). Over the twenty years from the first regional cerebral blood flow (rCBF) in Lund in 1965, CBF studies have been made in almost every aspect of clinical neurology and neurosurgery. The importance of stroke and subarachnoid hemorrhage in relation to human disability in the Western world is well established and it could have been hoped that the capacity to measure blood flow in focal regions of the brain, or individual hemispheres, or even in the whole brain would vastly enhance our capacity to treat these diseases. One could be forgiven for supposing that research workers and clinicians alike would be disappointed at the apparently scant influence that such measurements have had upon therapeutic measures, but this would be to close one's eyes to the renaissance of understanding of the cerebral circulation.

The twenty years since 1965 have seen as much progress and understanding of the cerebral circulation as the twenty years following the Franco–Prussian War saw in the understanding of cortical localization and functional control of the motor and sensory systems by the brain. It is no exaggeration to say therefore that the safety and expeditiousness of modern neurosurgery has been vastly increased by cerebral blood flow studies, quite apart from their direct influence on individual cases.

There have been three main thrusts of CBF research in clinical neurosurgery. The most obvious, and that which we have concerned with primarily in our institution has been in relation to subarachnoid hemorrhage. The second main thrust has related to obliterative vascular disease, most particularly since revascularization operations by extracranial to intracranial bypass became possible, and the third interest has related to phenomenology and prognosis in head injury.

The techniques available for modern CBF analysis are described in other parts of this book, but clinical application has demanded that external collimation be invariably employed. Relatively few centers have felt it worthwhile to attempt direct cortical measurement during surgery (Brock, Hadjidimos, Schürmann, Ellger, & Fischer, 1969) and the majority have confined themselves to pre- and postoperative analyses in relation to the diseases in which they have an interest. The few exceptions will be mentioned (Pickard, Matheson, Patterson, & Wyper, 1980). While in certain circumstances the use of the arterial route for tracer injection has seemed justified, there is little doubt that the utility of CBF measurements in clinical neurosurgery have been vastly enhanced by the development of inhalational or intravenous methods.
These have enabled repetitive measurements to be made on the same patient and have in many clinics reawakened interest in blood-flow measurement.

CURRENTLY PREFERRED TECHNIQUES

Highly focal blood-flow measurements using multiple closely collimated detectors were first used by us with the intra-arterial injection method (Symon et al., 1972; Wilkinson et al., 1969). While some of the results obtained with this method will be mentioned, it suffered from two major drawbacks in relation to neurosurgical patients. In the first place, repeated arterial injections were not thought justified in the majority of clinics in the course of evolution of a neurosurgical problem, and in the second place, measurement in such machines demanded that the patient be moved to the machine, which was in itself a major consideration in an unstable and seriously sick neurosurgical patient.

The problem of repetitive measurements was largely solved by the development of inhalational and intravenous technology. It has emerged that by far the most convenient method of study has been the use of the intravenous bolus technique pioneered by Austin et al. (Austin, Horn, Rouhe, & Hayward, 1972), using a small number of scintillation detectors over the two hemispheres, a further scintillation detector being placed in the expired airway from a face mask, measuring the activity in the patient's expired air. Expired air activity is a close approximation to the arterial concentration because of the high solubility of the gaseous isotope commonly used, ^{133}Xenon, in air. Satisfactory counts of around 200,000/min can be obtained with the use of 10–15 mC of Xenon dissolved in 0.5 ml of normal saline injected into a forearm drain in a rapid bolus.

Attempts to multiply the number of detectors are of relatively little use, and most neurosurgical units now present their multiple detector measurements as a hemispheral mean. Observations in our own department comparing a simple one-detector-per-hemisphere system with a five-detector hemisphere system have shown in acute circumstances of subarachnoid hemorrhage, no advantage to the multidetector system, although it is true that only by this method will small focal areas of ischemia be detected (Jabre, Symon, & Redmond, work in progress). Nevertheless the simplicity of a whole hemispheral technique and the many artifacts possible such as the see-through effect in a completely nonperfused area under one detector leading to entirely false regionalization, render the small number of detectors most useful in clinical circumstances.

There are undoubted disadvantages to the intravenous method, sheared to some extent by the inhalational system, in particular, the calculation of the end-expiratory curve may be extremely difficult in restless patients, or in those with an irregular breathing pattern, and attempts to obtain regional blood-flow measurements under those circumstances force a choice between abandoning the measurement or recourse to the intra-arterial methodology.

The development of simple portable blood flow machinery (Novo Instruments, Bagsvaerd, Denmark) and the use of the intravenous method have made it possible to study acutely ill neurosurgical patients repetitively, day by day. Comparison of the 10-detector and 2-detector systems have been made (Jabre, Symon, & Redmond, work in progress) and our present feeling is that the whole hemispheral measurement, centering the probe over the somatosensory cortex, is of maximum utility, at any rate in the circumstances of subarachnoid hemorrhage. Such counterplacement enables correlation with, for example, somatosensory evoked response measurements (Rosenstein, Wang, Symon, & Suzuki, in press) and centers the assessment on the most immediately clinically relevant vascular tree in the brain, that of the middle cerebral artery.

Where the measurements are concerned with depiction of suitability for bypass procedures, then more focal measurement using a multidetector system may be essential (Schmiedek et al., 1976), but these patients do not present the same management problems as acutely ill patients with subarachnoid hemorrhage, and may be readily moved to the large detector machines.

In the circumstances of carotid endarterectomy or carotid ligation (Sundt, 1983) where cerebral blood flow is being used as a predictor, either of the necessity for shunts, or for the safety of a carotid ligation, then a simple hemispheral detection system is entirely adequate.

It is worth pointing out that the greater the number of detectors the greater the amount of isotope necessary since multiple detectors, in order to achieve collimation, require internal baffles and a good deal of shielding, cutting down their sensitivity, and requiring an increase in Xenon dose to achieve statistically significant count rates. Particularly where one is aiming to measure repetitively, and this has been one of the great advances in recent years, the expense of Xenon becomes a real problem and the more economical the method, the more likely it is to be worthwhile and generally used.

Modern bedside portable machinery contains its own computer analysis, mak-

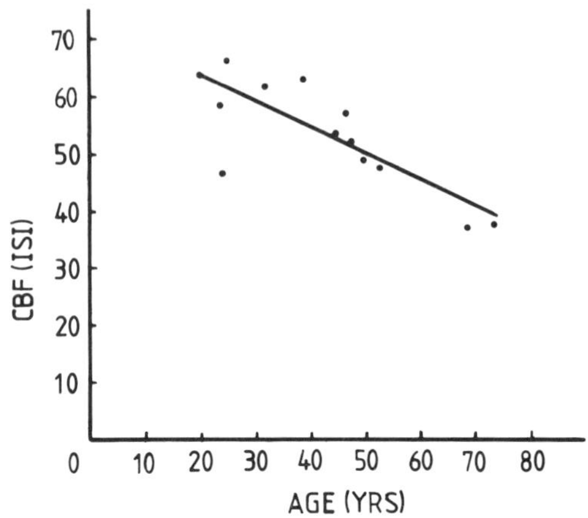

FIGURE 9.1. Correlation between age and blood flow determined by a single counter in each hemisphere in normal individuals. (From Rosenstein, Suzuki, Symon, & Redmond, *Neurosurgery, 15,* 522, 1984; with permission).

ing available fast and slow components and an initial slope index. This last, pioneered by Risberg, Ali, Wilson, Wills, and Halsey (1975) largely avoids problems of compartmental slippage which, particularly in the circumstances of rapidly developing ischemia, make comparison between one base flow and the next extremely difficult if, for example, a quantity of fast clearing tissue falls very rapidly. The evident day-to-day increase or decrease, for example, as weight gray, indicate that pathophysiological changes within the compartments render the attribution of fast and slow components to particular facets of the nervous system meaningless, and the averaging predominantly fast measurements, of Risberg et al. as the initial slope index (ISI) have proved in our hands most stable and satisfactory. The present ISI calculations run from 0.5 to 1.5 minutes and in our control studies we have found estimation of CBF in relation to age to display the familiar characteristics elsewhere reported (Rosenstein, Suzuki, Symon & Redmond, 1984), (Fig. 9.1).

CBF AND SUBARACHNOID HEMORRHAGE

The problems of subarachnoid hemorrhage have been pretty well defined by a series of cooperative studies over the years. The natural course of a patient with subarachnoid hemorrhage has been shown to be a triphasic one, some patients dying very rapidly within the first 24 hours of hemorrhage, some dying over the first few weeks, and others going on to prolonged survival (Alvord, Loeser, Bailey, & Copass, 1972; Graff, 1971), although recent work (Winn et al., 1981) indicated that there remains a gradual decline of survivors with recurrent hemorrhage at the rate of between 2% and 3% per year, following rupture of an aneurysm and initial, apparent complete recovery. The average aim of neurosurgery has been to operate on patients within the first few weeks of hemorrhage, or more recently within the first few days of hemorrhage, to intervene before recurrent hemorrhage causes the patient's death.

One of the predominant factors of prognosis is subarachnoid hemorrhage therefore is the time of the patient from the initial hemorrhage. The second is the condition of the patient at the time the operation is undertaken. A variety of grading systems have been suggested but that most commonly used is that of Hunt and Hess (1968), shown in Table 9.1. Operation on patients in good grades results in most clinics in the mortality of around 3% (grades 1 to 3), as is shown in the sample of some 300 personal cases. In poor grades, however, the mortality tends to be high, and one of the aims of CBF studies over the years has been to try to sort out, particularly in the grade 3 cases, how the determinant factors for prognosis in this particular group may be assessed and perhaps improved.

One of the main complications of subarachnoid hemorrhage is the phenomenon of cerebral vasospasm, a phenomenon initially described angiographically (Allcock & Drake, 1963), as shown in Fig. 9.2, where gross diminution of the angiographically visualized lumen of the main cerebral vessels is evident. This is often associated with clinical signs, as Du Boulay has shown, most particularly in relation to the middle cerebral artery (Du Boulay, Marshall, Merory, & Symon, 1980), and it appears that the determinant factors of the association of vasospasm and physical signs are the extent of the basal vasospasm and the efficiency of collateral circulation in the particular patient. There are significant problems in the attribution of clinical features to vasospasm since the matching between the angiographic picture and clinical features may not be very close (Ferguson, Harper, Fitch, Rowan, & Jennett, 1972; Millikan, 1975; Pitts et al., 1979; Symon et al., 1972). One of the aims of CBF analysis in cases with subarachnoid hemorrhage is therefore to access hemispheral perfusion distal

TABLE 9.1
The Hunt and Hess Grading System

Category	*Criteria*
Grade I	Asymptomatic, or minimal headache, and slight neck stiffness
Grade II	Moderate to severe headache, neck stiffness, no neurological deficit other than cranial nerve palsy
Grade III	Drowsiness, confusion, or mild focal deficit
Grade IV	Stupor, moderate to severe hemiparesis, possible early decerebrate rigidity and vegetative disturbances
Grade V	Deep coma, decerebrate rigidity, moribund appearance

Source: After Hunt and Hess, *J. Neurosurg., 28,* 14.

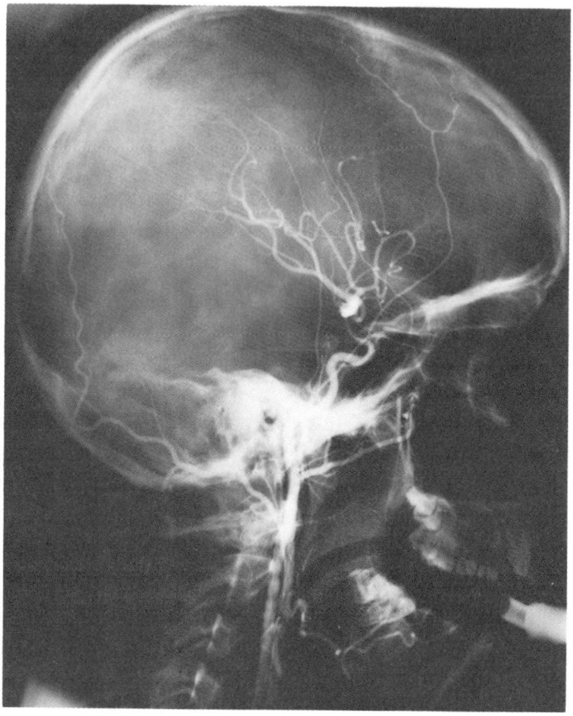

FIGURE 9.2. The angiographic picture of vasospasm. The patient was a 22-year-old woman with a terminal carotid artery aneurysm in grade IV at the time of angiography. There was a history of at least two hemorrhages, the first 2 weeks before, the second 3 days before. Extensive narrowing of the Circle of Willis in relation to the aneurysm is evident.

to apparent vascular constriction. The timing of the onset of vasospasm is interesting also, as it has been clearly established now that vasospasm reaches its maximum between 7 and 10 days (Kagström, Greitz, Hanson, & Galera, 1966) after the initial hemorrhage and then decrements over the course of about 3 weeks (Du Boulay, 1963).

We have tended therefore to describe vasospasm in two aspects: angiographic vasospasm and clinical vasospasm. There is a tendency to use the term "clinical vasospasm" for the picture of the deterioration following subarachnoid hemorrhage, not apparently associated with recurrent bleeding, but it is more exact to describe this as transient, or progressive neurological dysfunction following subarachnoid hemorrhage and to attribute it to vasospasm only if angiographic evidence is produced. Many clinics will not consider re-angiogram in patients under such circumstances and transient, or progressive neurological disturbance is thus the more exact description. The association between vasospasm and the initial severity of the hemorrhage has now been clearly established by a number of CT studies (Bell, Kendall, & Symon, 1980; Fisher, Kistler, & Davis, 1980), indicating that these phenomena of transient, or progressive, neurological disturbance associated with constriction of the arteries are most frequent when there is extensive blood around the basal cisterns.

The contribution of CBF measurements to the understanding of the phenomenon of vasospasm has been quite considerable. Heilbrun, Olesen, and Lassen (1972) initially showed that, following subarachnoid hemorrhage, there was a paralysis of autoregulation which lasted for some weeks. It is general experience that this disturbance of autoregulation need not be diffuse over the hemisphere but that it commonly involves the territory of the affected artery. Vasospasm which is clinically productive is usually associated with some focal ischemic deficit and there is a clear association in a number of papers (Ishii, 1979; Pitts et al., 1979; Symon et al., 1972) between focal ischemic deficit and diminished cerebral blood flow.

CBF analysis has also been helpful in establishing clinical correlations of the threshold concepts of ischemia established in animals. It has been known for some years that cortical perfusion may be reduced in the experimental primate to around 20 ml/100g/min from a normal of 54 ml/100g/min before synaptic electrical activity in the cortex fails, as assessed by the amplitude of the primate positive/negative wave of the somatosensory evoked response (Branston, Symon, Crockard, & Pasztor, 1974), (Fig. 9.3). Such an SEP virtually disappears by the time CBF has reached 14 ml/100g/min, and the half-value of this decline, 16 ml/100g/min, has been suggested by us as the threshold of blood flow for

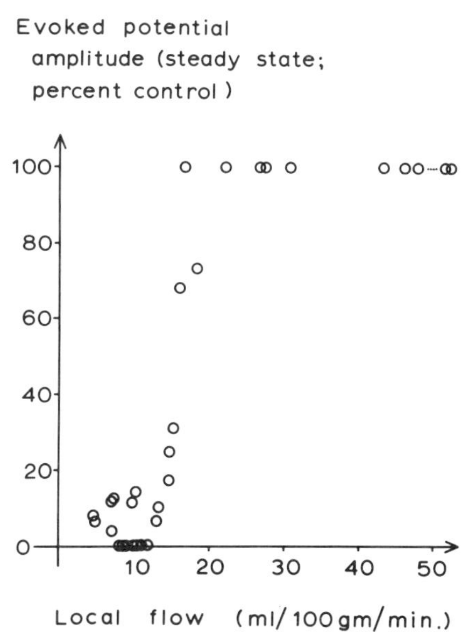

FIGURE 9.3. The steady state amplitude of a somatosensory evoked response plotted against steady state blood flow in experimental ischemia in the primate. (From Branston, Symon, Crockard, & Pasztor, *Exper. Neurol., 45,* 202, 1974; with permission).

electrical failure. Similar findings have been established by other workers (Heiss, Hayakawa, & Waltz, 1976; Sharbrough, Messick, & Sundt, 1973; Trojaborg & Boysen, 1973). In the same way, threshold for the maintenance of ionic homeostasis, estimated by flux of potassium into the extracellular space, and of calcium from the extracellular into the intracellular space (Astrup, Symon, Branston, & Lassen, 1977; Branston, Strong, & Symon, 1977), has indicated that such ionic changes occur at flow values of around 10 ml/100g/min. A persuasive association between these lower flow values and the early onset of infarction (at 2 hours) was suggested by Morawetz, DeGirolami, Ojemann, Marcoux, and Crowell (1978), and although it seems clear from more recent investigations (Jones et al., 1981) that even higher flow values just below the electrical threshold may be associated with infarction, rather longer ischemia is necessary to produce the infarct at these higher flows.

In neurosurgery, direct correlation between these acute experimental studies and acute CBF changes, either induced by preoperative vascular occlusion, or by the rapidly changing dynamics of evolving vasospasm in subarachnoid hemorrhage, establish flow and functional correlates which are very similar to our primate data.

Our clinical experience has indicated that Xenon studies at the bedside show a clear association between electrical function and CBF. The usual functional analysis in the clinic in our hands has been the measurement of transmission time of an evoked response from the neck to the cerebral cortex in the two hemispheres, enabling interhemispheral correlation. This measurement of central conduction time from the N14 peak at C2 to the N20 peak at the cortex to somatosensory evoked response stimulation from median nerve, has indicated that slowing of conduction time from its normal values of 5.4 ± 0.4 ms (SD) to outside two standard deviations, occurs when hemispheral CBF falls below 30 ml/100g/min (Rosenstein, Wang, Symon, & Suzuki, in press), (Table 9.2). Our primate work indicated that the delay in central conduction time attended flow levels measured in the primate brain by hydrogen clearance, in the region of the electrical threshold, (Hargadine, Branston, & Symon, 1980) the differences between this level and the levels in humans, probably relate more to the poor collimation of the bedside Xenon method which looks not only at ischemic tissue but at a fairly wide area of the hemisphere. Nevertheless the association between functional impairment was evidenced by conduction delay, and diminished cerebral perfusion, is highly significant.

It is our present clinical practice therefore to determine, in the subarachnoid hemorrhage patient, repetitive measurements of conduction time as an assessment of function associated with bedside observations of the clinical state, and repetitive measurements of hemispheral CBF taken over the somatosensory cortex by the intravenous Xenon elution method.

Good correlations have been obtained between the two systems, and in the circumstances of a grade 3 patient with mild hemispheral signs or perhaps some-

TABLE 9.2

Correlation of Hemispheral Cerebral Blood Flow and Grade at the Time of Admission

*Grade**	*No. of Patients (SD)*	*Mean* CBF_{isi}	*% Mean* CBF_{isi} *Expected for Age*	*Mean Arterial Pressure (mm Hg)*	*Mean* pCO_2 *(Torr)*	*Mean PBD***
I	3	51.0 ± 8.4	106.0 ± 27.8	105.4 ± 8.3	40.3 ± 5.7	7.3 ± 4.0
II	6	45.9 ± 2.4	90.8 ± 5.0	113.6 ± 27.1	36.0 ± 5.6	4.3 ± 2.9
III	4	42.3 ± 5.3	82.9 ± 19.4	86.7 ± 3.1	37.8 ± 8.3	3.8 ± 1.0
IV	5	33.3 ± 5.7	70.0 ± 11.1	109.5 ± 22.7	34.8 ± 2.9	8.6 ± 3.0

Figures are means ± standard deviation (SD).

*Hunt and Hess, 1968.

**PBD = Post bleed day. Represents the time in days from the time of hemorrhage to time of the first CBF study on admission.

Source: Data obtained by single hemispherical counter (Novo Cerebrograph 2a; from Rosenstein, Suzuki, Symon, & Redmond, *Neurosurgery, 15,* 523, 1984; with permission).

what drowsy, the presence of CBF above 30 and normal conduction time has indicated to us that operation may be proceeded forthwith. Where CBF is very low then pause for reflection might be indicated, but if CBF is low and conduction normal, then we have tended to go on the functional study and operate early. Where conduction is low and CBF is normal we have tended to feel that this represents the relative luxury perfusion of threatened ischemia and, particularly if the clinical signs point to hemispheral deficit in association with high blood flow but quite low conduction, then it is probable that an unstable state exists in the hemisphere and caution should be observed.

A cardinal rule in the utility of such predictions of course is the establishment of norms of behavior of CBF.

Since the advent of the bedside blood-flow system, we have endeavored to establish what the usual reaction of the hemisphere to craniotomy might be. It has emerged from our recent work (Jabre, Symon, & Redmond, work in progress) that a normally perfused hemisphere, disturbed, for example, for nonvascular tumor as, for example, a pituitary tumor at the basal skull, will often show a reactive hyperemia over the first few days. This was first pointed out in relation to subarachnoid hemorrhage (Merory et al., 1980) in a group of cases in which the postoperative hyperemia or ''first-day peak,'' was tentatively ascribed to patients with a good outcome. This has been sustained in our subsequent work, in subarachnoid hemorrhage reactive hyperemia or the ''first-day peak'' has been shown to be typical of patients who will go on to have a satisfactory clinical course. The assumption is that this is the normal behavior of the hemisphere and represents normal vascular reactivity.

Those patients who show a decline in CBF immediately postoperatively for a few days tend to develop hyperemia somewhat later and the prognosis in these cases is not quite so satisfactory. Strangely enough patients with extensive hemispheral tumors who have had major resections and whose course has been troubled, also tend to show loss of the first-day peak and it appears therefore that this phenomenon may not be specific to subarachnoid hemorrhage at all, but may represent much more the normal preservation of vascular reactivity in the circumstances of craniotomy.

Protracted observations of the behavior of CBF following subarachnoid hemorrhage have been reported by Meyer and his collagues (1983), using the large multidetector system, which of course demands the patient be moved and which render it rather more difficult to carry out frequently repeated measurements particularly in the sick patient. Once again it has been observed that in a proportion of subarachnoid hemorrhage cases reactive hyperemia occurs with a gradual falloff in perfusion over the first few weeks following subarachnoid hemorrhage, but this in our good prognosis cases has not been the norm. We have tended to find restoration of normal blood flow and reactivity in a stable form by the end of 10 days following subarachnoid hemorrhage.

Persistence of significantly low flow focally in the area of the aneurysm-bearing artery has been present in a number of observations. Many years ago using the intra-arterial method, we (Symon et al., 1972) showed significantly reduced flow in anterior communicating artery aneurysms around the periphery of the hemisphere at 10 days, at the time of the postoperative angiographic study, and similar significantly reduced blood flow in the center of the hemisphere in middle cerebral artery aneurysms. This indicates that focal flow reductions may persist for some time, not necessarily in association with clinical findings, and in our more recent studies associated with normalization of electrical potential activity indicating that these reduced flows, though significant, are not necessarily below the functional threshold (Wang, Cone, Symon, & Costa e Silva, 1984).

As onc might expect, CBF measurements have been shown to bear some relationship to clinical grading. In our own case, we have been able statistically to distinguish between grades 1 to 3 and the more severe patients in grade 5, but undoubtedly the most valuable access to prognosis in subarachnoid hemorrhage has been the capacity repetitively to measure CBF and to relate it to other repetitive analyses such as the functional studies.

Where focal hemispheral deficit has followed subarachnoid hemorrhage and perhaps operation, then remedial measures to restore perfusion have to be undertaken. From primate experience (Hope, Branston, & Symon, 1978) we have concluded that the best maneuver under these circumstances is to raise the systemic blood pressure in the presence of the diminished autoregulation, secondary to the reduced vasoreactivity following subarachnoid hemorrhage or operation (Kosnik & Hunt, 1976). Our general method is to give a modest fluid load of 500 ml to a litre of 10% Rheomacrodex (molecular weight 40,000) in saline, together with Meteraminol or Levophed, aiming to raise the systemic blood pressure by 30–40 torr at peak level (Symon, 1978). This maneuver demands, as a prerequisite of its employment, that the state of swelling of the hemisphere be assessed by CT scan. Focal low density following a subarachnoid hemorrhage or intracranial operation is fairly common and undoubtedly represents some water accumulation in the tissue, but, in the absence of shift so that the area of diminished permeability does not establish itself as a space-occupying lesion, we have found induced hypotension to be quite safe. Where the area of reduced density on CT scan is associated with hemispheral swelling and mid-line shift we have concluded that we are approaching the circumstances described by Langfitt and his associates many years ago (1965) in which induced hypotension might very well blow more water into the area of diminished permeability and early attempts to restore neurological dysfunction associated with such a CT picture by induced hypotension led invariably to drastic swelling of the hemisphere.

We would consider therefore that such a CT picture absolutely precludes the use of hypervolemic hypertension in the postoperative phase. Under appropriate circumstances, we have satisfactorily increased hemispheral perfusion in a

TABLE 9.3
A Series of Cases Studied During the Evolution of Transient or Progressive Neurological Deficit with Appropriate Blood Flow Measurements

Cases	Admission Grade	Base-line CBF_{isi} Right hemisphere	Base-line CBF_{isi} Left hemisphere	Expected Normal Mean CBF_{isi} for Age	Time of Deficit PBD/POD*	Type of Deficit	CBF_{isi} at Time of Onset of Deficit R hemisphere	CBF_{isi} at Time of Onset of Deficit L hemisphere	% Decrease in Flow R hemisphere	% Decrease in Flow L hemisphere	CBF_{isi} after Volume Expansion R hemisphere	CBF_{isi} after Volume Expansion L hemisphere	% Increase in Flow R hemisphere	% Increase in Flow L hemisphere	Mean Blood Pressure (mm Hg) Before treatment	Mean Blood Pressure (mm Hg) After treatment	Outcome
Preoperative cases																	
1	III	42	52	44.5	6/–	Stupor, hemiparesis, global aphasia	39	33	–7%	–36.5%	—	—	—	—	—	—	Died 18 hrs after the onset of deficit
2	I	45	39	52	9/–	Confusion, hemiparesis	34	30	–24.4%	23.1%	46	39	+35.3%	+30.0%	98.7	95.3	Deficit resolved; remainder of course uncomplicated
Postoperative cases																	
1	III	44	46	47	5/1	Aphasia	44	34	0%	–26.1%	44	42	0%	+23.5%	86	116.7	Deficit resolved; remainder

																of course uncomplicated
2	II	47	44	50	8/5	Confusion, decline in mental status	28	31	−40.4%	29.5%	43	39	+53.6%	+25.8%	96.7	96.7	Deficit resolved; remainder of course uncomplicated
3	II	46	47	46	17/5	Confusion	31	31	−32.6%	−31.9%	39	39	+25.8%	+25.8%	102.7	108	Confusion improved; transferred to psychiatric hospital for treatment of long-standing manic-depressive illness
4	II	42	45	50	5/1	Stupor, hemiparesis	35	37	−16.7%	−17.8%	44	45	+25.7%	+21.6%	100	100	Deficit resolved; remainder of course uncomplicated

*POD = Postoperative day
PBD = Postbleed day
Source: From Rosenstein, Suzuki, Symon, & Redmond, *Neurosurgery 15,* 522, 1984.

number of instances (Table 9.3), and it seems that under these circumstances fairly frequently repeated cerebral blood-flow measurements are of value in aiding the progress of therapy.

THE ASSESSMENT OF VASOREACTIVITY AS A PREDICTOR OF SUITABILITY FOR OPERATION

The presence of disordered vascular reactivity in certain cases of subarachnoid hemorrhage has been known for many years (Nornes, Knutzen, & Wikeby, 1977; Pickard, Boisvert, Graham, & Fitch, 1979; Yamamoto et al., 1979). More recently, some surgeons have attempted to assess the capacity of the damaged circulation to react and to use this as a predictor of suitability for operation. One of the first to do this was Mullan and his coworkers (Mullan, Hanlon, & Brown, 1978), who induced hypotension preoperatively in an endeavor to establish whether or not autoregulation remained.

A similar approach has been adopted by Pickard et al. (Pickard, Matheson, Patterson, & Wyper, 1980), who established that in a group of 25 cases, one could separate out those in whom induced hypotension by halothane resulted in a considerable reduction in hemispheral perfusion and those in which there was very little change. The latter group did well, the former group did badly. Pickard has extended these observations to peroperative assessment of blood flow during aneurysm surgery, but because of the time necessary for the calculation of the curves and the inevitable complication of Xenon inhalation in the circumstances of anesthesia, this is a method which is not generally adopted. The results are of very considerable interest to other neurosurgeons however, and in our own case have enabled us to correlate our functional studies by continuous peroperative measurement of somatosensory evoked response with the probable influence of operation on the cerebral circulation. These studies presently in progress may well yield valuable prognostic criteria, for example for the utility of temporary vascular occlusion during aneurysm surgery (Symon & Vajda, in press).

CBF IN HEAD INJURY

Several major studies have been made in head-injured patients (Bruce et al., 1973; Enevoldsen, Cold, Jensen, & Malmros, 1976; Fieschi, Battastini, Beduschi, Boselli, & Rossanda, 1974; Ovargaard & Tweed, 1974) revealing wide variations in cerebral blood flow. The demonstration of extremely high blood flow in the comatose patients led to the evolution of the syndrome of luxury perfusion, where the cerebellar metabolic rate for oxygen was very low, and high CBF during coma indicated an uncoupling of the two (Lassen, 1966). The syndrome is characterized by cerebral hyperemia, excessive blood flow relative to the brain's metabolic requirements. It appeared possible that the hyperemia was due to impaired CBF reactivity, autoregulation being abolished secondary to ischemia or hypoxic damage. The suggestion was that such hyperemia could be responsible for disruption of the blood-brain barrier and edema formation (Overgaard & Tweed, 1976). The syndrome of vasomotor paralysis was introduced by Langfitt and his coworkers (Langfitt, Weinstein, & Kassell, 1965) to explain brain swelling and intracranial hypotension in experimental studies of cerebral compression and trauma, and has been utilized by other workers, including ourselves, as a reason for avoiding hypervolemic hypoperfusion in circumstances of possible vasomotor paralysis following subarachnoid hemorrhage or aneurysm surgery.

Brain trauma has been shown to impair autoregulation (Lewelt, Jenkins, & Miller, 1980; Miller, Stanek, & Langfitt, 1972; Reivich, Marshall, & Kassell, 1968) and studies of these derangements of the cerebral circulation in association with trauma have been made in a number of centers in an attempt to elucidate the relationship between such CBF change and pathophysiology.

A particularly useful study by Obrist and his associates (Obrist, Langfitt, Jaggi, Cruz, & Gennarelli, 1984) in which 75 adult patients were studied after closed head injury, described eight detector measurements using the intravenous elution method with ^{133}Xe. The patients were serially studied within 96 hours of trauma, a somewhat late interval in the view of a number of observers, but repeatedly observed until death or recovery. Correlation with arteriovenous oxygen differences permitted assessment of the balance between metabolism and blood flow and provided estimates of $CMRO_2$.

This group demonstrated that two groups of patients could be clearly separated, one who exhibited hyperemia on one or more examinations and one group who had a consistently reduced flow during the illness. Hyperemia may be defined as a normal or supernormal CBF in the presence of coma, and arteriovenous oxygen differences in these cases indicated the presence of luxury perfusion, that is a metabolic uncoupling, the CBF being higher than apparent requirements for oxygen. All patients during coma showed a significant depression in $CMRO_2$. Hyperemia was found at all age levels and there was a significant association between hyperemia and the occurrence of intracranial hypotension defined as an intracranial pressure above 20 mmHg. Patients with reduced flow however, although they showed no evidence of local cerebral ischemia hut revealed the expected coupling of CBF and metabolism, CBF and metabolism being correspondingly depressed in parallel. Interestingly in this study the reactivity of the circulation to hyperventilation, that is the expected reduction with lowered pCO_2, was present in both groups, the hyperemic group being slightly more reactive. Significantly in 10 patients with low flow, hyperventilation resulted in widening of the arteriovenous oxygen difference, suggesting the possibility of ischemia under these circumstances. Obrist and his colleagues (Obrist et al., 1984) suggested that the utility of the repetitive measurements was used as a guide to the use of dehydrating agents to lower intracranial pressure, and as a guide to the use of hyperventilation.

Intracranial hypotension is known, as they pointed out, as the most critical problem in the management of head injury evidenced by several reports of poor outcome in relation to ICP change. Experimental evidence and the clinical evidence reported in these most recent studies indicate that the circulatory factors have a very important influence on intracranial hypotension, particularly when hyperemia can be established. The clear evidence of impaired oxygen availability secondary to hyperventilation in cases who have shown relatively normal CBF after head injury, indicates that this commonly accepted and across-the board, applied method of management of the airway may in certain circumstances be undesirable.

Within the circumstances of the intensive-care unit also, there have been several studies indicating the utility of relatively simple hemispheral blood-flow measurements as a guide to therapeutic intervention in patients with raised intracranial pressure secondary to head injury. There seems little doubt that the bedside flow apparatus now available will enable more generalized use of the technique in the intensive-care unit and should increase the appropriateness of therapeutic intervention in head injury.

rCBF AND REVASCULARIZATION

The assessment of established cerebrovascular pathology by isotope elution methods has been bedeviled by a number of interpretative difficulties. Chief among these have been collimation problems, which have blurred the presence of small, low-flow areas or, at worst, have enabled the registration of apparently normal blood flow through completely necrotic tissue in the look-through phenomenon (Hansen, Anderson, & Sundt, 1975). Further problems occur in the intra-arterial technique, where the isotope bolus may be dispersed in consequence of partial obstruction to the afferent circulation leading to considerable difficulties in the interpretation of curves (Nilsson, Cronqvist, & Ingvar, 1979).

It has become clear that the inhalation or intravenous techniques avoid certain pitfalls of the intra-arterial injection techniques, and reports from Risberg et al. (Risberg, Halsey, Wills, & Wilson, 1975) and from Norving et al. (Norving, Nilsson, & Risberg, 1982) have shown hemispheral asymmetry of a significant degree in patients with significant afferent vascular disease or occlusion. The presence of a truly ischemic focus is clearly of less significance and much more difficult to assess because of collimation problems.

It has been suggested that a deficiency of CO_2 response (Norving et al., 1982) could predict the efficiency of collateral circulation, and indeed the concept of a cerebrovascular reserve (Halsey, Morawetz, & Blauenstein, 1982) now seems a reasonable yardstick both in preoperative assessment and in postoperative therapeutic analysis. Sundt (Sundt, 1983; Sundt et al., 1981) has long been a proponent of peroperative assessment of cerebral blood flow during carotid endarterectomy. Sundt believes that the Mayo Clinic demonstration, found also by

Trojaborg and Boysen (1973), of a correlation between electroencephalographic abnormalities and blood flow significantly below 20 ml/100g/min, the human correlation of the threshold concept established in animals (Branston, Symon, Strong, & Hope, 1978), justifies use of internal shunts during carotid endarterectomy. Indeed, he has stated that very low blood flows, below 5 ml/100g/min, or circumstances where there has been a traumatic and catastrophic change in the EEG will demand immediate shunting before the endarterectomy itself, in contrast to his usual practice of clearing the plaque before the situation of the shunt and using the shunt only to enable more time to be taken to apply a patch graft from the saphenous vein, thus lengthening the period of available tolerance of cross-clamping.

Others have disagreed with this philosophy, notably Ferguson (1982), who in a review of a number of series of endarterectomy procedures, pointed out that the reported stroke mortality rates were indeed somewhat lower in situations where shunts had not been used. The controversy cannot be regarded as settled, but one of the main problems bedeviling the argument has been the relative lack of availability of portable blood-flow units to enable more centers to collect the data. This situation has now been resolved with the development of relatively inexpensive units suitable for peroperative use and we may expect further reports of correlation of ischemic tolerance and blood flow in the future.

Blood-flow analyses have also been used in relation to the superficial temporal middle cerebral artery bypass procedure. Austin early reported (Austin, Laffin, & Hayward, 1974) with the intravenous bolus technique that a 25% reduction in gray-matter blood flow in the frontal area on the side of the lesion in cases of internal carotid artery occlusion or stenosis occlusion of the internal carotid or middle cerebral artery in the head, not amenable to endarterectomy, justified the extracranial to intracranial bypass procedure. He reported in a series of 35 cases a significant increase in postoperative blood flow which correlated with improved psychometric testing and decreased the frequencies of transient ischemic attacks. Similar increases in flow are reported by Laurent, Lawner, and O'Connor, in 1982 who attempted to regionalize some of their findings pointing out that areas of lowest blood-flow preoperatively had the greatest increase in blood-flow postoperatively. They and others (Meyer et al., 1982) commented on the frequency of bilateral reduction in blood flow in extensive cerebrovascular disease and on the fact that successful revascularization by EC/IC bypass frequently increased blood flow on both sides of the brain.

A more recent careful study by Dorsch (Dorsch, Compton, & Collins, work in progress) of 60 patients with cerebrovascular disease confirmed significantly lower blood flow in the hemisphere on the lesion side but found that extra and intracranial bypass surgery had little effect on blood flow where preoperative blood flow was not significantly below the expected norm for age. However, if preoperative blood flow was more than one standard deviation below the center of the normal range, then a significant postoperative increase in blood flow could be detected. It is probably worth pointing out that the majority of authors in an assessment of blood flow have used hemispheral means, although Gratzl et al. (1976) claimed the best results and indeed regarded as the prime indication, a focal reduction in CBF in the selection of patients for extracranial to intracranial bypass surgery.

There seems little doubt that the simple peroperative methods of hemispheral blood flow now available will be more widely applied during carotid endarterectomy procedures following the guidelines of Sundt and his colleagues of the Mayo Clinic. The place of regional multicollimator rCBF analysis in the assessment of patients for superficial temporal and middle cerebral anastomoses cannot be regarded as yet as completely certain. Criteria for operation differ from center to center, and the effects of the procedure remain to be revealed by the breakdown of a large multicenter trial still in progress. It seems, however, that only by the correlation of flow, electrical function, and arterial pathology will we obtain valid criteria for submission of patients to surgery. The wide availability of relatively simple blood-flow machinery should enhance this scheme of data collection appreciably.

REFERENCES

Allcock, J. M., Drake, C. G. (1963). Postoperative angiography in cases of ruptured intracranial aneurysms. *J. Neurosurg.*, *20*, 752–759.

Alvord, E. C., Loeser, J. D., Bailey, W. L., & Copass, M. K. (1972). Subarachnoid haemorrhage due to ruptured aneurysms. A simple method of estimating prognosis. *Arch. Neurol.*, *27*, 273–284.

Astrup, J., Symon, L., Branston, N. M., & Lassen, N. A. (1977). Cortical evoked potential and extracellular K^+ and H^+ at critical levels of brain ischaemia. *Stroke*, *8*(1), 51–57.

Austin, G., Horn, N., Rouhe, S., & Hayward, W. (1972). Description and early results of an intravenous radioisotope technique for measuring regional cerebral blood flow in man. *Eur. Neurol.*, *6*, 43–51.

Austin, G., Laffin, D., & Hayward, W. (1974). Physiologic factors in the selection of patients for superficial temporal artery-to-middle cerebral artery anastomosis. *Surgery*, *75*(6), 861–868.

Bell, B. A., Kendall, B. E., & Symon, L. (1980). Computed tomography in aneurysmal subarachnoid haemorrhage. *J. Neurol. Neurosurg. Psychiat.*, *43*, 522–524.

Branston, N. M., Strong, A. J., & Symon, L. (1977). Extracellular potassium activity, evoked potential and tissue blood flow: Relationship during progressive ischaemia in baboon cerebral cortex. *J. Neurol. Sci.*, *32*, 305–321.

Branston, N. M., Symon, L., Crockard, H. A., & Pasztor, E. (1974). Relationship between the cortical evoked potential and local cortical blood flow following acute middle cerebral artery occlusion in the baboon. *Exper. Neurol.*, *45*, 195–208.

Branston, N. M., Symon, L., Strong, A. J., Hope, D. T. (1978). Measurements of regional cortical blood flow during changes in extracellular potassium activity evoked by direct cortical stimulation in the primate. *Exper. Neurol.*, *59*, 243–253.

Brock, M., Hadjidimos, A. A., Schürmann, K., Ellger, M., & Fischer, F. (1969). Brain tumor. In M. Brock, C. Fieschi, D. H. Ingvar, N. A. Lassen, & K. Schürmann (Eds.). *Cerebral blood flow* (pp. 169–171). New York: Springer–Verlag.

Bruce, D. A., Langfitt, T. W., Miller, J. D., Schutz, H., Vapalahti, M. P., Stanek, A., Goldberg, H. I. (1973). Regional cerebral blood flow, intracranial pressure, and brain metabolism in comatose patients. *J. Neurosurg., 38,* 131–144.

Dorsch, N. W. C., Compton, J. S., Collins, L. (work in progress). The effect on cerebral blood flow of extracranial to intracranial bypass surgery for cerebral ischaemia.

Du Boulay, G. (1963). Distribution of spasm in the intracranial arteries after subarachnoid haemorrhage. *Acta Radiol.* (Stockh.), *1,* 257–266.

Du Boulay, G. H., Marshall, J., Merory, J., Symon, L. (1980). The location of spasm and its relation to symptoms. In R. H. Wilkins (Ed.), *Cerebral Arterial Spasm* (pp. 394–396). Proc. 2nd. Intl. Workshop, 1979. Baltimore: Williams and Wilkins.

Enevoldsen, E. M., Cold, G., Jensen, F. T., Malmros, R. (1976). Dynamic changes in regional CBF, intraventricular pressure, CSF pH and lactate levels during the acute phase of head injury. *J. Neurosurg., 44,* 191–214.

Ferguson, G. G. (1982). Intra-operative monitoring and internal shunts: Are they necessary in carotid endarterectomy? *Stroke, 13*(3), 287–289.

Ferguson, G. G., Harper, A. M., Fitch, W., Rowan, J. O., & Jennett, B. (1972). Cerebral blood flow measurements after spontaneous subarachnoid haemorrhage. *Eur. Neurol., 8,* 15–22.

Fieschi, C., Battastini, N., Beduschi, A., Boselli, L., & Rossanda, M. (1974). Regional cerebral blood flow and intraventricular pressure in acute head injuries. *J. Neurol. Neurosurg. Psychiat., 37,* 1378–1388.

Fisher, C. M., Kistler, J. B., Davis, J. M. (1980). Relation of cerebral vasospasm to subarachnoid haemorrhage, visualised by computerised tomographic scanning. *Neurosurgery, 6,* 1–9.

Graaf, C. J. (1971). Prognosis for patients with non-surgically-treated aneurysms. Analysis of the cooperative study of intracranial aneurysms and subarachnoid haemorrhage. *J. Neurosurg., 35,* 438–443.

Gratzl, O., Schmiedek, P., Spetzler, R., Steinhoff, H., Klassen, A. C., Chou, S. N., & Resch, J. A. (1976). Clinical experience with extra-cranial arterial anastomosis in 65 cases. *J. Neurosurg., 44,* 313–324.

Halsey, J. H., Morawetz, R. B., Blauenstein, U. W. (1982). The hemodynamic effect of STA–MCA bypass. *Stroke, 13*(2), 163–167.

Hansen, E. J., Jr., Anderson, R. E., & Sundt, T. M., Jr. (1975). Comparison of ^{85}krypton and ^{133}xenon cerebral blood flow measurements before, during, and following focal incomplete ischemia in the squirrel monkey. *Circ. Res., 30,* 703–712.

Hargadine, J. R., Branston, N. M., & Symon, L. (1980). Central conduction time in primate brain ischaemia—A study in baboons. *Stroke, 11*(6), 637–643.

Heilbrun, M. P., Olesen, J., & Lassen, N. A. (1972). Regional cerebral blood flow studies in subarachnoid haemorrhage. *J. Neurosurg., 37,* 36–44.

Heiss, W. D., Hayakawa, T., & Waltz, A. G. (1976). Cortical neuronal function during ischemia. Effects of occlusion of one middle cerebral artery on single-unit activity in cats. *Arch. Neurol., 33,* 813–820.

Høedt–Rasmussen, K., Sveinsdottir, E., & Lassen, N. A. (1966). Regional cerebral blood flow in man determined by intra-arterial injection of radioactive inert gas. *Circ. Res., 18,* 237–247.

Hope, D. T., Branston, N. M., Symon, L. (1978). Potential beneficial effects of induced hypertension in acute cerebral ischaemia. *J. Neurol. Neurosurg. Psychiat., 41*(2), 185–190.

Hunt, W. E., & Hess, R. M. (1968). Surgical risk as related to time of intervention in the repair of intracranial aneurysms. *J. Neurosurg., 28,* 14–20.

Ishii, R. (1979). Regional cerebral blood flow in patients with ruptured intracranial aneurysms. *J. Neurosurg., 50,* 587–594.

Jabre, A., Symon, L., Redmond, S. (work in progress). A comparative study of the portable regional CBF monitor and the portable mean hemispheral CBF monitor: Advantages and disadvantages in clinical practice.

Jones, T. H., Morawetz, R. B., Crowell, R. M., Marcoux, F. W., FitzGibbon, S. J., DeGirolami, U., Ojemann, R. G. (1981). Thresholds in focal cerebral ischaemia in awake monkeys. *J. Neurosurg., 54,* 773–782.

Kagström, E., Greitz, T., Hanson, J., & Galera, R. (1966). *Changes in cerebral blood flow after subarachnoid haemorrhage.* Proceedings of the third International Conference on Neurological Surgery, International Congress Series Foundation No. 110, pp. 629–633. Amsterdam: Excerpta Medica.

Kosnik, E. J., & Hunt, W. E. (1976). Post-operative hypertension in the management of patients with intracranial aneurysms. *J. Neurosurg., 45,* 148–149.

Langfitt, T. W., Weinstein, J. D., & Kassell, N. F. (1965). Cerebral vasomotor paralysis produced by intracranial hypertension. *Neurology, 15,* 622–641.

Lassen, N. A. (1966). The luxury perfusion syndrome and its possible relation to acute metabolic acidosis localised within the brain. *Lancet, 2,* 1113–1115.

Lassen, N. A., Høedt–Rasmussen, K., & Sørensen, S. C., Skinhøj, E., Cronquist, S., Bodforss, B., & Ingvar, D. H. (1963). Regional cerebral blood flow in man determined by krypton^{85}. *Neurology, 13*(9), 719–727.

Laurent, J. P., Lawner, P. M., O'Connor, M. (1982). Reversal of intracerebral steal by STA–MCA anastomosis. *J. Neurosurg., 57,* 629–632.

Lewelt, W., Jenkins, L. W., & Miller, J. D. (1980). Autoregulation of cerebral blood flow after experimental fluid percussion injury of the brain. *J. Neurosurg., 53,* 500–511.

Merory, J., Thomas, D. J., Humphrey, P. R. D., Du Boulay, G. H., Marshall, J., Ross Russell, R. W., Symon, L., & Zilkha, E. (1980). Cerebral blood flow following surgery for recent subarachnoid haemorrhage. *J. Neurol. Neurosurg. Psychiat., 43,* 214–221.

Meyer, C. H. A., Lowe, D., Meyer, M., Richardson, P. L., & Neil–Dwyer, G. (1983). Progressive change in cerebral blood flow during the first three weeks after subarachnoid haemorrhage. *Neurosurgery, 12,* 58–76.

Meyer, J. S., Nakajima, S., Okabe, T., Amano, T., Centeno, R., Lee, Y. Y., Levine, J., Levinthal, R., & Rose, J. (1982). Redistribution of cerebral blood flow following STA–MCA by-pass in patients with hemispheric ischemia. *Stroke, 13*(6), 774–784.

Miller, J. D., Stanek, A., & Langfitt, T. W. (1972). Concepts of cerebral perfusion pressure and vascular compression during intracranial hypertension. *Prog. Brain Res., 35,* 411–432.

Millikan, C. H. (1975). Cerebral vasospasm and ruptured intracranial aneurysm. *Arch. Neurol., 32,* 433–449.

Morawetz, R. B., DeGirolami, U., Ojemann, R. G., Marcoux, F. W., & Crowell, R. M. (1978). Cerebral blood flow determined by hydrogen clearance during middle cerebral artery occlusion in unanaesthetised monkeys. *Stroke, 9,* 143–149.

Mullan, S., Hanlon, K., & Brown, F. (1978). Management of 136 consecutive supratentorial berry aneurysms. *J. Neurosurg., 49,* 794–804.

Nilsson, B., Cronqvist, S., & Ingvar, D. H. (1979). Regional cerebral blood flow (rCBF) studies in patients to be considered for extracranial-intracranial bypass operation: In J. S. Meyer, H. Lechner, & M. Reivich (Eds.). *Cerebral vascular diseases 2* (pp. 295–300). International Congress Series No. 449. Amsterdam: Excerpta Medica.

Nornes, H., Knutzen, H. B., & Wikeby, P. (1977). Cerebral arterial blood flow and aneurysm surgery. Pt. 2: Induced hypotension and autoregulatory capacity. *J. Neurosurg., 47,* 819–827.

Norving, B., Nilsson, B., & Risberg, J. (1982). rCBF in patients with carotid occlusion. Resting and hypercapnic flow related to collateral pattern. *Stroke, 13*(2), 155–162.

Obrist, W. D., Langfitt, T. W., Jaggi, J. L., Cruz, J., & Gennarelli, T. A. (1984). Cerebral blood flow and metabolism in comatose patients with acute head injury. *J. Neurosurg., 61,* 241–253.

Overgaard, J., & Tweed, W. A. (1974). Cerebral circulation after head injury. Pt. 1: Cerebral blood flow and its regulation after closed head injury with emphasis on clinical correlations. *J. Neurosurg., 41,* 531–541.

———. (1976). Cerebral circulation after head injury. Pt. 2: The effects of traumatic brain oedema. *J. Neurosurg., 45,* 292–300.

Pickard, J. D., Boisvert, D. P. J., Graham, D. I., & Fitch, W. (1979). Late effects of subarachnoid haemorrhage on the response of the primate cerebral circulation to drug induced changes in arterial blood pressure. *J. Neurol. Neurosurg. Psychiat., 42,* 899–903.

Pickard, J. D., Matheson, M., Patterson, J., & Wyper, D. (1980). The prediction of late ischaemic complications after cerebral aneurysm surgery by the intra-operative measurement of cerebral blood flow. *J. Neurosurg., 53,* 305–308.

Pitts, L. H., McPherson, B., Wyper, D. J., Jennett, B., Blair, I., & Cook, M. B. D. (1979). Effects of vasospasm on cerebral blood flow after subarachnoid haemorrhage. In R. H. Wilkins (Ed.). *Cerebral arterial spasm* (pp. 333–337). Proceedings of the Second International Workshop. Baltimore: Williams and Wilkins.

Reivich, M., Marshall, W. J. S., & Kassell, N. (1968). Effects of trauma upon cerebral vascular autoregulation. In J. F. Toole, J. Moossy, & R. Janeway (Eds.). *Cerebral vascular diseases* (pp. 91–100). New York: Grune & Stratton.

Risberg, J., Ali, Z., Wilson, E. M., Wills, E. Z., & Halsey, J. H. (1975). Regional cerebral blood flow by 133-Xenon inhalation. *Stroke, 6,* 142–148.

Risberg, J., Halsey, J. H., Wills, E. L., & Wilson, E. M. (1975). Hemispheric specialization in normal man studied by bilateral measurements of the regional cerebral blood flow. A study with the 133-Xenon inhalation technique. *Brain, 98,* 511–524.

Rosenstein, J., Suzuki, M., Symon, L., & Redmond, S. (1984). Clinical use of portable bedside cerebral blood flow measurements in the management of aneurysmal subarachnoid haemorrhage. *Neurosurgery, 15*(4), 519–525.

Rosenstein, J., Wang, A., Symon, L., Suzuki, M. (in press). Relationship between hemispheral CBF, CCT, and clinical grade in aneurysmal subarachnoid haemorrhage. *J. Neurosurg.*

Schmiedek, P., Gratzl, O., Spetzler, R., Steinhoff, H., Enzenbach, R., Brendel, W., Marguth, F. (1976). Selection of patients for extra-intracranial arterial bypass surgery based on rCBF measurements. *J. Neurosurg., 44,* 303–312.

Sharbrough, F. W., Messick, J. M., Jr., Sundt, T. M. (1973). Correlation of continuous electroencephalograms with cerebral blood flow measurements during carotid endarterectomy. *Stroke 4,* 674–683.

Sundt, T. M., Jr. (1983). The ischemic tolerance of neural tissue and the need for monitoring and selective shunting during carotid endarterectomy. *Stroke, 14*(1), 93–98.

Sundt, T. M., Sharbrough, F. W., Piepgras, D. G., Kearns, T. P., Messick, J. M., O'Fallon, W. M. (1981). Correlation of cerebral blood flow and encephalographic changes during carotid endarterectomy with results of surgery and hemodynamics of cerebral ischemia. *Mayo Clin. Proc., 56,* 533–543.

Symon, L. (1978). Disordered cerebral vascular physiology in aneurysmal subarachnoid haemorrhage. *Acta Neurochir., 41,* 7–22.

Symon, L., Ackerman, R., Bull, J. W. D., Du Boulay, E. P. G. H., Marshall, J., Rees, J. E., & Ross Russell, R. W. (1972). The use of the Xenon clearance method in subarachnoid haemorrhage. Post-operative studies with clinical and angiographic correlation. *Eur. Neurol., 8,* 8–14.

Symon, L., & Vajda, J. (in press). Surgical experiences with giant intracranial aneurysms. *J. Neurosurg.*

Trojaborg, W., & Boysen, G. (1973). Relation between EEG, regional cerebral blood flow and internal carotid artery pressure during carotid endarterectomy. *Electroenceph. Clin. Neurophysiol., 34,* 61–69.

Wang, A. D., Cone, J., Symon, L., & Costa e Silva, I. E. (1984). Somatosensory evoked potential monitoring during the management of aneurysmal subarachnoid haemorrhage. *J. Neurosurg., 60,* 264–268.

Wilkinson, I. M. S., Bull, J. W. D., Du Boulay, G. H., Marshall, J., Ross Russell, R. W., &

Symon, L. (1969). Regional blood flow in the normal cerebral hemisphere. *J. Neurol. Neurosurg. Psychiat., 32,* 367–378.

Winn, H. R., Berga, S. L., Richardson, A. E., Jane, J. A., Waldman, M. T., O'Brien, W. M. (1981). The natural history of vertebral basilar (VBA) aneurysms (abstract). *Stroke, 12,* 120.

Yamamoto, M., Meyer, J., Naritomi, H., Sakai, F., Yamaguchi, F., & Shaw, T. (1979). Noninvasive measurement of cerebral vasospasm in patients with subarachnoid hemorrhage. *J. Neurol. Sci., 43,* 301–311.

10 Regional Cerebral Blood Flow in Psychiatric Disorders

Jarl Risberg and Lars Gustafson
Departments of Psychiatry I and Psychogeriatrics, University Hospital, Lund, Sweden

The interest for studying regional cerebral blood flow (rCBF) in mental disorders has increased during recent years but the number of active centers is still small. The majority of CBF laboratories are devoted to neurological disorders such as stroke. The reasons for this difference between psychiatry and neurology are easy to find. The rCBF methodology belongs to a type of investigation techniques, which since long is familiar and natural for the neurologist and neurosurgeon to use. Moreover, the study of cerebrovascular disorders by rCBF is very logical and tempting from a basic science point of view, since the study aims at the primary cause and localization of the disease. For the psychiatrist, the method is new and strange and thus very few psychiatric clinics have independent laboratory facilities. Among the disorders labeled "psychiatric" only a few, e.g., multi-infarct dementia (MID) and some organic confusional states are considered to be primarily caused by a vascular disturbance. The flow changes found in the psychiatric disorders are in general reflections of the coupling between function, metabolism, and blood flow.

The flow disturbances seen will thus not enlighten us about the primary cause of the disease, but will mirror the functional consequences of the illness. Some researchers might find this less challenging than exploring basic pathophysiological mechanisms. It is, however, the conviction of the present authors that mapping of cortical function by rCBF has a great potential for increasing our knowledge about the disease process of several mental disorders. As will be discussed in detail later, recent results indicate that rCBF data are of considerable clinical value for evaluation of single cases, especially patients with symptoms of dementia. In this chapter a review will be given of current knowledge regarding rCBF in organic dementia, affective disease, and schizophrenia. The emphasis will be on studies using noninvasive rCBF technology. Some previously unpublished data from our laboratory will also be described.

ORGANIC DEMENTIA

Dementing disorders of middle and old age such as Alzheimer's Disease (AD) have been the focus of increasing interest during recent years. The need for further research in this field is very obvious. Changes of the age distribution in the industrialized countries make these disorders one of the major health problems for the decades to come. In spite of considerable research efforts the pathogenesis and etiology of the majority of the dementing illnesses are still unknown. Patients suffering from dementia are often difficult to evaluate, especially in the early stages of the disease. Psychogenic factors may interfere in a complex way with the disturbances caused by the organic brain disease. Sometimes mental disorders like affective disease cause conditions which mimic dementia (''pseudodementia''; Kiloh, 1961). Mapping of cortical functional changes by means of rCBF might thus be a valuable aid for the clinician in the investigation of the patient.

Global CBF Changes

It has been known for many years that the average cerebral blood flow and metabolism are reduced in *organic dementia* (Frackowiak et al., 1981; Freyhan, Woodford, & Kety, 1951; Gustafson & Risberg, 1974; Hachinski et al., 1975; Ingvar & Gustafson, 1970; Lassen, Feinberg & Lane, 1960; Lassen, Munck, & Tottey, 1957; Lavy, Melamed, Bentin, Cooper, & Rinot, 1978; Munck & Lassen, 1957; Obrist, Chivian, Cronqvist, & Ingvar, 1970; Perez, Mathew, Stump, & Meyer, 1977; Risberg & Gustafson, 1983; Simard, Olesen, Paulson, Lassen, & Skinhøj, 1971; Tachibana et al., 1984; Yamaguchi, Meyer, Yamamoto, Sakai, & Shaw, 1980). This reduction has been demonstrated by means of various measurement techniques and for primary degenerative as well as for cerebrovascular dementia. No consistent differences between the organic dementia disorders have been reported regarding the size of the reduction. The amplitude of the diminution seems to depend mainly on the severity of the dementia symptoms (Gustafson & Risberg, 1974; Hagberg & Ingvar, 1976). The size of the flow diminution can thus not be used for differential diagnosis but might be useful in the study of the course of the disease in the single patient (Risberg, 1980).

Regional CBF Changes

Recent neuropathological investigations have demonstrated marked regional accentuations of the cortical atrophy in AD (Brun & Englund, 1981; Brun &

Gustafson, 1970). A consistent pattern of degeneration has also been found in dementias of the Pick type (PD) (Gustafson, Brun, & Ingvar, 1977; Ingvar, Brun, Hagberg, & Gustafson, 1978) and by definition multi-infarct dementia (MID) involves focal processes (Hachinski et al., 1975). Focal changes of flow are thus expected from the neuropathological data and such changes have also been reported in several studies. Most investigations have reported parietal, temporal and sometimes also frontal decreases of flow in presenile or senile AD (Gustafson & Risberg, 1974; Gustafson & Risberg, 1979; Obrist et al., 1970; Ingvar & Gustafson, 1970; Perez et al., 1977; Risberg & Gustafson, 1983; Simard et al., 1971). In PD, the most marked flow decreases have been found in frontal and fronto-temporal regions (Gustafson et al., 1977; Gustafson & Risberg, 1979; Risberg & Gustafson, 1983), while multi-infarct dementia has been coupled to right–left asymmetries and spotty flow abnormalities (Gustafson & Risberg, 1979; Risberg & Gustafson, 1983; Yamaguchi et al., 1980). A close coupling between the symptoms of the patient as evaluated by psychiatric ratings and psychometric testing and the pattern of rCBF abnormalities has also been demonstrated (Gustafson & Risberg, 1974; Hagberg & Ingvar, 1976).

These consistent findings of specific patterns of flow abnormalities in the major organic dementia disorders have pointed to the possible clinical usefulness of rCBF data for differential diagnosis of dementia. In our laboratory, we have studied rCBF in dementia disorders for several years using the ^{133}Xe inhalation technique (Obrist, Thompson, King, & Wang, 1967; Obrist, Thompson, Wang, & Wilkinson, 1975; Risberg, Ali, Wilson, Wills, & Halsey, 1975). Recent results from our ongoing longitudinal study will now be presented.

The Demented Patients

Data from 121 patients with symptoms of organic dementia pertaining to our longitudinal study will be presented. At present autopsy has been performed in 38 out of 44 deceased patients in this group. The control group consisted of 20 healthy, male subjects (age 51 ± 6) (Risberg & Hagstadius, 1983).

The 121 patients were classified into 4 subgroups on the basis of results from clinical ratings of symptoms of dementia (Gustafson & Nilsson, 1983; Gustafson & Risberg, 1974):

1. Presenile Alzheimer's disease (AD), $n = 28$.
2. Senile dementia of the Alzheimer type (SDAT), $n = 27$.
3. Pick's disease (PD) or dementia with fronto-temporal degeneration, $n = 22$.
4. Multi-infarct dementia (MID), $n = 44$.

To be classified as presenile or senile (onset of symptoms before or after 65 years respectively) dementia of the Alzheimer type the patient had to display the clinical characteristics of the disease: slow progression, dysmnesia, dyspraxia, dysgnosia, and increased muscular tension (Gustafson & Nilsson, 1982). Patients suffering from PD (also called dementia with frontotemporal degeneration) were recognized by symptoms of personality changes (lack of insight, disinhibition etc.) and language disturbances (logorrhea and verbal stereotypy developing into mutism) (Gustafson & Nilsson, 1982). Patients with an ischemic score (Hachinski et al., 1975) greater than eight points were diagnosed as cases of MID. Patients who could not clearly be classified as belonging to any of the groups were not included in the study.

THE rCBF MEASUREMENTS

The rCBF measurements were made by conventional ^{133}Xe inhalation methodology (Obrist et al., 1967; Obrist et al., 1975; Risberg et al., 1975). Since the method is described in detail in other chapters of the present volume, only a short description of the specific features of our system will be given.

Radiation was recorded by 32 scintillation detectors placed in parallel in two detector holders positioned at the right angle to the lateral surfaces of the subject's head. The detectors had ¾″ by ¾″ NaI (T1) crystals and the lead collimators were 20 mm deep and had a diameter of 20 mm. Sixteen detectors, grossly localized, as shown in Fig. 10.1, covered each hemisphere. The curves were analyzed by the conventional algorithm for two-compartmental analysis developed by Obrist et al. (1975), with the addition of a correction routine for the air-passage artifact (Risberg, 1980). All results presented here will be based on the original 2–3 min ISI of Risberg et al. (1975). This parameter is preferred, due to its yet-unsurpassed reliability and immunity to compartmental slippage.

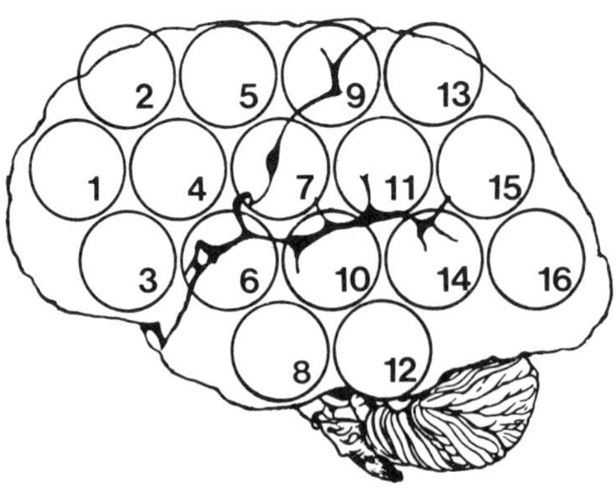

FIGURE 10.1. Approximate localization of the 16 detectors covering each hemisphere.

TABLE 10.1
Mean Hemispheric Flow Values (ISI) in Patients with Alzheimer's Disease, Pick's Disease, MID, SDAT, and in Normal Subjects

Diagnosis	*n*	*Age*	*ISI* Right	*ISI* Left	pCO_2 (mm Hg)
AD	28	64 ± 6	34.4 ± 6.1	33.6 ± 5.8	37.0 ± 5.0
PD	22	62 ± 8	37.3 ± 6.7	36.8 ± 6.9	36.1 ± 3.1
MID	44	68 ± 9	35.8 ± 7.1	35.4 ± 6.9	35.9 ± 4.5
SDAT	27	76 ± 7	33.5 ± 6.2	33.5 ± 5.9	36.5 ± 3.5
Normals	20	51 ± 6	44.9 ± 7.6	44.0 ± 7.5	38.0 ± 3.4

Clinical Diagnosis Compared with rCBF

The hemispheric mean CBF results for the four demented groups and the control group are shown in Table 10.1. The mean flow levels were, as expected, significantly ($p<0.01$ and less) lower for all the dementia groups, compared with the control group. None of the differences between the different dementia groups were statistically significant. It is also evident from the SD values that a consid-

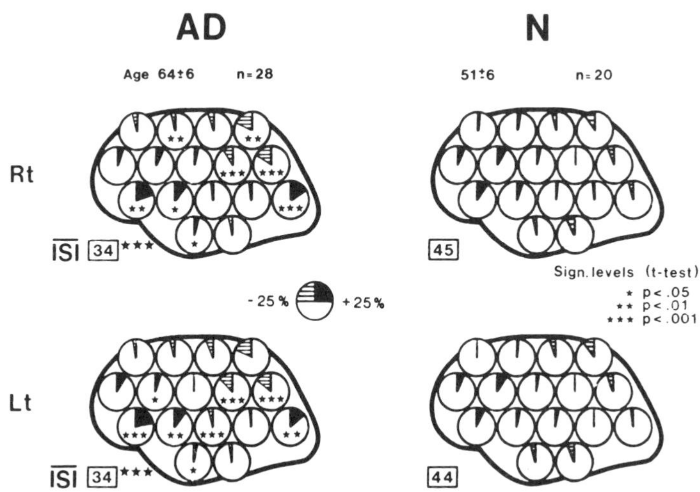

FIGURE 10.2. Comparison of rCBF (ISI-parameter) in a group of patients with presenile Alzheimer's disease (AD, clinical diagnosis) and a normal control group (N). The hemispheric averages are shown in the boxes. Clock symbols indicate regional values in percent of hemispheric mean. A black shadowing indicates a regional value above and a striped field a value below the hemispheric average (90° = 25%). Note the significantly (by t-test) lower distribution values in parietal and parieto-temporal regions for the demented group.

erable overlap between the demented patients and the normal subjects exists, despite the fact that the latter group was somewhat younger. Thus several patients with the clinical diagnosis of organic dementia have flow values within the normal range. The discriminative power of this parameter is therefore limited. Further analysis of the data will be based on the regional distribution of flow values, which is independent of the absolute level.

Comparisons between the control group and the different dementia groups regarding regional flow patterns (regional values in percent of the hemisphere average) are shown in Figs. 10.2–10.5. When comparing AD with the normal group, significantly lower values were seen in parietal, parieto-temporal and parieto-occipital regions of both hemispheres. Higher distribution values, indicating relatively better preserved areas, were seen in frontotemporal and occipital areas.

When the SDAT group was compared with the normals, the findings were rather similar to those made for the AD group (Fig. 10.3). The only differences were that the SDAT group showed diminutions in superior frontal regions and the parieto-occipital decreases were less marked than in AD. A markedly different abnormality of the flow pattern was found in PD (Fig. 10.4). Here the distribution flow values were significantly lower in frontal regions of both hemispheres with better preserved values occipitally. The MID group showed less distinct abnormalities, compared with the other dementia groups. The distribu-

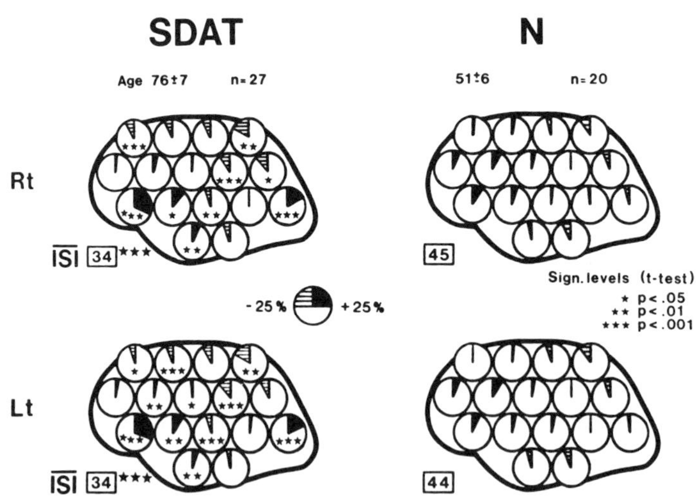

FIGURE 10.3. Comparison of rCBF in a group of patients with senile dementia of the Alzheimer type (SDAT, clinical diagnosis) and a normal control group (N). Symbols as in Fig. 10.2. Note the lower distribution values in parieto-temporal and superior frontal regions in the demented group.

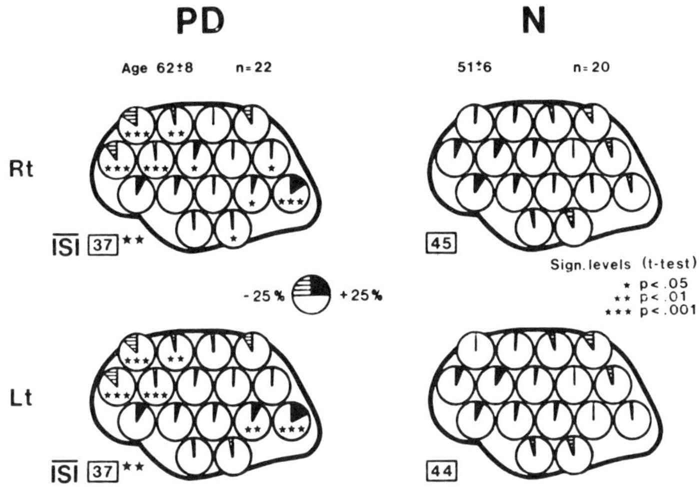

FIGURE 10.4. Comparison of rCBF in a group of patients with Pick's disease (PD, clinical diagnosis) and a normal control group (N). Symbols as in Fig. 10.2. Note the significantly lower distribution values in frontal regions.

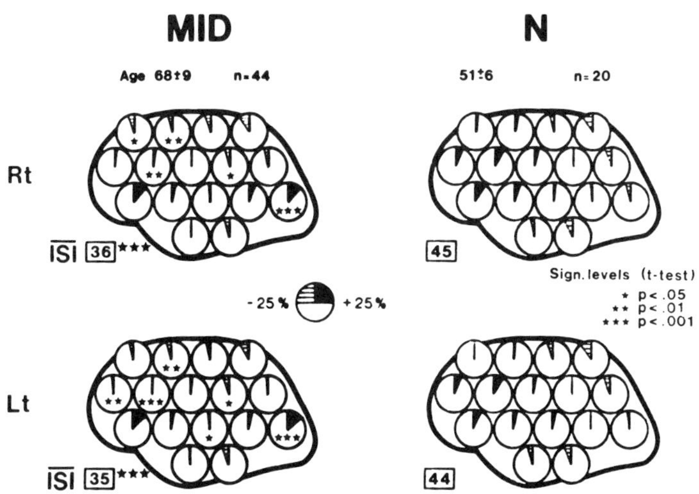

FIGURE 10.5. Comparison of rCBF in a group of patients with multi-infarct dementia (MID, clinical diagnosis) and a normal control group (N). Symbols as in Fig. 10.2.

tion flow values were close to the mean in many of the regions, which might be expected since the flow abnormalities in this group showed great interindividual variation. The characteristic right-left asymmetries and spotty flow abnormalities seen in the individual cases will disappear in the calculation of the group mean. However, as indicated in Fig. 10.5 regional analysis did reveal significantly lower values in some frontal and parieto-temporal areas.

Further statistical analysis of the data was made by means of stepwise discriminant analysis (BMDP7M), again using only the relative distribution flow values. The computer was forced to use the same regions in both hemispheres. The results are shown in Fig. 10.6. The demented patients were correctly classified in 81–96% of the cases while 0–10% of the normals were erroneously classified. Excellent results were obtained for the AD and PD groups, while some errors were made in the MID and SDAT groups. The computer used three to five regions of both hemispheres for the discriminant function. The regions selected were in general those showing the most significant group differences by t-test (Figs. 10.2–10.5). These results point to the possibility of direct computer aid in the interpretation of rCBF patterns for differential diagnosis of dementia.

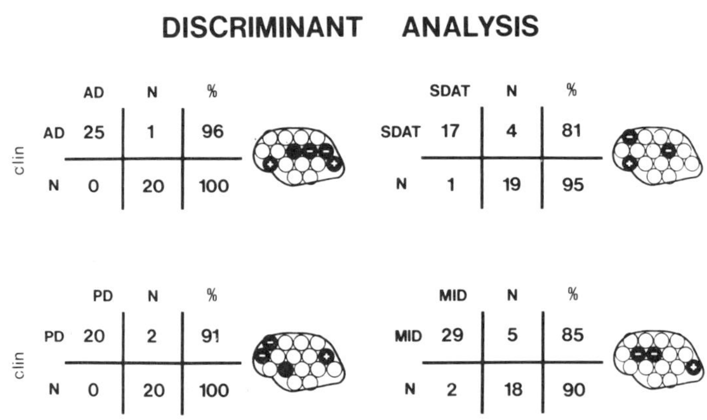

FIGURE 10.6. Stepwise discriminant analysis (BMDP7M) between four groups of patients with organic dementia (AD = presenile Alzheimer's disease, SDAT = senile dementia of the Alzheimer type, PD = Pick's disease, MID = multi-infarct dementia) and a normal group (N) based on the distribution flow values (regional value in percentage of hemispheric average). Columns show classification by the computer and the percentage of correctly classified subjects. The black regions are the ones used by the computer for the discriminant function. The computer was forced to use the same regions in both hemispheres. The sign of the difference in distribution flow value between the groups in the regions utilized is also indicated (one region in the AD and one in the PD group showed no significant difference).

Diagnosis by Autopsy Compared with rCBF

Yearly re-examinations have been made routinely in the present group and thus the time period between the last rCBF measurement and autopsy was less than 1 year in most of the patients. Many of the patients had had several rCBF measurements throughout the progression of their disease. A diagnostic subgrouping of the patients was made based on rCBF data. The main emphasis was on the latest results in the series, but some consideration was also given to earlier findings. The diagnosis was made by manual clinical evaluation of rCBF results. The criteria for distinguishing diagnostic categories were derived from the findings described and from previous research (Gustafson et al., 1977; Gustafson & Risberg, 1979; Risberg & Gustafson, 1983). To be classified as a case of AD or SDAT the patient has to display focal decreases in parietal, parieto-temporal, and parieto-occipital areas of both hemispheres.

The criterion for a focal decrease was a distribution value (percentage of hemispheric mean) which was at least 2 SD below the normal mean value for that region (Prohovnik, Håkansson, & Risberg, 1980; Risberg & Hagstadius, 1983). Such focal decreases had to be seen in at least two regions of each hemisphere. A part of the typical AD-SDAT feature was also focal decreases in superior frontal regions, which commonly were seen in the later measurements in the series and more often in SDAT than in AD. Relatively better preserved flow in occipital, frontotemporal, and central regions was also considered to be a typical finding,

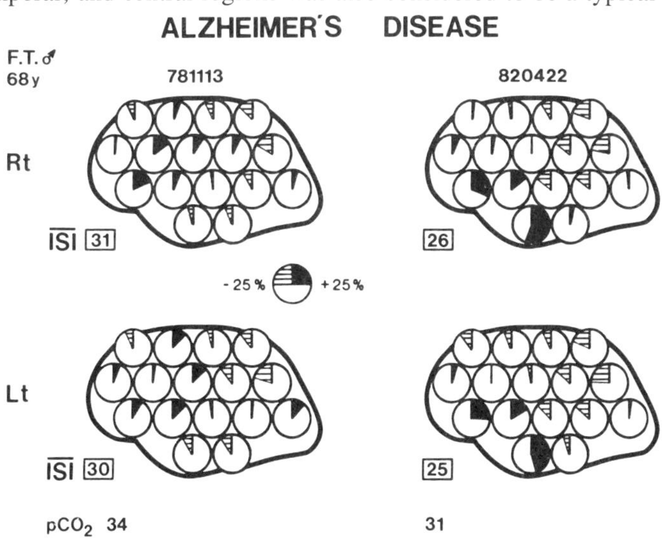

FIGURE 10.7. Repeated rCBF measurements in a case of progressing Alzheimer's disease. Symbols as in Fig. 10.2. Note the accentuated focal pathology of postcentral regions in the second study. The diagnosis was verified at autopsy.

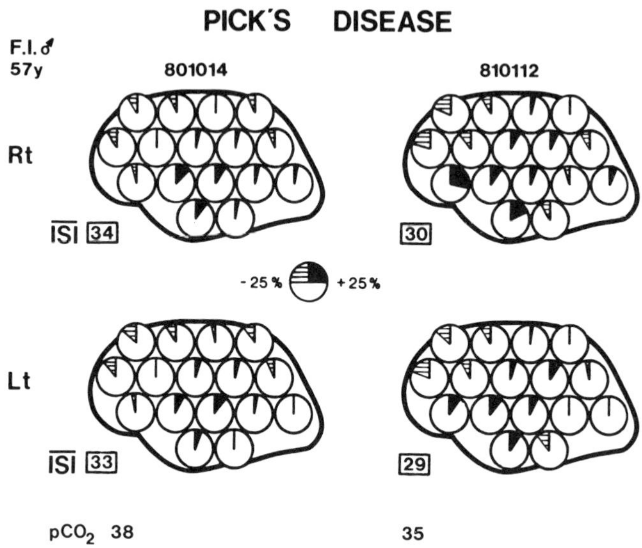

FIGURE 10.8. Repeated rCBF measurements in a case of rapidly progressing Pick's disease. Symbols as in Fig. 10.2. Note the accentuated focal pathology in frontal regions in the later study. The diagnosis was verified at autopsy.

together with a general symmetry and "smoothness" of the rCBF pathology. No differentiation between AD and SDAT was made, however, on the basis of rCBF data. The age of the patient at time of onset of symptoms, before or after 65 years of age, was used as the customary criterion. Typical progressive changes in one case of AD are shown in Fig. 10.7.

The criteria for classification as PD were focal decreases in frontal regions, together with better preserved values in posterior parts of the hemispheres. As with AD–SDAT a focal decrease had to be seen in at least two regions of each hemisphere and the flow abnormality should be generally symmetrical, smooth, and with gradual changes from focal disturbance to better perfused regions. Typical changes in a single case of PD are shown in Fig. 10.8.

The criteria for MID were the occurrence of right–left asymmetries and spotty and irregular focal flow abnormalities. An asymmetry of more than 5% for the hemispheric averages and more than 10% for homologous regional values was considered to be pathological (Prohovnik et al., 1980). At least two regions of each hemisphere had to show this type of pathology. A typical case of MID is shown in Fig. 10.9.

The definite diagnosis based on the neuropathological investigation (made by Dr. Arne Brun, Department of Pathology, University of Lund) has been obtained in 38 out of 44 deceased patients. In Fig. 10.10., the rCBF diagnosis made according to the criteria which have been described, and the diagnosis by autopsy

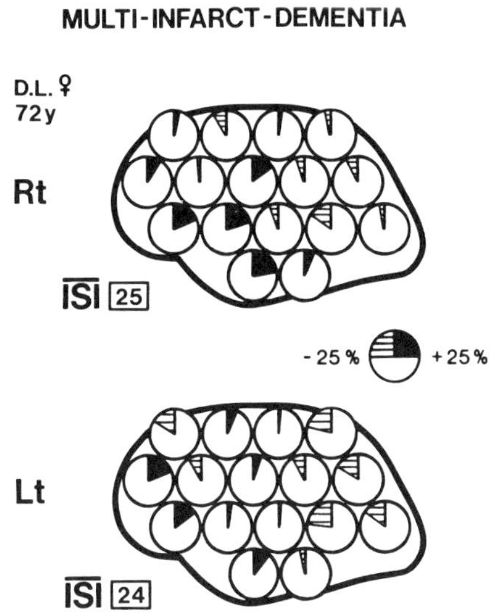

FIGURE 10.9. Results from a rCBF study in a case of multi-infarct dementia (verified at autopsy). Symbols as in Fig. 10.2. Note the asymmetrical and spotty flow abnormalities.

are compared. There are only four disagreements. Correct diagnosis by rCBF was thus achieved in about 90% of the patients. Two of the four erroneously classified patients belonged to the AD–SDAT groups according to autopsy, but the rCBF data suggested a diagnosis of MID. However, in these cases autopsy did show evidence of cerebrovascular disease in addition to pathology of Alzheimer type. Two cases of MID were misdiagnosed as AD and SDAT.

Comments

The results presented are in agreement with previous findings of a global CBF decrease with marked and systematic regional accentuations cited in the intro-

rCBF-diagnosis

Neuropathol.-diagnosis	AD	SDAT	PD	MID
AD	7			1
SDAT		10		1
PD			6	
MID	1	1		11

FIGURE 10.10. Neuropathological diagnosis compared with diagnosis by rCBF in 38 deceased patients. Abbreviations as in Fig. 10.6.

duction. The patterns of flow decreases demonstrated are also in good agreement with the patterns of accentuated atrophy of the superficial cortical layers found in recent neuropathological investigations (Brun & Englund, 1981; Brun & Gustafson, 1976; Gustafson et al., 1977; Ingvar et al., 1978).

No previous study has, however, shown the correspondence between the diagnosis by autopsy and rCBF diagnosis for a group of patients of the present size. The agreement must be considered satisfactory. However, it has to be pointed out that the rCBF data utilized were quite optimal. In many patients serial data were available throughout the progression of the disease and in most patients results from a rather advanced stage of the disease close in time to the death of the patient were available. Many of the rCBF results were thus grossly abnormal and easy to interpret. In early stages of the diseases, the rCBF changes will be more subtle and errors in the interpretation will occur to a larger extent. The clinical usefulness of rCBF for diagnosis of the very early stages of organic dementia will be the subject of further research by our group.

The relatively large number of patients (n = 22) with presumed or verified PD might be surprising since it is considered to be a rare disorder. The large material is due to the fact that we have been actively searching for patients with dementia dominated by symptoms of frontal lobe dysfunction within a fairly large region of southern Sweden. Patients with PD are thus overrepresented in our material. There are also indications of a geographical variation of dementia of the Pick type with relatively higher frequency in some regions of the Scandinavian countries (Sjögren, Sjögren, & Lindgren, 1952). The lower frequency in other countries, e.g., the United States, might also be due to misdiagnosis.

The present results demonstrate the validity of using rCBF for differential diagnosis between the major organic dementia disorders. This points to a role for the method as a part of the routine battery of investigations used in the often difficult clinical evaluation of patients displaying symptoms of dementia. We will now review findings regarding some other psychiatric disorders, which also might involve symptoms of dementia, before discussing the general clinical potential of rCBF measurements in psychiatry.

AFFECTIVE DISEASE

Fairly few studies of rCBF have been made in patients with manic or depressive disorders. The first observations were made by Wilson, Schieve, and Scheinberg (1952), who utilized the Kety–Schmidt technique in a study of 10 depressed patients. Normal CBF and metabolic values were reported. No studies of affective disorders using intra-arterial ^{133}Xe injection technique have been reported. Three studies of depression utilizing the inhalation technique have, however, been published. Mathew et al. (1980) reported a mean CBF level for 13 depressed patients, which was somewhat lower than for a matched control group. The mean gray-matter flow value, 75 ± 11 ml/100 g/min can, however, not be considered to be a pathologically low value since several studies of healthy subjects of similar age have reported values in this range (Blauenstein, Halsey, Wilson, Wills, & Risberg, 1977; Obrist et al., 1975; Prohovnik et al., 1980). Gur et al. (1984) recently reported normal mean CBF levels and regional flow patterns in 14 medicated unipolar depressives during resting conditions. These findings are in good agreement with the results from our series. We have not found any consistent differences between depressed patients, manic patients, and normal control subjects when the effects of age, arterial pCO_2 and medication have been corrected for (Gustafson, Risberg, & Silfverskiöld, 1981; Silfverskiöld, Gustafson, Johanson, & Risberg, 1979; Silfverskiöld, Gustafson, & Risberg, 1984a). Recent results from our study are shown in Fig. 10.11. Both patient groups had no or very little medication and were fairly close in age to the normal reference group. To be included in the manic group the patients had to show at least two of the following symptoms: elated mood, flight of ideas, reduced need for sleep, and hyperactivity. No patients with chronic psychosis, addiction, or significant neurological defects were included. The depressed group was studied before treatment with ECT and displayed depressive symptoms with risk of suicide, nutritional problems, and severe psychomotor retardation.

It is evident from the figure that the rCBF results are very similar in the three groups regarding mean flow levels and regional flow patterns. Normal rCBF results are seen also in the subgroup of depressed patients who display symptoms of pseudodementia. This is an important observation which opens a possibility of using rCBF for different diagnosis between pseudodementia and organic dementia. This is discussed in more detail later.

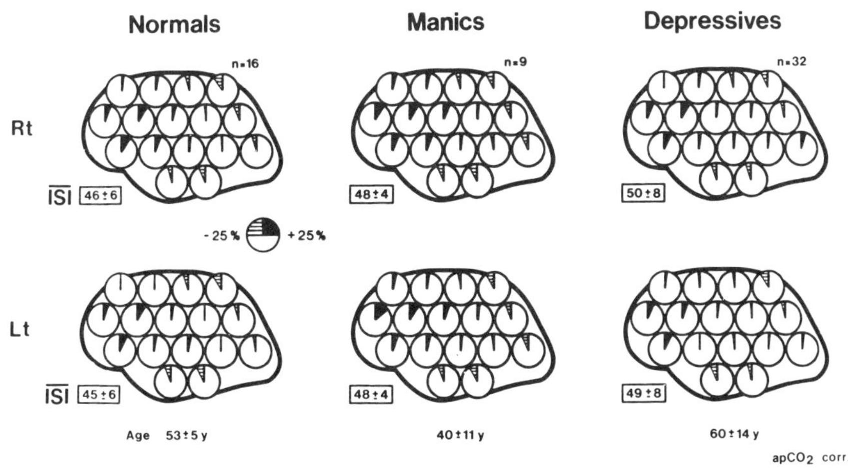

10.11. Comparison of rCBF in manic patients, depressed patients, and normal subjects. Symbols as in Fig. 10.2. None of the differences was statistically significant.

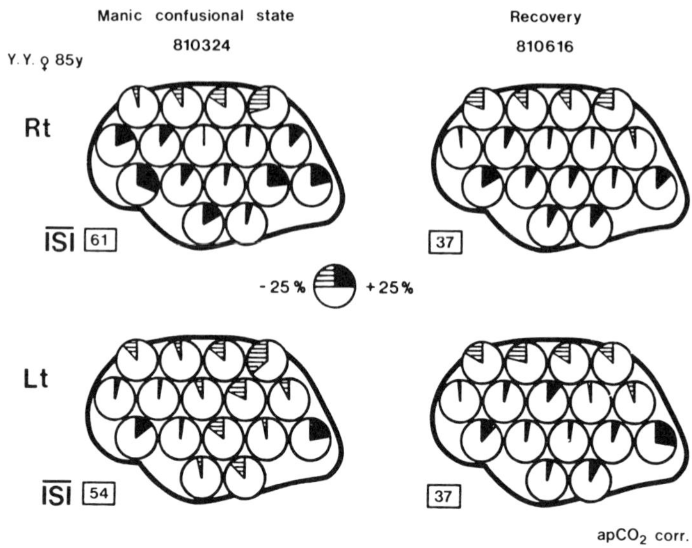

FIGURE 10.12. Repeated rCBF measurements in a case of manic confusion. Symbols as in Fig. 10.2. The patient had for the last 25 years suffered from recurrent manic-like episodes with elated mood, hyperactivity, continuous singing or talking, and reduced sleep. rCBF was measured at three of these episodes with consistent findings. In the manic confusional state the patient had an elevated flow level, especially in posterior and fronto-temporal regions of the right hemisphere. At recovery the flow level was slightly subnormal but symmetrical and without gross focal pathology. (Adapted from Silfverskiöld et al., 1984b.)

When examining the single patients with affective disease, it is evident that a small subgroup exists in which the affective disease is linked to an organic brain disease which also involves rCBF pathology (Silfverskiöld, Gustafson, & Risberg, 1984b). This pathology might be a pronounced but reversible hemispheric asymmetry of flow as is exemplified in the case illustrated in Fig. 10.12. This interesting subgroup of patients in which an affective disturbance is likely to be caused by an organic brain disease will be the subject of further research by our group.

SCHIZOPHRENIA

Brain function in schizophrenic patients has been studied by a variety of methods and with increasing interest during recent years. The first CBF study was published by Kety and collaborators (1948). Using the nitrous-oxide technique, they found a normal whole brain-blood flow. Hoyer and Oesterreich (1975) measured also global CBF and they demonstrated interesting relations between the flow level and the clinical picture. Patients with productive symptoms such as hallucinosis had an elevated level, while patients with nonproductive or negative symptoms such as inactivity had lower values than the normal controls.

The exploration of regional CBF in schizophrenia started with the work of Ingvar and Franzén (1974), who used the intra-arterial ^{133}Xe method. They demonstrated a normal mean hemispheric flow level in younger patients as well as in chronic patients with very long duration of the disease. In the latter group, a marked deviation from the normal flow distribution was found with relatively low frontal and high post-central flow values. (Franzén & Ingvar, 1975) The patients thus showed hypofrontality, in contrast to the normal hyperfrontal pattern (Prohovnik et al., 1980). The younger group with short duration of the disease showed only a tendency to a less hyperfrontal distribution compared to the controls. Interesting relations between symptomatology and rCBF distribution were also reported. Productive symptoms were correlated with high values in post-central regions while negative symptoms like inactivity and isolation were coupled to a pronounced hypofrontality.

Recent studies using the ^{133}Xe inhalation technique have given somewhat conflicting results. Mathew, Duncan, Weiman, and Barr (1982) and Ariel and collaborators (1983) reported somewhat lower mean values in schizophrenic patients compared with controls, but only the latter study reported relatively greater reduction in anterior areas. In contrast Mubrin, Knezević and Lazić (1982) and Gur et al. (1983) found no difference between schizophrenic patients and normal subjects regarding the mean flow level. Mubrin and collaborators reported hypofrontality in the elderly of the schizophrenics while Gur and collaborators could not find any differences between patients and normals regarding flow pattern during resting. The latter authors did, however, report interesting differences between the groups when activation procedures were applied. These findings are reviewed in another chapter of the present volume (Maximilian & Brawanski, 1987).

Fig. 10.13 shows preliminary findings from an ongoing study by our group (Warkentin et al., 1984). The study involves patients with acute schizophrenia and schizo-affective (cycloid) psychosis, which are studied at admission, during treatment, and at discharge. These groups are compared with chronic schizophrenic patients and with normal age- and sex-matched controls. There were no significant differences in mean flow level between the schizophrenic patients and the controls. (The lower value for the chronic schizophrenic patients is within the normal range for this age; Hagstadius & Risberg, 1983.) A marked hypofrontality and hyperposteriority was seen in the chronic schizophrenic group, confirming the earlier findings by Ingvar and Franzén (1974). For the acutely ill group only a tendency to less marked hyperfrontality compared with the normals was noticed. Fig. 10.14 shows changes of the hyperfrontality (frontal values as a percentage of the hemispheric mean) from admission to discharge.

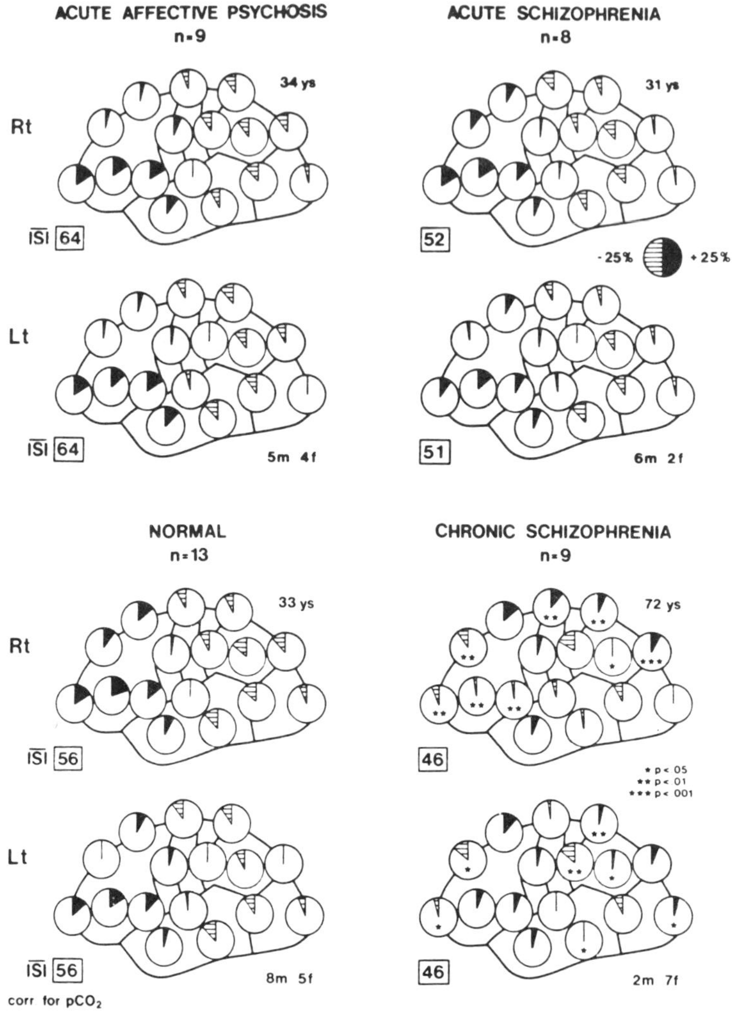

FIGURE 10.13. Preliminary results from rCBF measurements in acute and chronic psychosis. Patients with acute schizo-affective (cycloid) psychosis and acute schizophrenia are compared to normal age- and sex-matched controls and to patients with chronic schizophrenia (average 20 years of illness). The detectors were placed in a helmet and the .5 −1.5 min ISI was used. Symbols as in Fig. 10.2 except that 180° in the clock symbols indicates a 25% difference from the hemispheric mean. (Adapted from Warkentin et al., 1984.)

FRONTAL PERCENT (ISI)

		Affective Psychosis n=9	Schizophrenia n=8	Normal n=13	Cnronic Schizophrenia n=9
Admission	Right	106 ±3.2	106 ±1.8	107 ±1.7	100 ±4.6
	Left	105 ±3.4	104 ±2.9	105 ±2.9	101 ±5.2
Discharge	Right	106 ±2.7	104 ±1.4		
	Left	105 ±2.2	105 ±1.8		

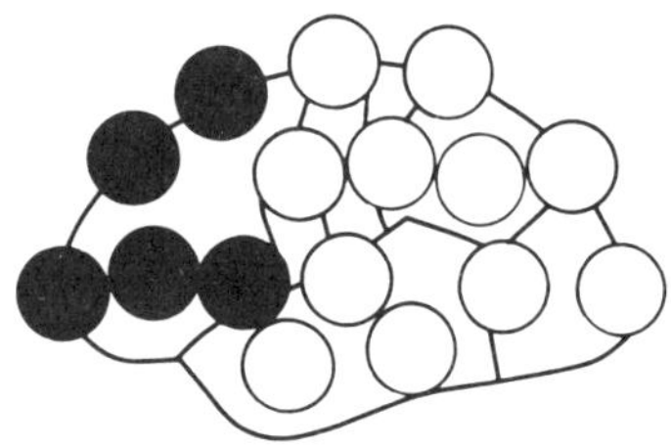

FIGURE 10.14. Frontal (black regions) percentage of the hemispheric mean in three psychotic groups and in a normal control group. Note the absence of hyperfrontality in the chronic group and the tendency to decrease of right frontal flow in the acute schizophrenic group at discharge. (Adapted from Warkentin et al., 1984.)

There is a tendency for the schizophrenic patients to show lower values in right frontal regions at discharge, compared with admission. This change is seen in parallel to a marked reduction of the psychotic symptoms following the treatment period. This indicates that the hypofrontality seen in some schizophrenic groups might be more related to the treatment of the disease by, e.g., neuroleptics, than to the disease itself. As a matter of fact, it has been demonstrated that haloperidol induces a hypofrontal flow pattern after 2 weeks of medication (Nilsson, Risberg, Johanson, & Gustafson, 1977).

It seems likely that the varying results reported by different groups are due to differences in the selection, clinical status, and medication of the patients studied. As Hoyer and Oesterreich (1975) demonstrated, the presence of productive symptomatology is linked to the flow level. Variations in symptomatology might thus explain why some groups find subnormal and other normal mean flow levels. The presence or absence of hypofrontality might also be linked to the symptoms displayed by the patients but seems also to be heavily influenced by the duration of the disease including treatment. It is obvious that further research is needed in this area.

THE CLINICAL USEFULNESS OF rCBF IN PSYCHIATRY

Findings regarding rCBF in some major psychiatric disorders have been reviewed. Several consistent observations of specific rCBF abnormalities have been made, e.g., in Alzheimer's disease. In addition to the scientific value of studying rCBF in these disorders, a routine clinical use of the method as an aid in the diagnostic and therapeutic work seems possible. When evaluating the rCBF method for such a clinical application, some general conditions which need to be met might be listed (Risberg & Gustafson, 1983):

1. The method has to provide valid and reliable information.
2. This information must be relevant for the care of the patient.
3. The hazards and discomfort for the patient, and the cost for obtaining the data, must be in balance with the clinical gain to be realized.
4. Similar information should not be obtainable with a less costly or hazardous technique.
5. The measurement procedure, and interpretation of results, must be reproducibly standardized.

Concerning the first condition there is today no doubt that brain-blood flow is realiably recorded by the modern noninvasive methods. It is obvious from data presented in this and other chapters of the present volume, that its precision and reproducibility is excellent (and generally superior to functional measures based on tomography).

The rCBF data are definitely of relevance for the care and treatment of the patient, especially if symptoms of dementia are present. Presence of the easily recognizable rCBF pathologies of AD–SDAT or PD might be information of crucial importance, as well as the finding of normal rCBF pointing to psychogenic, often treatable, factors (e.g., pseudodementia due to depression). Patients with diffuse encephalopathy, caused by, e.g., toxic agents such as alcohol and organic solvents, will have a diffuse decrease of rCBF without pronounced focal pathology (Berglund, 1981; Berglund & Risberg, 1981; Risberg & Hagstadius, 1983). It is of clinical importance to differentiate this group from other patients with sometimes similar symptoms which, however, are caused by a degenerative or vascular organic dementia disorder.

With present efforts to develop efficient therapies for the organic dementia disorders, an early and correct clinical diagnosis will become increasingly important in the future. In the present search for such therapeutic methods the rCBF method provides a valuable tool for the evaluation of the efficiency of the treatments, e.g., enhancement of cholinergic functions in Alzheimer's disease.

In psychiatric patients without symptoms of dementia, the clinical value of rCBF is more open to discussion. Further knowledge about the background of the rCBF changes in schizophrenia and other psychotic states might, however, make it possible to use the data for differential diagnosis and decisions about therapy. In affective disorders, the rCBF data might be of interest for diagnosing the subgroup of patients where the affective symptoms are likely to be caused by an organic brain disturbance (Fig. 10.12; Silfverskiöld et al., 1984b). Some data also indicate a possible usefulness of rCBF data for selection of patients for treatment by ECT and for elucidating the cortical changes caused by this type of therapy (Johanson, Risberg, Silfverskiöld, & Gustafson, 1979; Silfverskiöld et al., 1984a). Another area where the rCBF data are of potential clinical interest is the evaluation of confusional states in elderly patients. Our results indicate that organic (often cerebrovascular) and psychogenic factors interfere in a complex way in these patients.

The third condition on the list, which concerns the relationship between hazards, discomfort, and cost and the clinical gain, is certainly fulfilled by the method. The radiation risks can in practice be disregarded and everyone with practical experience of the noninvasive rCBF methods knows that the patient experiences very little discomfort. Provided the rCBF lab is being run in an efficient and regular way, the cost for a study can easily be kept at $100 or less. This is really a very low price for an investigation providing so crucial information. There is at present no less costly or hazardous method which can provide this information. There are, however, problems with the standardization of the measurement procedure, flow calculations and interpretation of the results. Hopefully, the present volume will provide a significant improvement on these points.

Ongoing methodological development will without doubt further increase the clinical and scientific value of the technique. The benefits obtained by improving the spatial resolution to about 1 cm are at present being explored in our laboratory with very positive results (Risberg & Hagstadius, 1984). Another chapter of this volume (Maximilian & Brawanski, 1987) describes rCBF changes seen in conjunction with different activation procedures. The present chapter has mainly been based on data from studies during the resting state. The addition of rCBF data from properly selected activation situations will add information of importance for the evaluation of brain function and dysfunction.

ACKNOWLEDGMENTS

This chapter was supported by the Swedish Medical Research Council (Projects 4969, 3950 and 4803), the Swedish Council for Humanistic and Social Science Research, the King Gustaf V and Queen Victoria's Foundation and the Thuring Foundation. The authors are indebted to Helena Fernö and Siv Karlson for preparation of the illustrations and to Maria Regnér for typing the manuscript.

REFERENCES

Ariel, R. N., Golden, C. J., Berg, R. A., Quaife, M. A., Dirksen, J. W., Forsell, T., Wilson, J., & Graber, B. (1983). Regional cerebral blood flow in schizophrenics. *Archives of General Psychiatry, 40,* 258–263.

Berglund, M. (1981). Cerebral blood flow in chronic alcoholics. *Alcoholism: Clinical and Experimental Research, 5,* 295–303.

Berglund, M., & Risberg, J. (1981). Regional cerebral blood flow during alcohol withdrawal. *Archives of General Psychiatry, 38,* 351–355.

Blauenstein, U. W., Halsey, J. H., Wilson, E. M., Wills, E. L., & Risberg, J. (1977). ^{133}Xenon inhalation method, analysis of reproducibility: Some of its physiological implications. *Stroke, 8,* 92–102.

Brun, A., & Englund, A. (1981). Regional pattern of degeneration in Alzheimer's disease: Neuronal loss and histopathological grading. *Histopathology, 5,* 549–564.

Brun, A., & Gustafson, L. (1970). Distribution of cerebral degeneration in Alzheimer's disease. *Archiv für Psychiatrie und Nervenkrankheiten, 223,* 15–33.

Frackowiak, R. S. J., Pozzilli, C., Legg, N. J., Du Boulay, G. H., Marshall, J., Lenzi, G. L., & Jones, T. (1981). Regional cerebral oxygen supply and utilization in dementia: A clinical and physiological study with oxygen-15 and positron tomography. *Brain, 104,* 753–778.

Franzén, G., & Ingvar, D. H. (1975). Abnormal distribution of cerebral activity in chronic schizophrenia. *Journal of Psychiatric Research, 12,* 199–214.

Freyhan, F. A., Woodford, R. B., & Kety, S. S. (1951). Cerebral blood flow and metabolism in psychoses of senility. *Journal of Nervous and Mental Disease, 113,* 449–459.

Gur, R. E., Skolnick, B. E., Gur, R. C., Caroff, S., Rieger, W., Obrist, W. D., Younkin, D., & Reivich, M. (1983). Brain function in psychiatric disorders. I. Regional cerebral blood flow in medicated schizophrenics. *Archives of General Psychiatry, 40,* 1250–1254.

———. (1984). Brain function in psychiatric disorders. II. Regional cerebral blood flow in medicated unipolar depressives. *Archives of General Psychiatry, 41,* 695–699.

Gustafson, L., Brun, A., & Ingvar, D. H. (1977). Presenile dementia: Clinical symptoms, pathoanatomical findings and cerebral blood flow: In J. S. Meyer, H. Lechner, & M. Reivich (Eds.). *Cerebral vascular disease* (pp. 5–9). Amsterdam: Excerpta Medica.

Gustafson, L., & Nilsson, L. (1983). Differential diagnosis of presenile dementia on clinical grounds. *Acta Psychiatrica Scandinavica, 65,* 194–209.

Gustafson, L., & Risberg, J. (1974). Regional cerebral blood flow related to psychiatric symptoms in dementia with onset in the presenile period. *Acta Psychicatrica Scandinavica, 50,* 516–538.

———. (1979). Regional cerebral blood flow measurements by the ^{133}Xe inhalation technique in differential diagnosis of dementia. *Acta Neurologica Scandinavica, 60*(Suppl. 72), 546–547.

Gustafson, L., Risberg, J., & Silfverskiöld, P. (1981). Cerebral blood flow in dementia and depression. *Lancet, 1,* p. 275.

Hachinski, V. D., Illif, L. D., Zilkha, E., Du Boulay, G. H., McAllister, V. L., Marshall, J., Ross Russel, R. W., & Symon, L. (1975). Cerebral blood flow in dementia. *Archives of Neurology, 32,* 632–637.

Hagberg, B., & Ingvar, D. H. (1976). Cognitive reduction in presenile dementia related to regional abnormalities in the cerebral blood flow. *British Journal of Psychiatry, 128,* 209–222.

Hagstadius, S., & Risberg, J. (1983). The effects of normal aging on the rCBF during resting and functional activation. *rCBF Bulletin, 6,* 116–120.

Hoyer, S., & Oesterreich, K. (1975). Blood flow and oxidative metabolism of the brain in patients with schizophrenia. *Psychiatria Clinica, 8,* 304–313.

Ingvar, D. H., Brun, A., Hagberg, B., & Gustafson, L. (1978). Regional cerebral blood flow in the dominant hemisphere in confirmed cases of Alzheimer's disease, Pick's disease and multi-infarct dementia: Relationship to clinical symptomatology and neuropathological findings. In R. Katzman, R. D. Terry, & K. L. Bick (Eds.). *Alzheimer's disease, senile dementia and related disorders of aging* (Vol. 7). New York: Raven Press.

Ingvar, D. H., & Franzén, G. (1974). Abnormalities of cerebral blood flow distribution in patients with chronic schizophrenia. *Acta Psychiatrica Scandinavica, 50,* 425–462.

Ingvar, D. H., & Gustafson, L. (1970). Regional cerebral blood flow in organic dementia with early onset. *Acta Neurologica Scandinavica, 46*(Suppl. 43), 42–73.

Johanson, M., Risberg, J., Silfverskiöld, P., & Gustafson, L. (1979). Regional cerebral blood flow related to acute memory disturbance following electroconvulsive therapy in depression. *Acta Neurologica Scandinavica, 60*(Suppl. 72), 534–535.

Kety, S. S., Woodford, R. B., Harmel, M. H., Freyhan, F. A., Appel, K. E., & Schmidt, C. F. (1948). Cerebral blood flow and metabolism in schizophrenia. *American Journal of Psychiatry, 104,* 765–770.

Kiloh, L. G. (1961). Pseudodementia. *Acta Psychiatrica Scandinavica,* (Suppl. 37), 336–351.

Lassen, N. A., Feinberg, I., & Lane, M. H. (1960). Bilateral studies of cerebral oxygen uptake in young and aged normal subjects and in patients with organic dementia. *Journal of Clinical Investigation, 39,* 491–500.

Lassen, N. A., Munck, O., & Tottey, E. R. (1957). Mental function and cerebral oxygen consumption in organic dementia. *Archives of Neurology and Psychiatry, 77,* 126–133.

Lavy, S., Melamed, E., Bentin, S., Cooper, G., & Rinot, Y. (1978). Bihemispheric decreases of regional cerebral blood flow in dementia: Correlation with age matched controls. *Annals of Neurology, 4,* 445–450.

Mathew, R. J., Duncan, G. C., Weiman, M. L., & Barr, D. L. (1982). Regional cerebral blood flow in schizophrenia. *Archives of General Psychiatry, 39,* 1121–1124.

Mathew, R. J., Meyer, J. S., Francis, D. J., Semchuk, K. M., Mortel, K., & Claghorn, J. L. (1980). Cerebral blood flow in depression. *American Journal of Psychiatry, 137,* 1449–1450.

Maximilian, V. A., & Brawanski, A. (1987). Neurofunctional and vascular challenge procedures during non-invasive rCBF measurements. (this volume).

Mubrin, Z., Knezević, S., & Lazić, L. (1982). Regional cerebral blood flow patterns in schizophrenic patients. A preliminary report. *rCBF Bulletin, 3.*

Munck, O., & Lassen, N. A. (1957). Bilateral cerebral blood flow and O_2 consumption in man by use of krypton 85. *Circulation Research, 5,* 163–168.

Nilsson, A., Risberg, J., Johanson, M., & Gustafson, L. (1977). Regional changes of cerebral blood flow during haloperidol therapy in patients with paranoid symptoms. *Acta Neurologica Scandinavica, 56*(Suppl. 64), 478–479.

Obrist, W. D., Chivian, E., Cronqvist, S., & Ingvar, D. H. (1970). Regional cerebral blood flow in senile and presenile dementia. *Neurology, 20,* 315–322.

Obrist, W. D., Thompson, H. K., King, C. H., & Wang, H. S. (1967). Determination of regional cerebral blood flow by inhalation of 133 xenon. *Circulation Research, 20,* 124–135.

Obrist, W. D., Thompson, H. K., Wang, H. S., & Wilkinson, W. E. (1975). Regional cerebral blood flow estimated by 133-xenon inhalation. *Stroke, 6,* 245–256.

Perez, F., Mathew, N. T., Stump, D. A., & Meyer, J. S. (1977). Regional cerebral blood flow, statistical patterns and psychological performance in multi-infarct dementia and Alzheimer's disease. *Canadian Journal of Neurological Sciences, 4,* 53–62.

Prohovnik, I., Håkansson, K., & Risberg, J. (1980). Observations on the functional significance of regional cerebral blood flow in "resting" normal subjects. *Neuropsychologia, 18,* 203–217.

Risberg, J. (1980). Regional cerebral blood flow measurements by ^{133}Xe-inhalation: methodology and applications in neuropsychology and psychiatry. *Brain and Language, 9,* 9–34.

Risberg, J., Ali, Z., Wilson, E. M., Wills, E. L., & Halsey, J. H. (1975). Regional cerebral blood flow by ^{133}xenon inhalation. Preliminary evaluation of an initial slope index in patients with unstable flow compartments. *Stroke, 6,* 142–148.

Risberg, J., & Gustafson, L. (1983). 133-Xe cerebral blood flow in dementia and in neuropsychiatry research: In P. L. Magistretti (Ed.). *Functional radionuclide imaging of the brain* (pp. 151–159). New York: Raven Press.

Risberg, J., & Hagstadius, S. (1983). Effects on the regional cerebral blood flow of long-term exposure to organic solvents. *Acta Psychiatrica Scandinavica, 67*(Suppl. 303), 92–99.

———. (1984). *Pilot experiments with high-resolution rCBF-technique.* Paper presented at the second Nordic meeting in Neuropsychology, Lund, Sweden.

Silfverskiöld, P., Gustafson, L., Johanson, M., & Risberg, J. (1979). Regional cerebral blood flow related to the effect of electroconvulsive therapy in depression. In J. Obiols, C. Ballús, E. Gonzalez, et al. (Eds.). *Biological psychiatry today* (pp. 1178–1183). Amsterdam: Elsevier.

Silfverskiöld, P., Gustafson, L., & Risberg, J. (1984a). Changes in regional cerebral blood flow during ECT. In B. Lerer, R. D. Weiner, & R. H. Belmaker (Eds.). *ECT: Basic mechanisms* (pp. 124–131). London: John Libbey.

———. (1984b). rCBF changes following seizures in two cases of organic affective syndrome. In M. Baldy-Mouliner, D. H. Ingvar, & B. S. Meldrum (Eds.). *Cerebral blood flow, metabolism and epilepsy* (pp. 39–43). London: John Libbey.

Simard, D., Olesen, J., Paulsen, O. B., Lassen, N. A., & Skinhøj, E. (1971). Regional cerebral blood flow and its regulation in dementia. *Brain, 94,* 273–288.

Sjögren, T., Sjögren, H., & Lindgren, A. G. H. (1952). *Morbus Alzheimer and Morbus Pick. A genetic, clinical and pathoanatomical study.* Copenhagen: Munksgaard.

Tachibana, H., Meyer, J. S., Kitagawa, Y., Rogers, R. L., Okayasu, H., & Mortel, K. F. (1984). Effects of aging on cerebral blood flow in dementia. *Journal of the American Geriatrics Society, 32,* 114–120.

Warkentin, S., Nilsson, A., Karlson, S., Flekkøy, K., Franzén, G., Gustafson, L., & Risberg, J. (1984). *Regional cerebral blood flow in schizophrenia and affective psychosis.* Paper presented at the second Nordic meeting in Neuropsychology, Lund, Sweden.

Wilson, W. P., Schieve, J. F., & Scheinberg, P. (1952). Effects of series of electric shock treatments on cerebral blood flow and metabolism. *Archives of Neurology and Psychiatry,* 68, 651–654.

Yamaguchi, F., Meyer, J. S., Yamamoto, M., Sakai, F., & Shaw, T. (1980). Noninvasive regional cerebral blood flow measurements in dementia. *Archives of Neurology, 37,* 410–418.

11 Cerebral Blood Flow in Infants and Children

Gorm Greisen
Department of Neonatology, Rigshospitalet, Copenhagen, Denmark

INTRODUCTION

During the last 10 years CBF in newborns has received considerable attention because important cerebrovascular pathology is seen in this period. The methods used for the study of CBF in newborn infants do not, however, match the clinical needs. A review is presented of studies of regulation of CBF, of CBF in various disease states, and of CBF in normal newborn infants. The available results are limited and often conflicting. Only a few studies of CBF in older children are available, but the methods used have been more conventional. It appears that resting CBF in children is about one-third higher than in adults, and that CBF is decreased in states of chronically impaired neural function.

The Newborn Period

Obstetrical and neonatal care have become more intensive and birth weight specific survival rates have improved uniformly during the last decades. The quality of survival is, therefore, of much concern and it is linked closely to neurodevelopmental outcome. The dominant perinatal brain pathology is vascular in origin: cerebral hemorrhage and ischemic/hypoxic encephalopathy (Pape & Wigglesworth, 1979).

Only a small portion of mental retardation or cerebral palsy in childhood is likely to originate in the perinatal period. In very low birth-weight infants, however, cerebral hemorrhage may occur in one of two cases. In survivors, severe neurodevelopmental handicap may be present in 10% (Stewart, Reynolds,

& Lipcomb, 1981), while as many as 50% may perform badly in school (Lloyd, 1984).

The immature brain is comparatively resistant to ischemic/hypoxic insult (Kjellmar, Karlsson, Olsson, & Rosen, 1974). Major asphyxia, hypotension, or hypoxia can usually be avoided during delivery and the immediate postnatal period. To explain the frequency of perinatal brain damage it has, therefore, been suggested that CBF regulation is less competent, compared with later in life (Wigglesworth & Pape, 1978).

In experimental newborn animals, resting CBF is lower than in adults of the same species; the more immature the animal is at birth, the lower the CBF (Vanucci & Hernandez, 1980). This low CBF corresponds to a low oxygen uptake (Hernandez, Brennan, Vanucci, & Bowman, 1978). Perfusion pressure/flow autoregulation has been demonstrated in fetal lambs (Tweed, Cote, Pash, & Lou, 1983), and in newborn puppies (Hernandez, Brennan, & Bowman, 1980). The range of autoregulation is adapted to the prevailing arterial blood pressure, but appears to be narrow, compared with adult animals and in fetal lamb it was interrupted by quite mild hypoxic stress (Tweed et al., 1983). The effect of CO_2 on the immature CBF has been suggested to be less marked, compared with the effect on adult CBF (Vanucci et al., 1980), and less marked in telencephalon, compared with the phylogenetically older diencephalon and rhombencephalon (Blomstrand, Karlsson, & Kjellmar, 1978). The effects of asphyxia (hypoxia, hypercarbia, acidosis, and hypotension) on the perinatal brain are complex, depending on the interaction of several protective mechanisms (Hernandez et al., 1981; Tweed et al., 1982). These mechanisms may be disrupted by prolonged partial asphyxia, resulting in decreasing CBF (Reivich, Brann, Shapiro, & Myers, 1971).

Clinical Research. Several methods for the estimation of CBF in human infants have been tried; some are special to newborns, others have been adapted, differences to their use from that in adults are briefly discussed.

The use of venous occlusion strain gauge plethysmography for measurement of CBF in human infants was reported by Cross et al. (1979). The compliance of the neonatal skull means that compression of the jugular veins results in an increase in cranial circumference. A measurement is taken as the mean of 3 to 10 manual bilateral compressions, each one lasting a few seconds. The infant must be quiet during the measurement. The validity depends on the correctness of the assumed relationship between head circumference and brain volume, on indirect estimation of vertebral flow, and on insignificance of extracranial flow. The result is an estimate of global CBF expressed in ml/100 g/min. The technique has not been validated, in humans or in experimental animals. The risks of the method relate to the increased cerebrovenous pressure, which, however, is probably less than that produced by the infant's own straining or crying.

Electrical impedance plethysmography has been used in adults and adapted for use in newborns. The transcephalic impedance, as measured by applying a small alternating current, is slightly pulsatile. The pulsatile waveform results from oppositely directed pulse-synchronous changes in cerebral blood volume, cranial volume, and displacement of cerebrospinal fluid. Several different indexes can be calculated from the waveform; for use in newborns there has been no attempt to estimate absolute values of CBF. This technique is very well suited for long-term monitoring. It has recently been compared with venous occlusion plethysmography and was judged to be as good (Costeloe, Smyth, Myrdoch, Rolfe, & Tizard, 1984). The method has only theoretical risks which are related to the small electrical currents used.

Study of cerebral circulation in the human newborn infant by Doppler ultrasound was first reported by Bada, Hajjar, Chua, and Sumner in 1980. Since then, a considerable number of studies have been published. The flow velocity in the anterior cerebral artery can be studied through the open anterior fontanel, or the carotids can be studied as in adults. Several indexes of cerebrovascular resistance and CBF can be calculated from the flow waveforms, but there has been no attempts to calculate absolute values of CBF. The Pourcelot pulsatility index (systolic flow velocity minus diastolic flow velocity, divided by systolic flow velocity), which is an index of cerebrovascular resistance has been mostly used. The validity of this pulsatility index has been questioned on theoretical gounds (Bejar, Merritt, Coen, Manning, & Gluck, 1982) and by animal studies (Batton, Hellman, Hernandez, & Maisels, 1983; Hansen, Stonestreet, Rosenkranz, & Oh, 1983). The validity of the indexes of CBF depends on the signal's being received from a single, straight, nondividing vessel, on the correctness of analysis of the received frequency shifts, on the knowledge of the angle between the ultrasound beam and the vessel under study, and on the knowledge of the relationship between arterial cross-sectional area and brain weight. We have found correlation coefficients between various Doppler ultrasound indexes and ^{133}Xenon clearance ranging from 0.41 to 0.82 (Greisen et al., 1984b). The method can potentially provide information on very fast or very brief changes in CBF. No side-effects of Doppler ultrasound in clinical use have, as yet, been demonstrated (NCRP, 1983).

The use of ^{133}Xenon clearance was first reported by Lou, Lassen, and Friis–Hansen in 1979. 0.5 mCi ^{133}Xenon was injected in the innominate artery, in the left common carotid artery or in the aortic arch during clinically indicated umbilical artery catherization. The slope from 15 to 60 sec after injection, multiplied by a partition coefficient of 0.8, was interpreted as gray-matter flow. Compared with the intracarotid technique used in adults, injection proximal to the internal carotid artery introduces the problems of recirculation and contribution to the countrates from extracranial tissues or from the airways. The applicability of this method is limited by its invasiveness.

Less invasive methods are now available. Ment et al. (1981) used a gamma camera to record the clearance of ^{133}Xenon, following 2 min of inhalation, from the head and chest. They used the chest clearance to generate a deconvoluted head curve, on which a slope was computed from 30 to 150 sec after inhalation. An intravenous injection method with external monitoring of the lung has been used by Younkin, Reivich, Jaggi, Obrist, and Delivoria–Papadopoulos (1982), and by ourselves (Greisen, 1984; Greisen et al., 1984a). With this technique, the problems of fitting a tight mask to an uncooperative infant and of sampling from the very small respiratory volume are avoided. The chest curves were corrected for chest wall contribution, the cranial clearance curves were analyzed according to the two-compartmental model and estimates of global CBF were obtained.

Compared with its use in adults, ^{133}Xe clearance in infants presents a number of problems. These are related mainly to the small physical dimensions, to the modest cortical representation in the clearance curves, and to frequent right-to-left shunting of blood past the lungs (Greisen et al., 1984a). On the other hand, we found that the Xenon blood–brain partition coefficient for newborn brain is identical for gray and white matter, and does not vary significantly with gestational age (Greisen, 1984). Patient radiation is a more serious consideration, compared with adults, although the dose involved is not excessive: For the intravenous technique we found total body radiation to be 0.2 mGy (20 mRad), less than of a plain X-ray of the chest (Greisen, 1984).

The use of positron emission tomography (PET) in newborn infants using labeled water was first reported by Volpe, Herscovitch, Perlman, and Raichle (1983). The spatial resolution is of the order of a few cu cm and thus not sufficient for full discrimination of cortex and white matter. A practical shortcoming is that PET scanning requires transport of the infant to the stationary equipment. For infants under intensive care, transportation may present a greater risk than radiation. Whole-body radiation dose was found to be 0.6 mGy (63 mRem).

Recently, the use of Xenon enhanced computerized tomography was reported (Manwarring, Kodak, Tarby, Johnson, & Suess, 1984). The resolution is better than for PET, but the low blood–brain partition coefficient in newborns is a drawback.

In conclusion, no ideal method for measuring CBF in the newborn infant has been developed. It is, therefore, necessary to consider the suitability of each method for every specific research problem, in view of the validity, specific biases, practicality, and patient risks.

Regulation of CBF in the Human Newborn. As yet, there is no evidence that regulation in the newborn differs qualitatively from that in adults, but studies are few and may not provide a full picture.

Marked decrease in CBF has been found in healthy, full-term infants during deep sleep when studied by venous occlusion plethysmography (Rahilly, 1980). The reduction was 25% compared with REM sleep. In the same study, a further decrease of 34% was found for an hour following breast-feeding. Both findings have been replicated (Dear, 1980; Mukhtar et al., 1982).

Marked decrease of CBF in healthy, full-term (Rahilly, 1980), and preterm (Leahy, Cates, MacCallum, & Rigatto, 1980) infants breathing 100% oxygen was found by venous occlusion plethysmography, the decreases were 33% and 15%, respectively. This was supported in the study of six healthy, term infants comparing venous occlusion and electrical impedance plethysmography (Costeloe et al., 1984); the decreases were 15% and 19%.

CO_2 sensitivity was demonstrated by breathing 2% CO_2 in healthy term (Rahilly, 1980) by venous occlusion plethysmography. The increase in CBF was 40%. In the similar study of healthy, preterm infants (Leahy et al., 1980), the CO_2 response was 7.8% per torr increase in alveolar CO_2 tension. In the study of six healthy infants (Costeloe et al., 1984), comparing venous occlusion plethysmography and electrical impedance plethysmography, the results were 2.4% per torr and 4.5 per torr, respectively. In nine preterm infants receiving an intravenous bolus of theophylline for recurrent apnea, pCO_2 as well as mean flow velocity, measured by Doppler ultrasound decreased significantly (Rosenkranz & Oh, 1984). Decreased cerebrovascular resistance as indicated by decreased pulsatility index of Doppler flow velocity waveforms was found in hypercapnia in six ventilated preterm infants (Daven, Milstein, & Gutrie, 1983).

The presence of pressure flow autoregulation in newborn infants has been more controversial. In a study of 19 stressed infants shortly after birth using the intra-arterial ^{133}Xenon clearance method (Lou et al., 1979), a striking correlation was found between gray-matter flow and systolic blood pressure. In two infants studied twice, ^{133}Xenon clearance changed proportionately to spontaneous blood pressure changes. From these data it was suggested that autoregulation may easily be lost in stressed, newborn infants and that this loss may be crucial in the pathogenesis of perinatal brain damage (Lou, Lassen, Friis–Hansen, 1979). In a Doppler ultrasound study of 32 preterm infants with varying degrees of respiratory illness (Ahmann et al., 1983), 50% were found to have arterial mean flow velocity varying proportionally to spontaneous blood pressure changes of five torr or more; in the remainder, flow velocities were unchanged or varied inversely with blood pressure. The changes in velocities were unrelated to the degree of perinatal asphyxia, respiratory distress, or subsequent cerebral hemorrhage. CBF measured by venous occlusion plethysmography was found to increase markedly in five very preterm, ill infants, who were transfused with resulting blood pressure increase (Milligan, 1980). All these infants subsequently developed cerebral hemorrhage. No study has demonstrated the absence or presence of pressure flow autoregulation in healthy newborn infants, although several authors have commented on the possibility of blood pressure changes being responsible for the CBF changes ascribed to other factors (Dear, 1980; Mukhtar, et al., 1982; Rahilly, 1980; Sankaran, Peters, & Finer, 1981).

Thus, available data are insufficient in outlining the competence of CBF regulation during the stresses of labor, birth, and the neonatal period. Due to methodological limitations, most confidence can be put on observations supported by studies using different methods. Pressing questions are related to the influence of hypoxia, hypercarbia, and hypocarbia on the pressure flow autoregulation in ill, preterm infants at risk of subsequent neurodevelopmental handicap. Other questions are related to the competence of the metabolism flow coupling in these infants, in view of the frequency of paroxysma electrical activity.

Cerebral Blood Flow in Specific Illnesses. The common illnesses of preterm infants are related to immaturity of the lungs, cardiovascular system, kidney, gut, and brain. Intensive care including mechanical ventilation, volume expansion, fluid, and electrolyte management, and intravenous nutrition is often required.

Respiratory distress is a common denominator of such multiple system illness in pretern infants. We found global CBF to be only 12 ml/100 g/min in ventilated, pretern infants studied during the first week of life by intravenous ^{133}Xenon clearance (Greisen, 1986). This was compared with a global CBF of 20 ml/100 g/min in similar, nonventilated infants. Studies of ventilated infants by venous occlusion plethysmography have not suggested decreased CBF (Milligan, 1980, 1981). But support of low CBF in respiratory distress has been found by Doppler ultrasound, demonstrating a complete cessation of flow in the superior sinus during positive pressure inspiration (Cowan & Thoresen, 1987), a decreased mean flow velocity in ventilated as compared with nonventilated infants (Ellison, Horn, Brown & Denny, 1986), and a higher pulsatility index in the anterior cerebral artery, compared with the median cerebral artery in infants with respiratory distress (Drayton & Burns, 1983). It is not clear if CBF is reduced by the mechanical ventilation as such, as a part of the multisystem, low-flow disease or as the result of a reduced cerebral metabolic rate.

A very fluctuating cerebral blood-flow velocity pattern was found in 27 of 52 ventilated, preterm infants (Perlman, McMenamin, & Volpe, 1983). The pattern correlated tightly with fluctuating blood pressure waveform, which in turn presumably was due to uncoordinated breathing efforts. It was inferred that volume flow fluctuated. It is, however, also possible that these beat-to-beat variations in cerebro-arterial inflow were taken up by the capacitance of the arterial system itself. In any case, later cerebral hemorrhage was much less frequent in the infants showing a stable pattern.

Patency of the arterial ductus is common in preterm infants and often complicates respiratory distress. Several studies by Doppler ultrasound have demonstrated an increased cerebral arterial pulsatility index in the presence of a patent arterial ductus (Lipman, Sewer, & Brazy, 1982; Martin, Snider, Katz, Peabody, & Brady, 1982; Perlman, Hill, & Volpe, 1981; Wilcox et al., 1983). This has been interpreted as signifying increased cerebrovascular resistance. But as even arterial pulse pressure is increased this may not be valid (Bejar et al., 1982).

However, in one study, mean flow velocity was also decreased (Ellison & Denny, 1982).

Pneumothorax is a serious complication of respiratory distress; if treatment is delayed the intrathoracic pressure may be very elevated, resulting in significant disturbance of central hemodynamics. The pulsatility index of Doppler flow velocity waveforms was found to be reduced (Hill, Perlman, & Volpe, 1982). It was assumed that pressure flow autoregulation was lost and the reduced pulsatility index was interpreted as increased cerebral blood flow caused by a narrow pulse pressure and increased mean arterial blood pressure. Similar decreases in the pulsatility index, mainly due to increased diastolic flow velocity, was reported in neonatal seizures and during endotracheal suctioning (Perlman & Volpe, 1983). In all those cases, it remains possible that the changes in cerebral blood-flow velocity waveform mainly reflect the changed central hemodynamics and increased sympathetic system tone, and that there is little change in volume flow.

Reduced Doppler ultrasound stroke distance and peak systolic flow velocity as well as increased pulsatility index were found in 11 term, polycythemic, otherwise healthy newborn infants (Rosenkrantz & Oh, 1982). All three variables were normalized along with whole blood viscosity and hematocrit values after partial exchange transfusion with plasmanate. Mean arterial blood pressure dropped slightly. These findings were interpreted as reflecting a decreased cerebrovascular resistance and an increased CBF, either as a result of the normalized viscosity or of the normalized oxygen carrying capacity.

Cerebral hemorrhage of prematurity (often called germinal layer hemorrhage or subependymal/intraventicular hemorrhage) appears to be a rather specific entity, developing in the periventricular germinal matrix, usually over the head of the caudate nucleus. From here it may rupture into the ventricular system. It has been hypothesized that such hemorrhage is the result of hyperperfusion during arterial hypertension (Lou et al., 1979). Ment et al. (1981), using the ^{133}Xe inhalation technique, demonstrated that CBF was higher on the side of the larger or only hemorrhage in 4 out of 5 infants. In a subsequent study using the same method, a 50% reduction in CBF was demonstrated in infants with hemorrhage, compared with those infants who never developed hemorrhage (Ment et al., 1984). In those who did not have a hemorrhage at the time of the study, but developed hemorrhage later, CBF was reduced by 25%. Very low regional CBF was found by PET scanning in large areas surrounding intraparenchymal hemorrhages (Volpe et al., 1983). When the effect of ventilation was taken into account, using intravenous ^{133}Xenon clearance, we found that 9 infants with small hemorrhages had higher CBF, compared with 33 without (Greisen, 1986). The evidence obtained by Doppler ultrasound is equally contradictory (Bada et al., 1979; Bada et al., 1982; Perlman & Volpe, 1982) and it seems probable that our current pathophysiological concepts are too simplistic.

In severe posthemorrhagic progressive hydrocephalus, high pulsatility index by Doppler ultrasound was found by Hill and Volpe (1982). Low global CBF and particularly low parieto-occipital regional CBF has recently been demonstrated by Xenon enhanced CT scanning (Manwarring et al., 1984).

Birth asphyxia affects preterm as well as term infants, but is a more dominant cause of morbidity and mortality in the term infants. The CBF changes are likely to be complex, and to differ during acute asphyxia and the postasphyxic period. Bada et al. (1979) reported decreased pulsatility index as measured by Doppler ultrasound, reflecting decreased cerebrovascular resistance in 12 term infants requiring ventilation for resusitation after birth. In contrast, Sankaran, Peters, and Finer (1981) found CBF as estimated by venous occlusion plethysmography, decreased in 7 similarly asphyxiated, term infants. CBF was decreased on Days 2 and 4; on Day 6, CBF was no longer significantly lower than in the control group of infants. Differences in blood pressure were not considered to play a role.

Reference Values. As a consequence of methodological constraints, there are no commonly agreed upon reference values for human newborns. In 16 healthy, term infants, 2 to 8 days after birth, the mean CBF obtained by venous occlusion plethysmography was 40.1 ml/100 g/min (range (22–59, Cross et al., 1979). In 24 healthy preterm infants of 34 weeks gestation, 2 to 24 days after birth, mean CBF obtained by the same method was 32.5 ml/100 g/min (range 16–50, Leahy et al., 1980). Using intravenous ^{133}Xenon clearance in 15 healthy, neurologically normal infants of 31 weeks gestation, 3 to 57 days after birth (Younkin et al., 1982), mean global CBF was found to 28 ml/10 g/min +/− 9 SD (CBF extrapolated to infinity, recalculated using our neonatal partition coefficient (Greisen, 1984). Using a similar technique in 11 preterm infants without respiratory distress, 31 weeks gestational age, 0 to 5 days after birth, we found mean CBF to 19.8 ml/100 g/min +/− 5.3 SD (Greisen, 1984).

Apart from the methodological problems, it is clear from the foregoing discussion, that there are several biological factors which may contribute to the variance within "reference" materials and among them. Gestational age, postnatal age, state of sleep, timing of feeding, possible immobilization stress are all likely to influence resting CBF in healthy infants. During the first days of life, hematocrit is usually high and hemoglobin dissociation curve shifted to the left, although both may vary much. Rapid changes in pCO_2 associated with handling the infant before and during CBF measurement may further contribute to the variation in the results.

Clinical Practice. There is, at present, no place for the measurement of CBF in the management of ill newborn infants. Low CBF (Lou & Skov, 1979) and low as well as high CBF (Ment et al., 1983) shortly after birth have been associated with poor neurodevelopmental outcome but it remains to be demonstrated that manipulation of CBF can improve outcome. Alternatively, change of

CBF values will have to be correlated to brain function, brain metabolism, or known brain pathology.

Later Infancy and Childhood

Older infants and children rarely present with cerebrovascular disease, and when they do, the pathophysiology is presumably akin to that seen in adults. Only a few studies of CBF in this age group have been reported.

The N_2O Kety–Schmidt technique has been used in four studies using groups of control children. Garfunkel, Baird, and Siegler (1954) studied 16 children with minor neurological illness and developmental quotients above 60. The age was 3 to 72 months. Sedation by seconal, atropine, and morphine was used, supplemented by penthotal in the most restless infants. The mean value was 61 ml/100 g/min (range 44–71). In the next study (Kennedy & Sokoloff, 1957), 9 healthy children aged 3 to 11 years were kept cooperative by projecting moving pictures, CBF was 106 ml/100 g/min +/− 10 SD, compared with 60 ml/100 g/min +/− 9 SD in 9 young adult males. In a study of the effects of malnutrition on cerebral metabolism, CBF was 90.3 ml/100 g/min in 5 normal or slightly malnourished children, less than 40 months of age (Mehta, Kalsi, Nain, & Menkes, 1977). The children were not sedated and most required some restraint during the study. By use of N_2O desaturation curve during induction of anesthesia for elective surgery in 70 neurologically normal children aged 11 days to 15 years, CBF was found to be 65 ml/100 g/min +/− 17 SD. There was no correlation between CBF and age.

In nine normal, resting children aged 7–15 years, mean CBF was 71 ml/100 g/min (Lou, Henriksen, & Brun, 1984). CBF was calculated from a 2-cm thick slice positioned 5 cm above the orbito-meatal line obtained by emission computed tomography after ^{133}Xenon inhalation.

In summary, none of the studies can pretend to yield reference values for children; neither sedation, restraint, nor distraction is acceptable. A possible overall interpretation is that resting CBF is somewhat higher in children than in adults and that this difference is diminished during sedation and accentuated during activation. This interpretation is supported by the cerebral metabolic rates of oxygen measured in the four studies using the arteriovenous differences.

Decreased CBF was demonstrated in chronic neural dysfunctions in four of the studies. In 14 children with severe mental retardation (developmental quotient below 30), CBF was reduced by 40% compared with the controls (Garfunkel et al., 1954) and in severe protein-calorie malnutrition (weight below 50% of standard for age), CBF was reduced by 25%, compared with controls (Mehta et al., 1977). In the study of 13 children with severe dysphasia or attention deficit disorder (Lou et al., 1984), global CBF was not lower than in the controls, but regional relative hypoperfusion of perisylvian and frontal lobe white matter, corresponded well to the clinical symptoms. Finally, regional CBF was reported to be low, corresponding to the angiomatas of the Sturge–Weber syndrome (Riela et al., 1984).

REFERENCES

Ahmann, P. A., Dykes, F. D., Lazzara, A., Holt, P. J., Giddens, D. P., & Carrigan, T. S. (1983). Relationship between pressure passitivity and subbependymal/intraventricular hemorrhage as assessed by pulsed Doppler ultrasound. *Pediatrics, 72,* 665–669.

Bada, H. S., Hajjar, W., Chua, C., & Summner, D. S. (1979). Noninvasive diagnosis of neonatal asphyxia and intraventricular hemorrhage by Doppler ultrasound. *J. Pediatr., 95,* 775–779.

Bada, H. S., Miller, J. E., Menke, J. A., Menten, T. G., Bashiru, M., Binstadt, D., et al. (1982). Intracranial pressure and cerebral arterial pulsatile flow measurements in neonatal intraventricular hemorrhage. *J. Pediatr., 100,* 291–296.

Batton, D. G., Hellman, J., Hernandez, & Maisels, M. J. (1983). Regional cerebral blood flow, cerebral blood velocity and pulsatility index in newborn dogs. *Pediatr. Res., 17,* 908–912.

Bejar, R., Merritt, T. A., Coen, R. W., Manning, F., & Gluck, L. (1982). Pulsatility index, patent ductus arteriosus, and brain damage. *Pediatrics, 69,* 818–821.

Blomstrand, S., Karlsson, K., & Kjellmar, I. (1978). Measurement of cerebral blood flow in the fetal lamb with a note on flow distribution. *Acta Physiol. Scand., 103,* 1–8.

Cavazutti, M., & Duffy, T. E. (1982). Regulation of local cerebral blood flow in normal and hypoxic newborn dogs. *Ann. Neurol., 11,* 247–257.

Costeloe, K., Smyth, D. P. L., Myrdoch, N., Rolfe, P., & Tizard, J. P. M. (1984). A comparison between electrical impedance and strain gauge plethysmography for the study of cerebral blood flow in the newborn. *Pediatr. Res., 18,* 290–295.

Cowan, F., & Thoresen, M. (1987). The effects of intermittent positive pressure ventilation on cerebral arterial and venous blood velocities in the newborn infant. *Acta Pædiatr. Scand., 76,* 239–247.

Cross, K. W., Dear, P. R. F., Hathorn, M. K. S., Hyams, A., Kerslake, D. McK., Milligan, D. W. A., Rahilly, P. M., & Stothers, J. K. (1979). An estimation of intracranial blood flow in the new-born infant. *J. Physiol., 289,* 329–345.

Daven, J. R., Milstein, J. M., & Gutrie, R. D. (1983). Cerebral vascular resistance in premature infants. *Am. J. Dis. Child., 137,* 328–331.

Dear, P. R. F. (1980). Effect of feeding on jugular venous blood flow in the normal infant. *Arch. Dis. Child., 55,* 365–370.

Drayton, M. R., & Burns, P. N. (1983). Cerebral blood flow in respiratory distress syndrome—Regional changes observed using duplex Doppler ultrasound. *Abstracts, the Neonatal Society.* London.

Ellison, P. H., & Denny, J. (1982). Cerebral blood flow measured by Doppler velocimeter in preterm infants with and without patient ductus arterisus. *Ann. Neurol., 12,* 224, (Abstract No. 86), *Child Neurology Society.*

Ellison, P., Horn, J., Brown, P., & Denny, J. (1986). Continuous wave ultrasound measure of neonatal cerebral blood flow. *Acta Pædiatr. Scand., 75,* 905–912.

Garfunkel, J. M., Baird, H. W., & Siegler, J. (1954). The relationship of oxygen consumption to cerebral functional activity. *J. Pediatr., 44,* 64–72.

Greisen, G. (1984). CBF in the newborn. Issues and methods with special reference to the intravenous 133-Xenon clearance technique. *rCBF Bull., 7,* 134–138.

———. (1986). Cerebral blood flow in preterm infants during the first week of life. *Acta Pædiatr. Scand., 75,* 43–51.

Greisen, G., Frederiksen, P. S., Mali, J., & Friis–Hansen, B. (1984a). Analysis of cranial 133-clearance in the newborn by the two-compartment model. *Scand. J. Clin. Lab. Invest., 44,* 239–250.

Greisen, G., Johansen, K., Ellison, P. H., Frederiksen, P. S., Mali, J., & Friis–Hansen, B. (1984b). Cerebral blood flow in the newborn infant: Comparison of Doppler ultrasound and 133-Xenon clearance. *J. Pediatr, 104,* 411–417.

Hansen, N. B., Stonestreet, B. S., Rosenkranz, T. S., & Oh, W. (1983). Validity of Doppler measurements of anterior cerebral artery blood flow velocity: Correlation with brain blood flow in piglets. *Pediatrics, 72,* 526–531.

Hernandez, M. J., Brennan, R. W., & Bowman, G. S. (1980). Autoregulation of cerebral blood flow in the newborn dog. *Brain Res., 184,* 199–202.

Hernandez, M. J., Brennan, R. W., Vanucci, R. C., and Bowman, G. S. (1978). Cerebral blood flow and oxygen consumption in the newborn dog. *Am. J. Physiol., 34,* R209–R215.

Hernandez, M. J., Hawkin, R. A., & Brennan, R. W. (1981). Sympathetic control of regional cerebral blood flow in the asphyxiated newborn dog. *J. Cereb. Blood Flow Metab., 1,* (Suppl. 1), 268–269.

Hill, A., Perlman, J. M., & Volpe, J. J. (1982). Relationship of pneumothorax to occurrence of intraventricular hemorrhage in the premature newborn. *Pediatrics, 69,* 144–149.

Hill, A., & Volpe, J. J. (1982). Decrease in pulsatile flow in the anterior cerebral arteries in infantile hydrocephalus. *Pediatrics, 69,* 4–7.

Kennedy, C., & Sokoloff, L. (1957). An adaptation of the nitrous oxide method to the study of the cerebral circulation in children; Normal values for cerebral blood flow and cerebral metabolic rate in childhood. *J. Clin. Invest., 36,* 1130–1137.

Kjellmar, I., Karlsson, K., Olsson, T., & Rosen, K. G. (1974). Cerebral reactions during intra-uterine asphyxia in the sheep. I. Circulation and oxygen consumption in the fetal brain. *Pediatr. Res., 8,* 50–57.

Leahy, F. A. N., Cates, D., MacCallum, M., & Rigatto, H. (1980). Effect of CO_2 and 100% O_2 on cerebral blood flow in preterm infants. *J. Appl. Physiol., 48,* 468–472.

Lipman, B., Serwer, G. A., & Brazy, J. E. (1982). Abnormal cerebral hemodynamics in preterm infants with patent ductus arteriosus. *Pediatrics, 69,* 778–781.

Lloyd, B. W. (1984). Outcome of very-low-birthweight babies from Wolverhampton. *Lancet, ii,* 739–741.

Lou, H. C., Henriksen, L., & Bruhn, P. (1984). Focal cerebral hypoperfusion in children with dysphasia and/or attention deficit disorder. *Arch. Neurol., 41,* 825–829.

Lou, H. C., Lassen, N. A., & Friis–Hansen, B. (1979). Is arterial hypertension crucial for the development of cerebral hemorrhage in premature infants? *Lancet, i,* 1215–17.

———. (1979). Impaired autoregulation of cerebral blood flow in the distressed newborn infant. *J. Pediatr., 94,* 118–121.

Lou, H. C., Lassen, N. A., Tweed, W. A., Johnson, G., Jones, M., & Palerhnuik, R. J. (1979). Pressure passive cerebral blood flow and breakdown of the blood brain barrier in experimental fetal asphyxia. *Acta Pediatr. Scand., 68,* 57–63.

Lou, H. C., & Skov, H. (1979). Low cerebral blood flow: A risk factor in the neonate. *J. Pediatr., 95,* 606–609.

Manwarring, K. H., Kodak, J. A., Tarby, T. J., Johnson, S. D., & Suess, D. M. (1984). Stable Xenon computed tomography in the assessment of neonatal intraventricular haemorrhage and posthaemorrhagic hydrocephalus. *Ann. Neurol., 16,* 411, (Abstract No. 117), *Child Neurology Society.*

Martin, C. G., Snider, R., Katz, S. M., Peabody, J. L., & Brady, J. P. (1982). Abnormal cerebral blood flow patterns in preterm infants with a large patent ductus arteriosus. *J. Pediatr., 101,* 587–593.

Mehta, S., Kalsi, H. K., Nain, C. K., & Menkes, J. K. (1977). Energy metabolism of brain in human protein- calorie-malnutrition. *Pediatr. Res., 11,* 290–293.

Ment, L. R., Duncan, C. C., Ehrenkranz, R. A., Lange, R. C., Taylor, K. J., Kleinman, C. S., et al. (1984). Intraventricular hemorrhage in the preterm neonate: Timing and cerebral blood flow changes. *J. Pediatr., 104,* 419–425.

Ment, L. R., Ehrenkrantz, R. A., Lange, R. C., Rothstein, P. T., & Duncan, C. C. (1981). Alterations in cerebral blood flow in preterm infants with intraventricular hemorrhage. *Pediatrics, 68,* 763–769.

Ment, R. L., Scott, D. T., Lange, R. C., Ehrenkranz, R. A., Duncan, C. C., & Warshaw, J. B. (1983). Postpartum perfusion of the preterm brain: Relationship to neurodevelopmental outcome. *Childs Brain, 10,* 266–272.

Milligan, D. W. A. (1980). Failure of autoregulation and intraventricular haemorrhage in preterm infants. *Lancet, i,* 896–898.

———. (1981). Positive pressure ventilation and cranial volume in newborn infants. *Arch. Dis. Child, 56,* 331–335.

Mukhtar, A. I., Cowan, F. M., & Stothers, J. K. (1982). Cranial blood flow and blood pressure changes during sleep in the human neonate. *Early Human Develop., 6,* 59–64.

National Council on Radiation Protection and Measurements. (1983). *Protection in nuclear medicine and ultrasound diagnostic procedures in children.* Bethesda, Md.

Pape, & K. E., & Wigglesworth, J. S. (1979). *Haemorrhage, ischaemia and the perinatal brain.* Clinics in developmental medicine (Nos. 69–70). London: Spastics International medical publications.

Perlman, J. M., Hill, A., & Volpe, J. J. (1981). The effect of patent ductus arteriosus on flow velocity in the anterior cerebral arteries: Ductal steal in the premature newborn infant. *J. Pediatr., 99,* 767–771.

Perlman, J. M., McMenamin, J. B., & Volpe, J. J. (1983). Fluctuating cerebral blood-flow velocity in respiratory distress syndrome. *N. Engl. J. Med., 309,* 204–209.

Perlman, J. M., & Volpe, J. J. (1982). Cerebral blood flow velocity in relation to intraventricular hemorrhage in the premature newborn infant. *J. Pediatr., 100,* 956–959.

———. (1983a). Seizures in the preterm infant: Effects on cerebral blood flow velocity, intracranial pressure, and arterial blood pressure. *J. Pediatr., 102,* 288–293.

———. (1983b). Suctioning in the preterm infant: Effects on cerebral blood flow velocity, intracranial pressure, and arterial blood pressure. *Pediatrics,* 329–334.

Rahilly, P. M. (1980a). Effects of sleep state and feeding on cranial blood flow of the human neonate. *Arch. Dis. Child, 55,* 265–270.

———. (1980b). Effects of 2% carbondioxide, 0.5% carbondioxide and 100% oxygen on cranial blood flow of the human neonate. *Pediatrics, 66,* 685–689.

Reivich, M., Brann, A., Shapiro, H., & Myers, R. E. (1971). Regional cerebral blood flow during prolonged partal asphyxia. *Research on Cerebral Blood Flow, Vth Salzburg Conference* (pp. 217–227). Vienna: Thoma.

Reivich, M., Brann, A. W., Shapiro, H., Rawson, J. & Sano, N. (1971). Reactivity of the cerebral vessels to CO_2 in the newborn rhesus monkey. *Europ. Neurol., 6,* 132–136.

Riela, A. R., Stump, D. A., Roach, E. S., Garcia, J. C., & McLean, W. T. (1984). Regional cerebral blood flow characteristics of the Sturge–Weber syndrome. *Ann. Neurol., 16,* 399, (Abstract No. 76.), *Child Neurology Society.*

Rosenkranz, T. S., & Oh, W. (1982). Cerebral blood flow velocity in infants with polycytaemia and hyperviscosity: Effects of partial exchange transfusion with plasmanate. *J. Pediatr., 101,* 94–98.

———. (1984). Aminophylline reduces cerebral blood flow velocity in low birth weight infants. *Am. J. Dis. Child., 138,* 489–491.

Sankaran, K., Peters, K., & Finer, N. (1981). Estimated cerebral blood flow in term infants with hypoxic-ischemic encephalopathy. *Pediatr. Res., 15,* 1415–1418.

Settergren, G., Lindblad, B. S., & Persson, B. (1980). Cerebral blood flow and exchange of oxygen, glucose, ketone bodies, lactate, pyruvate and amino acids in anesthetized children. *Acta Pediatr. Scand., 69,* 457–465.

Stewart, A. L., Reynolds, E. O. R., & Libscomp, A. P. (1981). Outcome for infants of very low birthweight: Survey of world literature. *Lancet, i,* 1038–1040.

Tweed, W. A., Cote, J., Pash, M., & Lou, H. (1983). Arterial oxygenation determines autoregulation of cerebral blood flow in the fetal lamb. *Pediatr. Res., 17,* 246–249.

Tweed, W. A., Cote, J., Wade, J. G., Gregory, G., & Mills, A. (1982). Preservation of fetal brain blood flow relative to other organs during hypovolaemic hypotension. *Pediatr. Res., 16,* 137–140.

Vanucci, R. C., & Hernandez, M. J. (1980). Perinatal cerebral blood flow. In *Perinatal brain insult.* Mead Johnson Symposium No. 17. Miami: Florida.

Volpe, J. J., Herscovitch, P., Perlman, J. M., & Raichle, M. E. (1983). Positron emission tomography in the newborn. Extensive impairment of regional cerebral blood flow with intraventricular hemorrhage and hemorrhagic cerebral involvement. *Pediatrics, 72,* 589–601.

Wigglesworth, J. S., & Pape, K. E. (1978). An integrated model for haemorrhagic and ischaemic laesions in the newborn brain. *Early Human Develop., 2,* 179–199.

Wilcox, W. D., Carrigan, T. A., Dooley, K. J., Giddens, D. P., Dykes, F. D., Lazzara, A., et al. (1983). Range-gated pulsed Doppler ultrasonographic evaluation of carotid arterial blood flow in small preterm infants with patent ductus arteriosus. *J. Pediatr., 102,* 294–298.

Younkin, D. P., Reivich, M., Jaggi, J., Obrist, W., & Delivoria–Papadopoulos, M. (1982). Noninvasive method of estimating newborn regional cerebral blood flow. *J. Cereb. Blood Flow Metab., 2,* 415–420.

12 Cerebral Blood Flow in Hematological Disorders

J. P. H. Wade
Senior Registrar in Neurology,
St. Bartholomew's Hospital, London

M. M. Brown
Registrar in Neurology,
National Hospital for Nervous Diseases, London

The Cerebral Blood Flow laboratory at the National Hospital, Queen Square, has worked in close collaboration with the department of hematology, St Thomas's Hospital over the past 6 years in an attempt to establish what abnormalities, if any, occur in the cerebral circulation in patients suffering from hematological disorders. Our initial interest concerned the polycythemias and was stimulated by the wealth of literature which has established a link between the incidence of cerebrovascular events and the height of the hematocrit, but the research has continued into a more theoretical analysis of some of the factors which appear to control cerebral blood flow.

CBF IN THE POLYCYTHEMIAS

Studies on patients in whom the hematocrit is above the generally accepted normal range form the basis of this section. There are several conditions characterized by an elevated hematocrit and these can be subdivided by means of red cell mass and other investigations into primary and secondary groups. Both groups can be further subdivided but unfortunately little nosological consensus exists and so it becomes necessary to define our terminology at this stage.

The *primary* group includes patients with primary proliferative polycythemia (or polycythemia rubra vera), idiopathic erythrocytosis and apparent polycythemia (Wetherley–Mein & Pearson, 1982). Primary proliferative polycythemia is a condition manifested by a red cell mass which exceeds the predicted value, based on the patient's height and weight (Nadler, Hidalgo, & Bloch, 1962) by 25% or more. In addition two or more of the following must be present: splenomegaly, leukocytosis, thrombocythemia, raised serum B12, or an elevated leukocyte alkaline phosphatase (Berlin, 1975). Patients with idiopathic erythrocytosis have an elevated red call mass but no underlying cause for polycythemia and features of primary proliferative polycythemia are not demonstrable (Pearson & Wetherley–Mein, 1979). Apparent polycythemia refers to a condition in which the red cell mass is not elevated but some combination of a definitely reduced or low normal plasma volume and a high normal red cell mass cause an elevation of hematocrit (Pearson, 1980). In the past, this condition has been variously referred to as Geisbock's disease (1905), relative (Lawrence & Berlin, 1952), stress (Damasheck, 1953) and spurious polycythemia (Weinreb & Shih, 1975), and pseudopolycythemia (Burge, Johnson, & Prankerd, 1975).

There is experimental evidence which suggests that the effect of an elevated hematocrit on cerebral blood flow is similar in patients with primary proliferative polycythemia, idiopathic erythrocytosis and apparent polycythaemia (Humphrey et al., 1979; Thomas et al., 1977b). Patients with primary proliferative polycythemia and idiopathic erythrocytosis undoubtedly suffer an increased risk of stroke and this can be related to the height of the hematocrit with other factors, such as thrombocythemia, being of secondary importance (Chievitz & Thiede, 1962; Modan & Modan, 1968; Pearson & Wetherley–Mein, 1979). It seems likely that the incidence of vascular occlusion is also high in patients with apparent polycythemia (Burge, Johnson, & Prankerd, 1975). Furthermore, there is some evidence to suggest that normal subjects with a mildly elevated hematocrit are at an increased risk from cerebral infarction (Kannel et al., 1972). The grouping together of patients with primary proliferative polycythemia, idiopathic erythrocytosis, and apparent polycythemia therefore seems justified in the context of this discussion, and the purely descriptive term *primary high hematocrit* is used to describe the group as a whole.

The causes of secondary polycythaemia include hypoxic chest disease, congenital heart disease, certain hemoglobin abnormalities and autonomous erythropoietin-producing lesions. With the exception of the latter group, these patients appear to tolerate high hematocrit values better than the primary group and less often present with strokes. However, they are of considerable theoretical interest and studies of cerebral blood flow have thrown some light on adaptive mechanisms within the cerebral circulation. They are therefore considered separately.

CBF in Patients with Primary High Haematocrit

It was Kety himself (1949) who first measured cerebral blood flow in a subject with polycythemia and he recorded a very low flow (22ml/100g/min) in a patient with a hematocrit of 0.63. Nelson and Fazekas (1956) studied another polycythemic patient and again found that cerebral blood flow was low at 27ml/100g/ min. They went on to repeat the measurement after the hematocrit had been reduced and found a considerable improvement in flow although interpretation was made difficult because the patient had suffered a stroke during the interim period. Eisenberg (1962), again using the Kety–Schmidt method, measured cerebral blood flow in normal subjects and compared base-line values with studies following acutely induced hypervolemia by either whole blood or albumin. Expansion of the intravascular compartment with whole blood was not associated with any increase in cerebral blood flow, but he reported a 32% increase in flow following expansion with a similar volume of 5% albumin solution. This discrepancy was explained by the reduction in hematocrit which accompanies hemodilution and suggests that changes in blood volume per se have no effect on cerebral blood flow.

Using a rather more sophisticated technique, Gottstein and Held (1969) arrived at similar conclusions when they measured flow changes produced by intravenous low molecular weight dextran in normal subjects. They also measured the cerebral consumption of oxygen and found it remained unchanged after hemodilution.

Thomas et al. (1977a) measured cerebral blood flow in 16 patients with either primary proliferative polycythemia or idiopathic erythrocytosis using the noninvasive intravenous ^{133}Xenon method, which allowed repeated studies during treatment to lower the hematocrit. The mean base-line cerebral blood flow was found to be considerably reduced at 37.9ml/100g/min when compared with their control value for flow fast of 69.1ml/100g/min. Flow improved by 73% following a reduction in mean hematocrit from 0.536 to 0.455, and this was associated with a 30% reduction in blood viscosity. They reported similar results in a group of 38 patients with hematocrit values in the high normal range (0.47–0.53), in whom polycythemia had been excluded. Again, a modest reduction in hematocrit (from a mean of 0.51 to 0.45) lead to a 50% increase in flow. They argued that since the oxygen-carrying capacity (calculated from the hemoglobin concentration) fell by less than 15%, the improvement in flow was due to the reduction in blood viscosity. Seven of the patients who had been complaining of lethargy lost their symptoms and a further 9, with transient ischemic attacks, improved considerably. The results from these studies imply that even a modest elevation in hematocrit produces a significant reduction in cerebral blood flow.

Humphrey et al. (1979), using the same technique to measure cerebral blood flow, published similar results in patients with apparent polycythemia. In their study, patients were subdivided into two groups on the basis of red cell mass and plasma volume measurements. In one group the red cell mass was at the upper limit of normal whereas in the other the plasma volume was reduced. The cerebral blood-flow response to lowering the hematocrit by venesection was similar in both groups which reinforces the contention that it is the elevated hematocrit itself, rather than the nature of the underlying condition, which is the important factor.

Following hemodilution, both the oxygen-carrying capacity and the viscosity of the arterial blood are reduced and either factor, be it alone or in combination, might be responsible for the increase in flow. In an experimental study on dogs, Haggendal, Nilsson, and Norback (1966) investigated these two factors by comparing the flow increase during carbon monoxide inhalation with that which followed acute hemodilution. In both situations the oxygen-carrying capacity is reduced but only hemodilution will lead to a fall in blood viscosity. When the degree of reduction in carrying of oxygen was taken into consideration, similar flow increases were observed and it was concluded that viscosity was not a primary determinant in setting cerebral blood flow. However, they were unable to demonstrate any flow change over the hematocrit range 0.30–0.60 and here the results are at variance with all the studies which have been performed on humans. The relevance of experimental work done on dogs must therefore be questioned.

Paulson et al. (1973) have performed similar experiments on awake humans which confirmed the important role of arterial oxygen content in determining cerebral blood flow. The increase in cerebral blood flow was more marked during carbon monoxide exposure than following hemodilution for a given drop in oxygen-carrying capacity and this may have been due to the left shift of the oxygen dissociation curve which occurs with carbon monoxide exposure and which adversely influences oxygen delivery to the tissues. The subjects chosen by Paulson et al. were all young and presumably healthy and age itself might have some bearing on the relationship between viscosity and flow.

Thomas et al. (1977b) have suggested that it is the older patients who are least able to maintain appropriate flow in the face of elevated blood viscosity; the implication is that the cerebral mechanisms which normally adapt to variations in blood viscosity diminish with age or in the presence of cerebrovascular disease. Indeed, Thomas et al. (1977b) and Humphrey et al. (1979) suggest that elevated hematocrit (and therefore increased blood viscosity when measured on whole blood in large bore viscometers) leads to a readjustment of the homeostatic mechanism which serves to couple cerebral blood flow to cerebral oxygen utilization. If this is true, then reducing the hematocrit should lead to more oxygen's being transported to the brain in a form which is available to the tissues. Henriksen, Paulson, and Smith (1981), however, failed to demonstrate a significant increase in oxygen transport to, or utilization by, the brain following acute hemodilution in six patients with neurological disease and marginally elevated hematocrit values.

One of the present authors has recently reported a study of 20 patients with primary high hematocrit, before and after venesection (Wade, 1983). The patients were elderly (mean age 61 years) and 7 had symptoms referrable to the central nervous system, 4 of whom had suffered either a completed stroke or transient ischemic attack. Cerebral blood flow was measured by the noninvasive procedure described by Thomas et al. (1979), arterial oxygen concentrations were measured directly with a Lex 02 Total 02 Content analyzer (Lexington Instruments) and oxygen dissociation curves were plotted on an Aminco Hem-O-Scan analyzer. Blood was also taken for viscosity measurements and these were performed in a coaxial cylindrical visocometer (Contraves Low Shear 30 Viscometer). Measurements were performed at a shear rate of 91 s-1 which, although considerably less than estimates of shear rates in the microcirculation (Kobari et al., 1984), is within the range at which blood behaves as a Newtonian fluid (Whitmore, 1968). Ideally, CMRO2 should have been measured on each occasion, but this would have involved jugular bulb catheterization and was not considered justified. However, measurements of arterial blood gases, arterial oxygen content, and the position of the oxygen dissociation curve permitted a reasonable examination of the oxygen transport mechanism. The investigation was repeated at least 5 days after the last venesection and the venesection regime consisted of weekly sessions during which 300 to 450 ml of blood were taken until the hematocrit was within the desired range.

The mean hematocrit for the group fell from 0.537 to 0.444 and the whole blood viscosity dropped predictably in that the correlation coefficient between hematocrit and whole blood viscosity was 0.926. The change in arterial oxygen content mirrored the reduction in hemoglobin and arterial pCO_2 and pH were not influenced by venesection. Overall, the product of mean cerebral blood flow and mean arterial oxygen content rose by an average of 11.0% ($P<0.001$) and this was considered physiologically significant because the position of the oxygen dissociation curve did not change. (Fig. 12.1)

For the group as a whole, therefore, venesection lead to a modest but significant increase in the amount of oxygen transported to the brain and it is tempting to suggest that elevated blood viscosity may be disrupting, or at least resetting, the coupling between cerebral blood flow and metabolism. Almost half the patients reported some improvement in mental function, which might imply a state of relative cerebral hypoxia, a suggestion given some support by the study of Willison et al. (1980). It was noted, however, that there were several patients in this study in whom venesection did not appear to influence transport of oxygen to the brain. Schmidt-Schonbein (1977) argues that hyperviscosity factors assume clinical significance only in the presence of an abnormal vascular bed with limited ability to dilate in response to metabolic stimuli. We therefore went on to assess the vasomotor reserve in patients with elevated hematocrit (and hence whole blood viscosity) before and after venesection, in 10 further subjects with primary high hematocrit (Wade, 1981). Three of the patients had primary proliferative polycythemia, three had idiopathic erythrocytosis and the remaining 4 had apparent polycythemia. Two out of the 10 subjects showed symptoms attributable to the central nervous system (vertebrobasilar transient ischemic at-

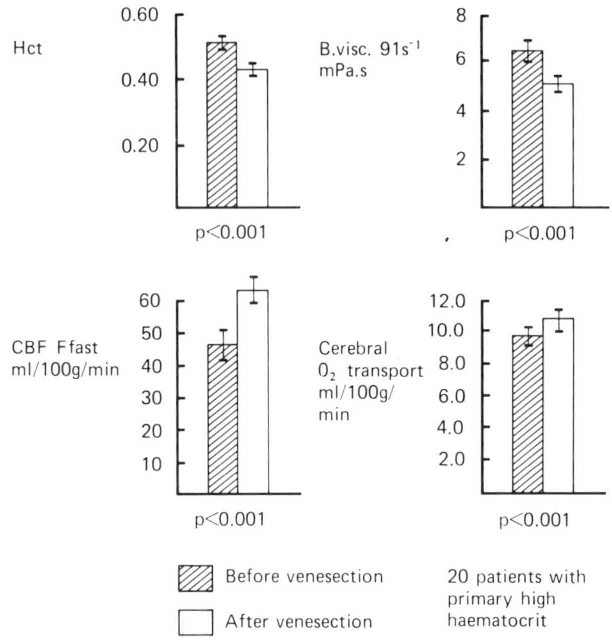

FIGURE 12.1. Hematocrit (Hct), Blood viscosity (B. visc), Cerebral blood flow (CBF) and Cerebral O_2 transport (CBF × arterial O_2 content) in 20 patients before and after venesection.

tacks), the remainder with incidental complaints and none had neurological signs at the time of investigation.

Hypercapnia was induced by the inhalation of 5% CO_2 in air and since many subjects found this uncomfortable, investigation time was limited to about 5 minutes. End-tidal CO_2 was monitored using a Godart infra-red CO_2 analyzer (capnograph) and ^{133}Xenon was given by injection after end-tidal CO_2 values had stabilized. This usually took about a minute, so only 4 minutes of the cerebral desaturation curves were obtained. A bicompartmental analysis was therefore impossible and the flow indexes given refer to the mean flow initial (F init). F init values were derived from the first minute of the clearance curves obtained after the point at which the mean count rate for the six cerebral detectors had fallen 10% from peak. The assumption here is that for the first minute, the mean slope of the deconvoluted clearance curve displayed on a semilogarithmic scale, is proportional to the mean cerebral blood flow. The results obtained using this method tend to reflect flow in the faster compartment of the brain. The partition coefficient is somewhat arbitary because the relative weight of gray and white matter perfused depends on the flow in each compartment and the relative mass of each tissue. However, a figure of 1.14 was used, based on the mean value calculated by Wyper, Lennox, and Rowan (1976). F init values were corrected for the patient's hemoglobin value according to Veall and Mallet's formula (1965).

The results clearly demonstrate that the ability of the cerebrovascular bed to dilate in response to an increase in arterial pCO_2 is not compromised by the presence of an elevated blood viscosity (Fig. 12.2). Indeed, the mean percentage of reactivity prior to venesection was 3.7 (SD 0.9) and the corresponding value after venesection was 3.5 (SD 1.2). Following venesection, the mean hematocrit was 0.458 and this reduction was associated with a significant increase in baseline cerebral blood flow. The reactivity of the cerebral vessels is thus independent of the blood viscosity value, and it is apparent that the cerebral blood vessels are not maximally dilated even when cerebral blood flow is low and the blood viscosity elevated.

We have subsequently studied three more polycythemic subjects in a study analogous to Henriksen and colleagues (1981), and have come up with remarkably similar results showing that the brain does not utilize more oxygen after hematocrit reduction (Fig. 12.3). The 3 subjects had primary proliferative polycythemia, and cerebral blood flow and CMRO2 were measured before and after venesection. Jugular venous oxygen tension and CMRO2 remained virtually

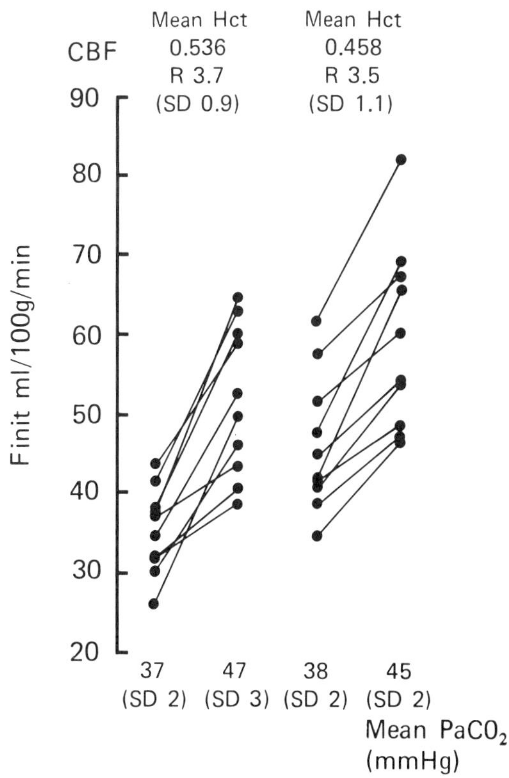

FIGURE 12.2. Reactivity of the cerebrovascular bed to 5% CO_2 in 10 subjects with primary high hematocrit before (mean Hct 0.536) and after (mean Hct 0.458) venesection.

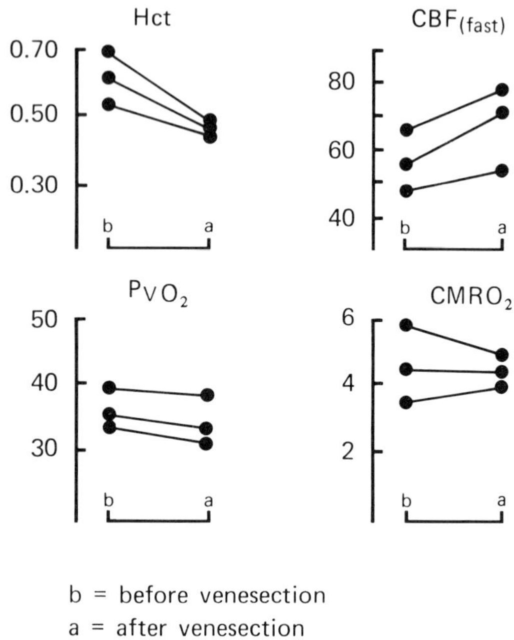

FIGURE 12.3. Hematocrit (Hct), cerebral blood flow (CBF), jugular venous oxygen tension (Pv O_2) and cerebral oxygen consumption ($CMRO_2$) in three subjects with primary proliferative polycythemia, before and after venesection.

constant, suggesting appropriate coupling of cerebral blood flow to CMRO2 at both hematocrit levels. These data appear at variance with the earlier finding of increased oxygen transport to the brain following hematocrit reduction in the 20 subjects with primary high hematocrit and explanations for this remain speculative. It should be noted, however, that flow values were corrected for changes in λ secondary to hemoglobin reduction according to the method described by Veall and Mallett (1965). This correction tends to exaggerate the flow increase following hematocrit reduction and is only correct if the hemoglobin value obtained from an arm vein reflects that in the cerebral microcirculation. Oldendorf et al. (1965) have cast some doubt on this and hematocrit correction could therefore lead to a systematic error creeping into the results.

Cerebral Blood Flow in Secondary Polycythaemia

Hypoxic Lung Disease. Patients with long-standing hypoxic lung disease may develop polycythemia in response to chronic hypoxia and it appears that the increase in red cell mass is quatitatively the same as that seen in normal subjects at high altitude (Shaw & Simpson, 1961), although in some subjects the erythropoeitic response appears exaggerated (Harrison, 1973). Controversy exists over the role of hematocrit reduction in the management of these patients and it is often argued that it is unwise to decrease the red cell mass in patients with polycythemia secondary to lung disease because the high hematocrit represents a compensatory response to hypoxia. The consensus favors moderate hematocrit reduction in subjects with grossly elevated levels, especially if right heart failure supervenes, because it has a beneficial effect on pulmonary vascular resistance (Harrison et al., 1973; Weisse et al., 1975). It becomes probable that the reduction in pulmonary vascular resistance is due to the improved flow characteristics of the blood and if so it may be a general effect when flow to other organs is considered.

Cerebral blood flow has been measured in patients with hypoxic lung disease by several workers. Patterson, Heyman, and Duke (1952) studied 9 patients with long-standing lung disease and found that cerebral blood flow, using the Kety–Schmidt technique, was some 35% higher than normal. Details of the patients' hematocrit values were not given but the mean hemoglobin level for the group was 14.6 g/dl, suggesting that they were not polycythemic. Patients with grossly elevated $PaCO_2$ values tended to have the highest cerebral blood flows although it was noted that the flow response to chronically elevated $PaCO_2$ was not of the same magnitude as that seen in normal subjects undergoing acute changes in $PaCO_2$. They were also able to measure CMRO2 and interestingly this did not significantly differ from their control value. In 1953, Scheinberg et al., using the same technique, found that cerebral blood flow and CMRO2 were both normal in 23 patients with chronic hypoxia secondary to lung disease. Their patients had less severe airways disease than did those of Patterson, Heyman, and Duke, and this probably explains the differing results. Hematocrit was not considered as an independent variable in determining cerebral blood flow and neither the hematocrit nor hemoglobin values are given in their paper. $PaCO_2$ correlated with cerebral blood flow ($r = 0.51$), whereas arterial oxygen saturation and pH did not.

In the final study, Skinhoj (1968), measured cerebral blood flow by the intracarotid ^{133}Xenon technique in eight patients with chronically deranged blood gases secondary to lung disease. He found that cerebral blood flow was either normal or high and demonstrated a correlation between cerebral blood flow and cerebrospinal fluid pH. He demonstrated that it was those patients with the highest arterial pCO_2 values who were least able to maintain normal CSF pH homeostasis. Thus, the relationship between $PaCO_2$ and CSF pH which exists in patients with severe hypercapnia (Huang & Lyons, 1966) may explain the correlation between cerebral blood flow and $PaCO_2$ noted by Scheinberg et al. (1953).

We have reported our findings in 12 patients with polycythemia secondary to chronic hypoxic lung disease and assessed the value of hematocrit reduction by repeating the measurements after venesection (Wade et al., 1981). Cerebral blood flow was determined by the intravenous ^{133}Xenon method but the technique had to be modified because the assumption that end-tidal Xenon reflects arterial values no longer holds true in patients with airways disease. A method of continuous arterial sampling was developed and subsequently validated by com-

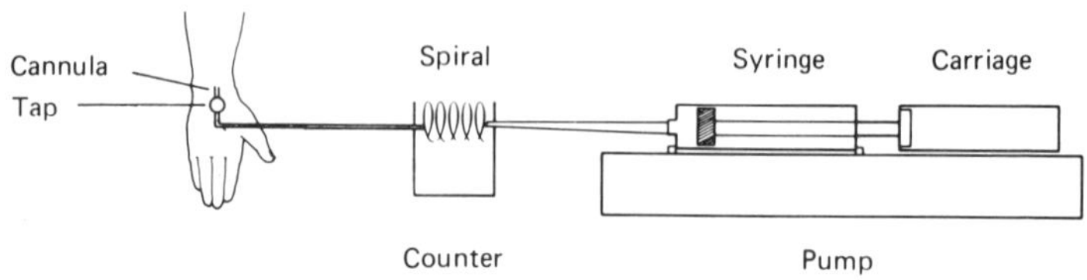

Patient	Finit ml/100g/min	
	Air curve data	Arterial curve data
1	36.2	33.2
2	43.8	42.4
3	69.4	66.9
4	37.3	37.6
5	49.5	46.1
6	32.6	31.5
Mean	44.8	43.0
S.D.	13.5	13.0

FIGURE 12.4. Cerebral blood flow (F init) in six subjects with normal lung function in whom end-tidal air and arterial $^{Xe}133$ counts were monitored simultaneously. Data from each were utilized by the computer to calculate F init values.

parison of cerebral blood-flow results in 6 normal subjects in whom end-tidal and arterial Xenon concentrations were measured simultaneously (Fig. 12.4). Arterial blood was withdrawn at a constant rate of 10ml/min, and with a dead space of about 2 ml, the transit time was of the order of 12 sec. Count rates at peak were approximately 300/sec. Since blood was removed at 10 ml/min investigation time was necessarily limited and only 4 minutes of the desaturation curves were monitored so only flow initial (F init) values were obtained.

Of the 12 patients studied, 11 gave a history consistent with the diagnosis of chronic bronchitis (Medical Research Council, 1965). The final subject had suffered poliomyelitis as a child with residual weakness of the chest wall muscles and diaphragm. Seven subjects had complained of severe generalized headache and three of those also suffered episodes of nocturnal confusion. All subjects had severe disturbances of their blood gases, the mean PaO_2 was 52 mmHg, mean $PaCO_2$ 56 mmHg and the mean pH was 7.37. The mean prevenesection F init was 39.1ml/100g/min and was significantly higher than the corresponding result obtained from the patients with primary high hematocrit. In Fig. 12.5, prevenesection values for hematocrit, blood viscosity, F init and cerebral oxygen transport (F init × arterial oxygen content) are compared between the two groups. The mean hematocrit and blood viscosity were significantly higher in the patients with secondary polycythemia. Despite this, mean prevenesection F init was 24% higher ($P<0.01$) and the difference in mean cerebral oxygen transport was also significant.

Venesection resulted in a reduction in hematocrit from a mean value of 0.613 to 0.495, and blood viscosity at 91 s-1 fell from 8.08 mPa.s to a postvenesection mean of 5.04. The F init rose by an average of 21% following venesection to a value of 47.2 (s.d. 10.9) ml/100g/min ($P<0.005$) although this did not occur in every patient (Fig. 12.6). Mean cerebral oxygen transport actually fell from 7.61 (s.d. 1.42)ml/100g/min to 7.26 (s.d. 1.75)ml/100g/min, but this was not statistically significant. None of the subjects felt worse after hematocrit reduction and six reported improvement in either headache or exercise tolerance or both. Two of the patients who had reported episodes of nocturnal confusion were considerably relieved and in one of these cerebral oxygen transport went up while in the other it fell.

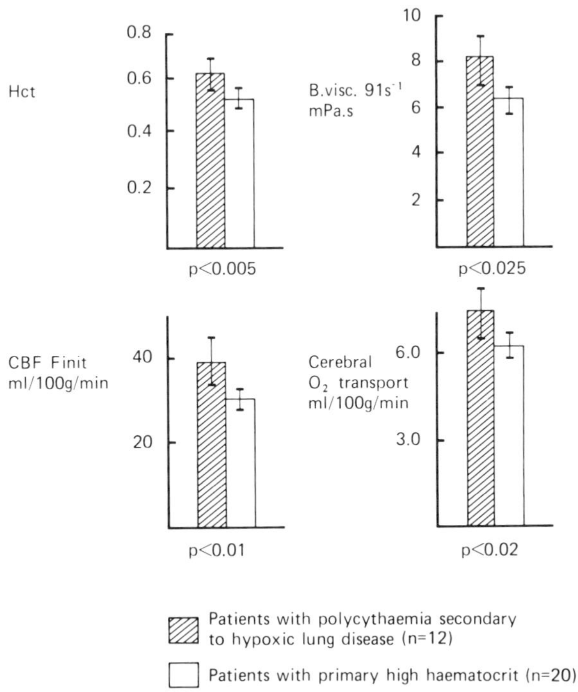

FIGURE 12.5. Hematocrit (Hct), blood viscosity (B. visc), cerebral blood flow (CBF) and cerebral oxygen transport (CBF × arterial O_2 content) in 12 subjects with polycythemia secondary to hypoxic lung disease and 20 subjects with primary high hematocrit.

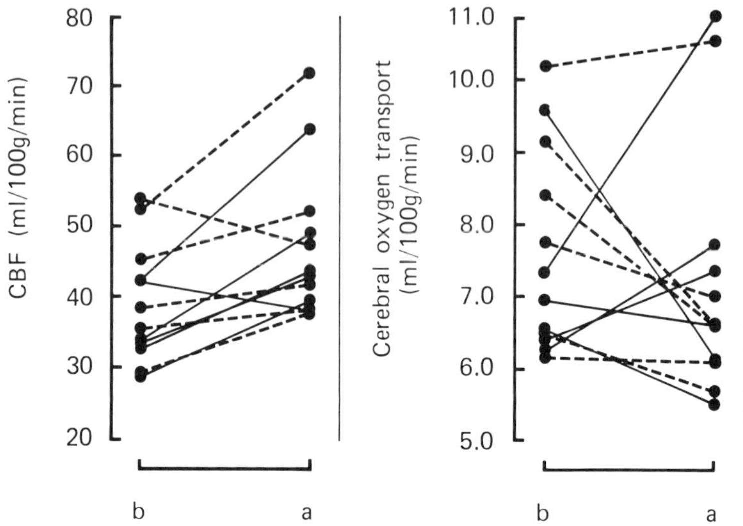

FIGURE 12.6. Cerebral blood flow (F init) and cerebral oxygen transport (cerebral blood flow × arterial oxygen content) in 12 subjects with polycythemia secondary to hypoxic lung disease before (b) and after (a) venesection. Subjects represented as continuous lines reported symptomatic improvement; those represented as discontinuous lines reported no change.

The data were not corrected for changes in $PaCO_2$ because there is considerable evidence that cerebral blood flow tends to normalize under conditions of chronic hypercapnia (Ekstrom-Jodal & Haggendal, 1969; Skinhoj, 1968). The study demonstrated that in patients with polycythemia secondary to hypoxic lung disease, cerebral blood flow is considerably higher than expected on the basis of the hematocrit alone. In addition, the fact that no simple relationship exists between change in cerebral blood flow and change in hematocrit serves to distinguish this group of patients from those in the primary high hematocrit group. Oxygen transport to the brain is maintained in patients with this type of secondary polycythemia despite the elevated hematocrit and is not generally improved by venesection. In the subjects in whom the symptoms of headache and/or drowsiness were improved, the lack of a consistent increase in cerebral oxygen transport suggests that the mental symptoms result from the adverse influence of other factors such as arterial pH, on cerebral metabolism, and this interpretation is supported by experimental work on EEG changes during acute respiratory acidemia in normal man (Meyer, Gotoh, & Tomita, 1966). Maintenance of overall flow when the hematocrit is elevated implies a dilated vascular bed, which could explain the headaches but this remains speculative in the absence of blood volume measurements.

CBF in Patients With Polycythemia Secondary to an Abnormal Hemoglobin Characterized by Increased Oxygen Affinity

Oxygen transport to the tissues depends on both the flow of blood and its oxygen content. The oxygen content of the blood is, in turn, a function of the hemoglobin concentration and the relative saturation of the hemoglobin with oxygen because very little oxygen is transported dissolved in the plasma. Although these factors determine the total amount of oxygen transported to the tissues, tissue oxygen availability also depends on the ability of hemoglobin to give up oxygen in the capillaries (Finch & Lenfant, 1972). During experimentally induced hypoxia, cerebral blood flow increases and this serves to ensure that as the arterial oxygen content falls, the product of cerebral blood flow and arterial oxygen content remains constant (Jones et al., 1981; Winso, 1971). However, even when the hemoglobin is 100% saturated, oxygen delivery to the brain will be adversely influenced if the bound oxygen is not available to the cerebral tissues.

Several hemoglobin variants have been described in which the primary abnormality is reflected by an increased oxygen affinity of the blood (Bellingham, 1976). Erythropoeisis is stimulated because less oxygen is available to the tissues over the physiological range of oxygen tensions and as a result, some of these

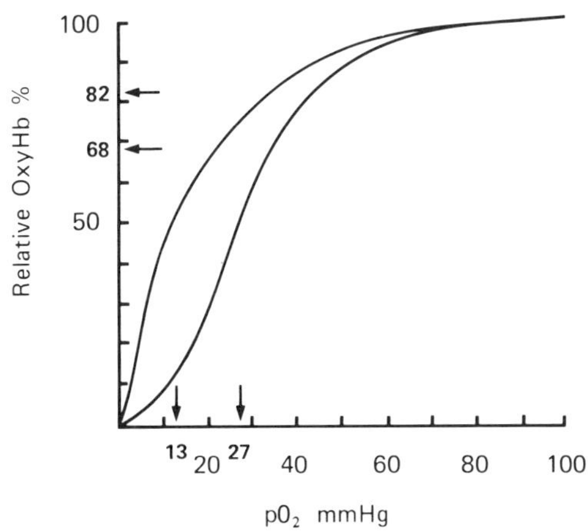

Whole blood oxygen dissociation curves. The curve on the left is from one of the subjects with the abnormal Hb. The other curve is from one of the patients in the control group. The arrows on the X axis indicate their respective P50 values. On the Y axis the percentage saturations at pO_2 35mmHg are shown.

FIGURE 12.7.

patients will develop polycythemia. The increase in hematocrit may compensate for the primary defect in oxygen delivery, but this compensation will only be effective if flow rates are maintained despite the elevated blood viscosity.

We have studied six subjects with erythrocytosis secondary to a hemoglobin variant characterised by increased oxygen affinity and the results are of theoretical interest to the discussion on the relative importance of oxygen delivery and blood viscosity in the control of cerebral blood flow (Wade et al., 1980). All the subjects were from the same family and had a hemoglobin variant known as hemoglobin Yakima, which was first described by Jones et al. (1967). Their mean hematocrit was 0.513 (s.d. 0.40) and their mean *P* 50 was 13.0 (s.d. 0.4) mmHg which differs markedly from the normal value for our laboratory which is 27.7 (s.d. 1.8) mmHg. The *P* 50 refers to the partial pressure of oxygen at which the hemoglobin is 50% saturated with oxygen and it is derived from the oxygen dissociation curve. Its physiological importance can be understood by reference to Fig. 12.7. The normal oxygen dissociation curve is seen below and the *P* 50 is within normal limits at 27 mm Hg. The curve is taken from one of the subjects with hemoglobin Yakima and is clearly left-shifted. If we assume a normal value

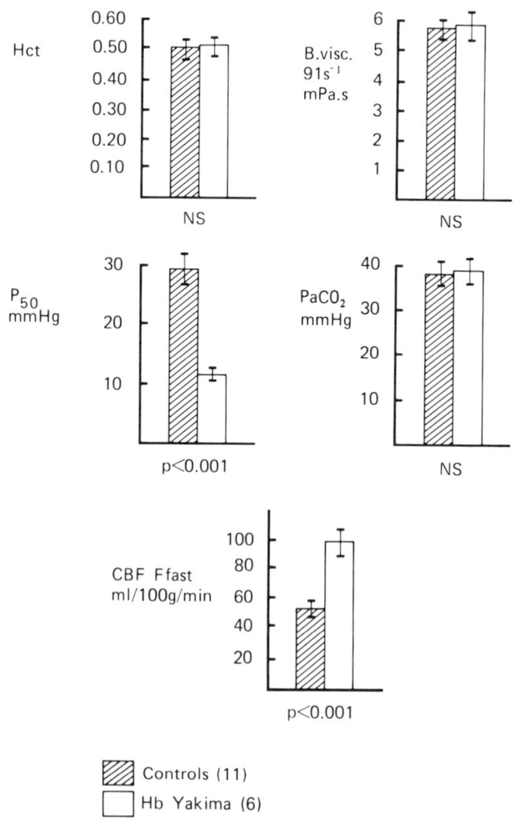

FIGURE 12.8. Hematocrit (Hct), blood viscosity (B. visc) P50 and $PaCO_2$ in 11 subjects with primary high hematocrit (controls) and 6 subjects with polycythemia secondary to hemoglobin Yakima.

for the cerebral tissue oxygen tension of around 35 mm Hg, then it will be apparent that normal hemoglobin has given up almost a third of its oxygen, while the abnormal hemoglobin remains over 80% saturated.

The results of the measurements of cerebral blood flow, blood viscosity and $PaCO_2$ are shown in Fig. 12.8. A comparative group of 11 patients with primary polycythemia are also included and the difference in cerebral blood flow is impressive. The mean F fast in the study group was 99.1 (s.d. 12.9) ml/100g/min, whereas in the control group the equivalent value was 54.8 (s.d. 8.5)ml/100g/min. The F unit measurements reflected a similar difference. Blood viscosity measurements were elevated to a similar degree in both groups; thus flow is increased despite the abnormal viscosity and clearly, oxygen delivery is a major factor in determining cerebral blood flow in this situation.

CEREBRAL BLOOD FLOW IN THE ANEMIAS

The converse rheological situation to polycythemia is anemia where the low hematocrit leads to a reduction in whole blood viscosity. Several workers have measured cerebral blood flow in the anemias, starting with Scheinberg (1951), who used the Kety–Schmidt method, and found that flow was some 50% higher in patients with pernicious anemia in whom the hemoglobin level was less than 7 g/dl. Heyman, Patterson, and Duke (1952), using a similar method, reported high flow values in patients with sickle cell anemia. Their results, from 18 patients, suggested an inverse relationship between the hemoglobin level and cerebral blood flow. Sickle cells differ rheologically from ordinary red blood cells in that they are less flexible and because flexibility may have some bearing on the flow characteristics of blood in the microcirculation, the group at the National Hospital, Queen Square, are currently interested in reassessing flow in patients with sickle cell disease. Preliminary and as yet unpublished data suggest that cerebral blood flow is increased and compatible with the reduced hemoglobin value.

Patients with spherocytosis also have abnormally rigid red blood cells and in a personal series of 11 subjects, again unpublished, it appears that flow is elevated with values of the same order as found in subjects with iron deficiency anemia. It, therefore, seems that abnormalities of red cell deformability do not lead to a disruption of the normal coupling between cerebral blood flow and cerebral oxygen utilization.

Brown has published data on cerebral blood flow and blood viscosity in 34 patients with iron deficiency anemia (1984). Cerebral blood flow (F fast) was significantly higher than in nonanemic controls, by a mean of 12ml/100g/min. Whole blood viscosity was reduced and he demonstrated that the inverse relationship which exists between hematocrit and blood viscosity in polycythemic subjects holds true in anemia. When Brown's data are combined with the 20

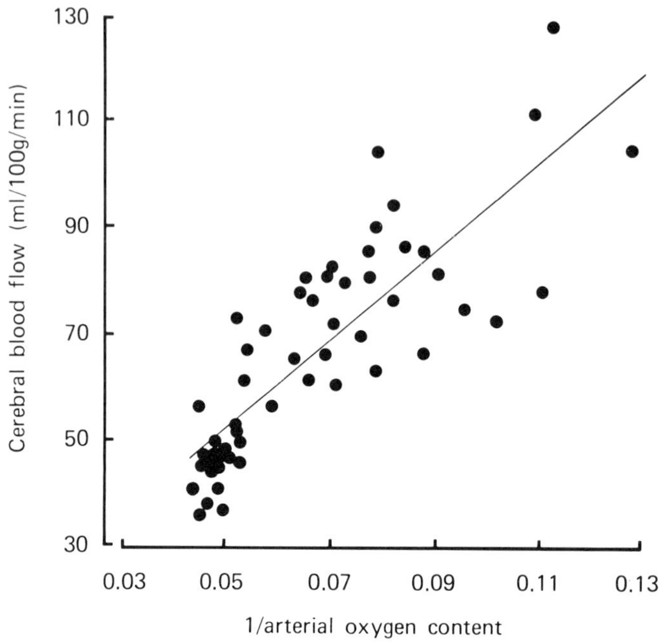

FIGURE 12.9. Cerebral blood flow (CBF) plotted against the reciprocal of arterial oxygen content in 54 subjects with polycythemia, normocythemia, and anemia.

patients with primary high hematocrit reported by Wade (1983), in whom cerebral blood flow was measured in the same laboratory using the same equipment, it is possible to demonstrate a close inverse relationship between cerebral blood flow and the reciprocal of arterial oxygen content (Fig. 12.9). The response to arterial oxygen content appears to be linear and is not attenuated at the polycythemic end of the scale, as would be predicted if elevated blood viscosity were disrupting the normal matching of flow and oxygen delivery.

CEREBRAL BLOOD FLOW IN THE LEUKEMIAS

Patients with leukemia may suffer from the "hyperviscosity syndrome" with cerebral symptoms such as deafness, vertigo, ataixa, seizures, visual disturbances, and a depression of consciousness (Davies–Jones, Preston, & Timperely, 1980). They tend to be patients with extreme elevations of white cell count and the condition responds to a reduction of blood viscosity achieved by leucopheresis (Preston et al., 1978b). Brown (1984) has demonstrated that the presence of an abnormal number of white cells influences in vitro blood viscosity measurements by a degree comparable with changes in the number of red cells. He went on to study cerebral blood flow in seven subjects with various leukemias (three with chronic myeloid, two with prolymphocytic, and two with chronic lymphocytic). The majority had only minor cerebral symptoms but one case, referred with a diagnosis of hyperviscosity, presented with blurred vision associated with retinal venous engorgement and scattered hemorrhages (case 2, Table 12.1). Whole blood viscosity (measured using a Contraves Low Shear 30 coaxial viscometer) was significantly higher then predicted on the basis of the hematocrit alone, but despite this, all but one of the subjects had a F fast value higher than would be expected on the basis of their hematocrit (Table 12.1). The increase in cerebral blood flow in leukemic patients was not explicable by variations in age or $PaCO_2$, which were similar to those found in the anemic subjects used to predict cerebral blood flow.

Thus elevated blood viscosity did not lead to a reduction in cerebral blood flow, indeed, some unidentified factor appeared to lead to an increase in flow values. This study suggests that the cerebral symptoms are not likely to be due to a generalized reduction in cerebral blood flow resulting directly from an increase in blood viscosity; it seems more probable that they are due to focal occlusions of small blood vessels by aggregates of white cells (McKee & Collins, 1974).

TABLE 12.1
Haemaglobin (Hb), White Cell Count (WCC), Whole Blood Viscosity (WBV) and Cerebral Blood Flow (CBF) in 7 Patients with Leukemia ("Predicted" whole blood viscosity refers to the blood viscosity value predicted on the basis of the subjects' hematocrit level. "Predicted" CBF levels refer to the levels expected on the basis of the hematocrit values [see text].)

	Cerebral Blood Flow in Leukaemia					
Patient	*HB gm/dl*	*WCC × 10^9/l*	*WBV at 94.5s^{-1} mPa.s*	*Predicted WBV mPa.s*	*CBV ml/100g/min*	*Predicted CBF ml/100g/min*
1	11.7	652	10.9[c]	4.0	69.7	68.0
2	7.3	475	7.3[c]	2.5	117.7[a]	92.0
3	5.9	424	4.2[c]	2.4	118.7	99.4
4	10.1	250	4.3[c]	3.3	82.2	76.7
5	9.5	244	3.6[b]	3.1	71.0	80.0
6	12.6	122	5.8[c]	4.1	85.2[a]	63.1
7	11.6	49	4.4[a]	3.9	88.2	68.4
Mean	9.8	317	5.8[a]	3.3	90.4[a]	78.2

[a] $p < 0.05$.
[b] $p < 0.01$.
[c] $p < 0.001$.

Patients with paraproteinemia may also suffer from the "hyperviscosity syndrome" and the cerebral symptoms are nearly always associated with an elevation of plasma viscosity (Preston et al., 1978a; Somer, 1975). This is particularly likely to occur if the paraprotein is IgM but abnormalities may also occur in both IgA and IgG myelomas (McGrath & Penny, 1976). As a result of the elevated plasma viscosity, the whole blood viscosity is higher than predicted on the basis of the hematocrit alone, and it has been suggested that the cerebral symptoms occur as a consequence of the reduced blood fluidity. This hypothesis received some support from a study by Humphrey et al. (1980) in which cerebral blood flow was found to be significantly lower in a group of 21 paraproteinemic subjects, than in a small group of anemic subjects without paraproteinemia. However, the two groups were not matched for arterial oxygen content and subsequent analysis suggested that the levels of cerebral blood flow found in the paraproteinemic patients of this earlier study could well be appropriate for their level of oxygen content.

Brown (1984) therefore studied a further 36 patients with a paraprotein band

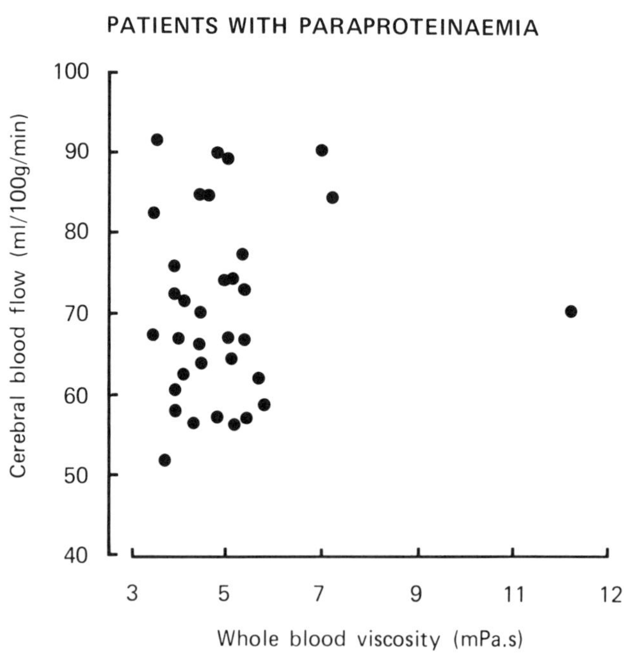

FIGURE 12.10. Cerebral blood flow (F fast) plotted against whole blood viscosity in 36 patients with paraproteinemia.

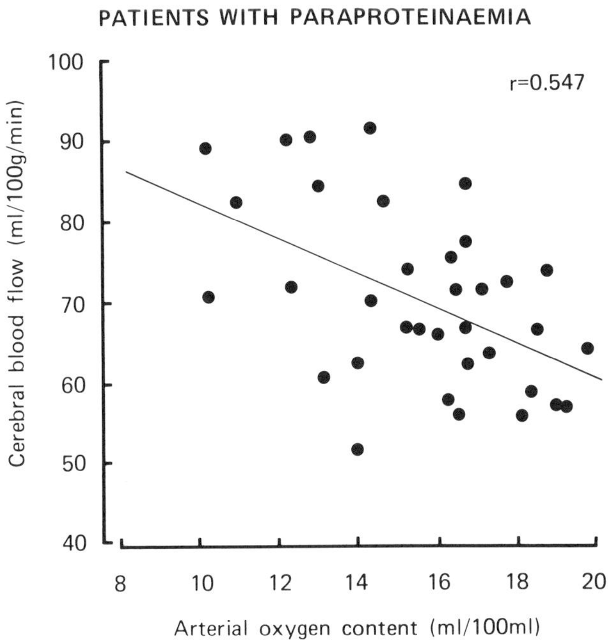

FIGURE 12.11. Cerebral blood flow (F fast) plotted against arterial oxygen content in 36 patients with paraproteinemia.

on serum electropheresis resulting from myeloma or macroglobulinemia. He excluded patients with abnormal electrolytes, elevated serum calcium, or deranged renal function. Sixteen subjects had macroglobulinemia (IgM paraproteinemia), 12 had IgG myeloma, and 8 patients had IgA meyloma. Seventeen of the patients had mild to moderate cerebral symptoms attributed clinically to hyperviscosity. Cerebral blood-flow measurements did not correlate with whole blood viscosity (Fig. 12.10) but a close relationship did emerge between cerebral blood flow and arterial oxygen content (Fig. 12.11). When the results in those subjects who had significant elevations of plasma viscosity were compared with those obtained from an anemic group without hyperviscosity, in whom the hemoglobin and arterial oxygen content values were similar but the whole blood viscosity measurements quite different, cerebral blood flow was found to be virtually identical (Table 12.2). It was not possible to correlate cerebral symptomatology with cerebral blood-flow measurements in individual cases and it therefore seems unlikely that the "hyperviscosity syndrome" is due to a generalized reduction in flow resulting only from an increase in blood viscosity. Thus it seems certain that other factors are involved. The importance of Brown's work is that in both the leukemias and the paraproteinemias, abnormalities of blood viscosity do not inevitably lead to a disruption of flow and a state of relative

TABLE 12.2
Hemoglobin (Hb), Age, Mean Arterial Blood Pressure (MABP), $PaCO_2$, Whole Blood Viscosity (WBV), Plasma Viscosity (PLV) and Cerebral Blood Flow (F fast) in 36 Subjects with Paraproteinemia and a Comparative Group of Subjects with Anemia ($N = 20$)

	Paraproteinaemia *(n = 36)*	*Anaemia* *(n = 20)*	
Hb (g/dl)	10.3 ± 2.0	10.3 ± 2.2	N.S.
Age (years)	62.0 ± 9.7	55.2 ± 15.9	N.S.
MABP (mmHg)	104 ± 19	105 ± 17	N.S.
pCO_2 (kPa)	4.8 ± 0.5	4.8 ± 0.6	N.S.
WBV at $94.5s^{-1}$ (mPa.s)	5.3 ± 1.9	3.8 ± 0.8	$p < 0.003$
PLV (mPa.s)	2.52 ± 1.35	1.44 ± 0.11	$p < 0.002$
CBF (ml/100g/min)	73.1 ± 11.4	74.6 ± 11.8	N.S.

cerebral ischemia; it provides firm evidence that the cerebral circulation autoregulates for fluctuations in blood viscosity in much the same way as it does for blood pressure.

DISCUSSION

Two main conclusions can be drawn from these studies. Firstly, it is clear that the arterial oxygen content is of fundamental importance in the regulation of cerebral blood flow in normal humans and secondly, it has become apparent that regulatory mechanisms serve to maintain an essentially "appropriate" CBF independently of alterations in blood viscosity. It therefore becomes necessary to review the clinical significance of whole blood viscosity measurements and to achieve this we must first consider the mechanics of the circulation. The following brief account owes much to the excellent reviews by Charm and Kurland (1974), Caro et al. (1978) and Schmidt-Schonbein (1981).

Mechanics of the Circulation

In the larger arteries, flow will show the influence of inertia, whereas in the microcirculation, flow is dominated by viscous forces. Viscosity is important only where the blood is being sheared and the boundary layer (i.e., that part of the fluid next to the vessel wall where shearing occurs) in large arteries is small, compared with the diameter of the vessel. The situation in the microcirculation is quite different; here viscous forces dominate because as vessel size diminishes the size of the boundary layer increases. The Reynolds number (*Re*) predicts the relative importance of inertial and viscous effects and can be defined by the following:

$$Re = \frac{\text{inertial forces}}{\text{viscous forces}} = \frac{Ud}{v}$$

where U = mean velocity, d = vessel diameter, and v = the kinematic viscosity of blood (i.e., viscosity/specific gravity). Flow in vessels where the Re value is greater than unity is dominated by the influence of inertia whereas flow where the Re value is less than unity is dominated by viscous forces. In practice, Re remains above unity in vessels down to the size of 100 um and thus, viscous forces have a minimal influence on flow in the larger arteries, while they are of critical importance in the microcirculation.

The importance of these viscous forces can be gauged from the finding that the main pressure drop in the systemic circulation occurs across the microcirculation (defined here as those vessels having a diameter of less than 100 um). The microcirculation includes the smaller arterioles, capillaries and venules, and it is here the flow rates are essentially determined by local pressure gradients and viscous forces. Vessel wall shear rates are probably in the region of 2000 s-1 (Kobari et al., 1984), which is certainly well above the value at which blood behaves as a Newtonian fluid in vivo. It is therefore reasonable to use Poiseuille's law as a basis for the analysis of blood flow in the resistance part of the circulation.

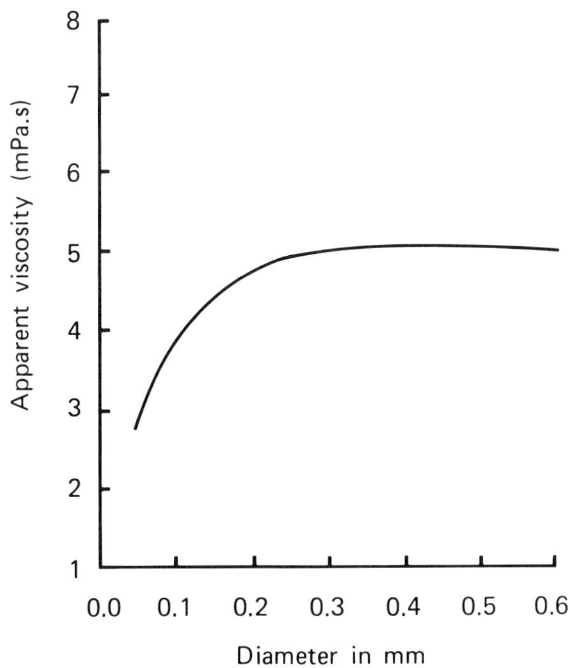

FIGURE 12.12. The Fahraeus–Lindqvist Effect. Apparent viscosity of blood falls in tubes of less than 300 μm diameter.

However, in this part of the circulation it is no longer possible to regard blood as a homogeneous fluid with the same properties it displays in the viscometer, and it becomes necessary to consider it as a suspension of red cells in plasma.

In vitro, and at low Re values (less than unity), red cells migrate toward the axis of the tube leaving a layer of plasma around the central core of red cells. The axial migration is more pronounced at high flow rates and when the cell to tube ratio is large, so the thickness of the cell free layer is greater in vessels of 100 um diameter or less. The red cells move along the center of the tube at relatively higher velocity than the plasma near the wall, leading to a reduction in the apparent hematocrit. The cell-free layer also establishes a sheath of relatively low viscosity fluid (plasma) at the wall and these two factors explain why the apparent viscosity of blood falls when flow in small tubes (less than 300 um) is considered (Fig. 12.12). The reduction in apparent viscosity in small tubes was first described by Fahraeus and Lindqvist in 1931 and still bears their name.

The diameter of the capillaries range from 10 um down to about 3 um and the unstressed diameter of the red cells is 7 um; thus red cells have to pass along them in single file. Under these circumstances, it has been suggested that the viscosity of plasma is the main determinant of flow (Schmidt-Schonbein, 1981). When the vessel size is smaller than that of the red cell, flow will also be related to the force required to deform the cell.

In Vivo Significance of In Vitro Viscosity Measurements

Whole blood viscosity measurements in vitro have shown that blood is a non-Newtonian fluid at low shear rates in that the apparent viscosity falls as the shear rate is increased. At rest, the red cells aggregate to form a tangled network and if the sample is subjected to a low shear stress (below a critical level), blood is believed to deform rather than flow. The critical shear stress required to establish flow is called the yield stress and this value is proportional to the volume of cells (hematocrit). It will also increase when the concentration of fibrinogen or globulin is high, because these proteins promote rouleaux formation.

As the shear rate is increased, the average length of the rouleaux decreases and with shear rates in excess of about 50 s-1 the red cells are present individually. This process is associated with a fall in the viscosity but it also seems probable that red cell deformation contributes to the non-Newtonian behavior of blood. At shear rates in excess of 100 s-1, viscosity does not fall with further increases in shear rate, unless the hematocrit is very high. Thus, with increasing hematocrit, blood viscosity at any particular shear rate increases and the shear rate above which Newtonian behavior is observed also rises.

Hematocrit is the single most important factor determining viscosity when blood is studied in conventional viscometers at low shear rates (less than 50 s-1) (Begg & Hearns, 1966). At higher shear rates it exerts a less pronounced effect and the viscosity of the suspending fluid (plasma) and the deformability of the red cells assume greater significance.

From the discussion on the mechanics of the circulation, it will be appreciated that the blood viscosity value, as measured by relatively large bore viscometers, is of limited value. Blood flow in the larger arteries is essentially governed by inertial forces and in the microcirculation, where viscous forces predominate, the apparent viscosity of blood depends not only on the shear rate but also on other variables such as vessel size, red cell deformability, and plasma viscosity. It should also be recalled that this is the part of the circulation where the mechanical energy of the heart is dissipated. In addition, in vitro, whole blood viscosity measurements may exaggerate the influence of hematocrit because they are performed on relatively large samples at relatively low shear rates.

The viscometric finding of a high viscosity resulting from an elevated hematocrit level may therefore reflect a potential rather than actual property of blood in the normal circulation. These potential properties may assume significance, however, under pathological conditions. For instance, tissue damage may be greater following a transient cessation of blood flow when the hematocrit is elevated because the increased yield stress value of blood might effectively inhibit restoration of flow.

The hemodynamic effects of elevated hematocrit may also be important when flow is chronically retarded and the vasomotor reserve of the vascular bed is exhausted. Such a situation may arise, for example, when the heart is malfunctioning or the feeding artery to a vascular bed is severely stenosed. Under these conditions, flow will be limited by the actual level of the apparent viscosity in the respective blood levels and might be improved by reducing this level. At high hematocrit values, the critical shear rate below which red cell aggregation occurs, will be increased and intravascular stagnation may result. This could lead to heterogeneous perfusion of the microcirculation with areas of stagnation effectively bypassed and the arrested circulation may allow coagulatory processes to take place. Support for this comes from the clinical observation made by Toghi et al. (1978), that the incidence of cerebral infarction is especially high in those patients who have a combination of severe arterial disease and elevated hematocrit.

It has also been established that the normal autoregulatory response to changes in perfusion pressure is disrupted in the region of a cerebral infarct and here regional cerebral blood flow passively follows changes in perfusion pressure (McHenry et al., 1974; Meyer et al., 1973). If the autoregulatory mechanisms which serve to compensate for changes in blood viscosity fail as well, then a reduction in viscosity may well improve local blood flow and potentiate oxygen delivery. This hypothesis could explain the clinical observation made by Harrison et al. (1981) that infarct size following carotid occlusion is in part dependent on the hematocrit value with larger infarcts occurring in subjects with elevated values.

Cerebral Blood Flow and Changes in the Arterial Oxygen Content

The cerebral circulation in normal man adapts to changes in whole blood viscosity arising from abnormal hematocrit (polycythemia), reduced red cell deformability (sickle cell disease) and elevated plasma viscosity (paraproteinemia). Cerebral blood flow remains "appropriate" and the oxygen demands of the tissues are met. When the arterial oxygen content falls, cerebral blood flow increases so that the product of flow and arterial oxygen content remains constant. This explains why the response of the circulation to a reduction in PaO_2 appears to be a threshold phenomenon, with very little increase in flow occurring until the PaO_2 drops below about 50 mmHg (Shimojyo et al., 1968; Winso, 1971) since hemoglobin remains almost 100% saturated (and hence the arterial oxygen content remains constant) over the PaO_2 range 50–100 mmHg (Fig. 12.7). Cerebral tissue oxygen tension is dependent on the arterial oxygen content and the cerebral blood flow, and the maintenance of constant PO_2 (other things being equal) would require the flow rate to be directly proportional to the arterial oxygen content, such that the product of the two remains constant. This prediction corresponds to the cerebral blood flow findings reported herein. It is beyond the scope of this review to discuss possible mechanisms whereby the cerebral vessels are regulated in response to changes in tissue PO_2.

SUMMARY

It seems prudent to conclude by summarizing the foregoing in a rather dogmatic way which will hopefully prove of interest to fellow workers:

1. In patients with a normal circulation, reducing whole blood viscosity by hematocrit reduction of plasma protein manipulation will not necessarily lead to an increase in oxygen transport to the brain.

2. In the individual case, cerebral blood flow will change in a predictable manner when the hematocrit is altered.

3. The arterial oxygen content frms the basis of the relationship between cerebral blood flow and hematocrit in normal humans; the circulation compensates for changes in blood viscosity.

4. The arterial oxygen content is essentially defined by the hemoglobin level and when cerebral blood flow is measured before and after a procedure which affects the hemoglobin concentration, we can only judge its physiological significance if both the CBF and Hb level are given.

5. Finally, all the studies reported in this chapter have concerned global cerebral blood flow and metabolism. Abnormalities of blood fluidity may affect the rate at which rCBF reflects regional substrate demands. Further studies on

rCBF during activation procedures may help explain why patients with elevated Hct values often complain of cognitive difficulties.

ACKNOWLEDGMENTS

We are indebted to the endowment fund of St. Thomas's Hospital and the Medical Research Council for providing funds. We would also like to thank Dr. D. J. Thomas and Dr. P. R. D. Humphrey for allowing us to use their data in compiling this review. The study would not have been possible without the continued assistance of Dr. T. C. Pearson and Professor G. Wetherley-Mein of St. Thomas's Hospital, Professor J. Marshall and Dr. R. W. Ross Russell of the National Hospital for Nervous Diseases and Dr. J. D. Richards of University College Hospital.

REFERENCES

Begg, T. B., & Hearns, J. B. (1966). Components of blood viscosity: The relative contribution of haematocrit, plasma fibrinogen and other proteins. *Clinical Science, 31,* 87–93.

Bellingham, A. J. (1976). Haemoglobins with altered oxygen affinity. *British Medical Bulletin, 32,* 234–238.

Berlin, N. I. (1975). Diagnosis and classification of the polycythaemias. *Seminars in Haematology, 12,* 339–351.

Brown, M. M. (1984). *The influence of pathological and therapeutic changes in blood viscosity on cerebral blood flow in man.* M.D. thesis, Cambridge University, England.

Burge, P. S., Johnson, W. S., & Prankerd, T. A. (1975). Morbidity and mortality in pseudopolycythaemia. *Lancet, 1,* 1266–1268.

Caro, C. G., Pedley, T. J., Schroter, R. C., & Seed, W. A. (1978). *The Mechanics of the Circulation.* Oxford, England: Oxford University Press.

Charm, S. E., & Kurland, G. S. (1974). *Blood Flow and the Microcirculation.* New York: Wiley.

Chievitz, E., & Thiede, T. (1962). Complications and causes of death in polycythaemia vera. *Acta Medica Scandinavica, 172,* 513–523.

Damasheck, W. (1953). Stress erythrocytosis. *Blood, 8,* 282–284.

Davies–Jones, G. A. B., Preston, F. E., & Timperely, W. R. (1980). *Neurological complications in clinical haematology.* Oxford, England: Blackwell Scientific Publications.

Eisenberg, S. (1962). Cerebral circulatory effects of acutely induced hypervolaemia in human subjects. *Circulation Research, 10,* 767–771.

Ekstrom–Jodal, B., & Haggendal, E. (1969). Cerebral blood flow (pp. 82–85). Eds. Brock, B., Fieschi, C., Ingvar, D. H., Lassen, N. A., and Schurmann, K. New York: Springer–Verlag.

Fahraeus, R., & Lindqvist, T. (1931). The viscosity of the blood in narrow capillary tubes. *American Journal of Physiology, 96,* 562–568.

Finch, C. A., & Lenfant, C. (1972). Oxygen transport in man. *New England Journal of Medicine, 286,* 407–415.

Geisbock, F. (1905). Die bedeuntung der blutdruckmessung für die artzliche praxis. *Deutsch Archive für Klinische Medizin, 83,* 363–409.

Gottstein, K., & Held, K. (1969). Cerebral blood flow (pp. 104–105). Eds. Brock, Fieschi, Ingvar, Lassen and Schurmann, K. New York: Springer–Verlag.

Haggendal, E., Nilsson, N. J., & Norback, B. (1966). Effect of blood corpuscle concentration on CBF. *Acta Chirurgica Scandinavica,* (Suppl. 364), 3–12.

Harrison, B. D. W. (1973). Polycythaemia in a selected group of patients with chronic airways obstruction. *Clinical Science, 14,* 563–570.

Harrison, B. D. W., Davis, J., Madgwick, R. G., & Evans, M. (1973). The effects of a therapeutic decrease in packed cell volume on the responses to exercise of patients with polycythaemia secondary to lung disease. *Clinical Science and Molecular Medicine, 45,* 833–847.

Harrison, M. J. G., Pollock, S., Kendall, B. E., & Marshall, J. (1981). Effect of haematocrit on carotid stenosis and cerebral infarction. *Lancet, 2,* 114–115.

Henriksen, L., Paulson, O. B., and Smith, R. J. (1981). Cerebral blood flow following normovolaemic haemodilution in patients with high haematocrit. *Annals of Neurology, 9,* 454–457.

Heyman, A., Patterson, J. L., & Duke, T. W. (1952). Cerebral circulation and metabolism in sickle cell and other chronic aneamias, with observations on the effects of oxygen inhalation. *Journal of Clinical Investigation, 31,* 824–828.

Huang, C. T., & Lyons, H. A. (1966). The maintenance of acid-base balance between cerebrospinal fluid and arterial blood gases in patients with chronic respiratory disorders. *Clinical Science, 31,* 273–284.

Humphrey, P. R. D., Du Boulay, G. H., Marshall, J., Pearson, T. C., Ross Russell, R. W., Slater, N. G. P., Symon, L., Wetherley–Mein, G., & Zilkha, E. (1980). Viscosity, cerebral blood flow and haematocrit in patients with paraproteinaemia. *Acta Neurologica Scandinavica, 61,* 201–209.

Humphrey, P. R. D., Marshall, J., Ross Russell, R. W., Wetherley-Mein, G., Du Boulay, G. H., Pearson, T. C., Symon, L., & Zilkha, E. (1979). Cerebral blood flow and viscosity in relative polycytheamia. *Lancet, 2,* 873–876.

Jones, R. T., Osgood, E. E., Brimhall, B., & Koler, R. D. (1967). Haemoglobin Yakima: 1. Clinical and biochemical studies. *Journal of Clinical Investigation, 46,* 1840–1847.

Jones, M. D., Traystman, R. J., Simmons, M. A., & Molteni, R. A. (1981). Effects of changes in arterial O_2 content on cerebral blood flow in the lamb. *American Journal of Physiology, 240,* H209–H215.

Kannel, W. B., Gordon, T., Wolf, P. A., & McNamara, P. (1972). Haemoglobin and the risk of cerebral infarction. *Stroke, 3,* 409–420.

Kety, S. S. (1949). The physiology of the human cerebral circulation. *Anesthesiology, 10,* 610–613.

Kobari, M., Gotoh, F., Fukuuchi, Y., Tanaka, K., Suzuki, K., & Uematsu, D. (1984). Blood flow velocity in the pial arteries of cats, with particular reference to the vessel diameter. *Journal of Cerebral Blood Flow and Metabolism, 4,* 110–114.

Lawrence, J. H., & Berlin, N. I. (1952). Relative polycythaemia—The polycythaemia of stress. *Yale Journal of Biological Medicine, 24,* 498–505.

McGrath, M. A., & Penny, R. (1976). Paraproteinaemia. Blood hyperviscosity and clinical manifestations. *Journal of Clinical Investigation, 58,* 1155–1162.

McHenry, L. C., West, J. W., Cooper, E. S., Goldberg, H. I., & Jaffe, M. E. (1974). Cerebral autoregulation in man. *Stroke, 5,* 695–706.

McKee, L. C., & Collins, R. D. (1974). Intravascular leukocyte thrombi and aggregates as a cause of morbidity and mortality in leukaemia. *Medicine* (Baltimore), *53,* 463–478.

Medical Research Council (1965). Definition and classification of chronic bronchitis. *Lancet, 1,* 775–778.

Meyer, J. S., Gotoh, F., & Tomita, M. (1966). Acute respiratory acidemia. Correlation of jugular blood composition and electroencephalogram during CO_2 narcosis. *Neurology, 16,* 463–474.

Meyer, J. S., Shimazu, K., Fakuuchi, Y., Ohuchi, T., Okamoto, S., Koto, A., & Ericsson, A. D. (1973). Impaired neurogenic cerebrovascular control and dysautoregulation after stroke. *Stroke, 4,* 169–186.

Modan, B., & Modan, M. (1968). Benign erythrocytosis. *British Journal of Haematology, 14,* 375–381.

Nadler, S. B., Hidalgo, J. U., & Bloch, T. (1962). Prediction of blood volume in normal human adults. *Surgery, 51,* 224–232.

Nelson, D., & Fazekas, J. F. (1956). Cerebral blood flow in polycythaemia vera. *Archives of Internal Medicine, 98,* 328–331.

Oldendorf, W. H., Kitano, M., Shimuzi, S., & Oldendorf, S. Z. (1965). Haematocrit of the human cranial pool. *Circulation Research, 17,* 532–539.

Patterson, J. L., Heyman, A., & Duke, T. W. (1952). Cerebral circulation and metabolism in chronic pulmonary emphysema. *American Journal of Medicine, 12,* 382–387.

Paulson, O. B., Parving, H. H., Olesen, J., & Skinhoj, E. (1973). Influence of carbon monoxide and of haemodilution on cerebral blood flow and blood gases in man. *Journal of Applied Physiology, 35,* 111–116.

Pearson, T. C. (1980). Who should you treat for polycythaemia? *British Journal of Hospital Medicine, 24,* 66–73.

Pearson, T. C., and Wetherley-Mein, G. (1979). The course and complications of idiopathic erythrocytosis. *Clinical and Laboratory Haematology, 1,* 189–196.

Preston, F. E., Cooke, K. B., Foster, M. E., Winfield, D. A., & Lee, D. (1978a). Myelomatosis and the hyperviscosity syndrome. *British Journal of Haematology, 38,* 517–530.

Preston, F. E., Sokol, R. J., Lilleyman, J. S., Winfield, D. A., & Blackburn, E. K. (1978b). Cellular hyperviscosity as a cause of neurological symptoms in leukaemia. *British Medical Journal, 1,* 476–478.

Scheinberg, P. (1951). Cerebral blood flow and metabolism in pernicious anaemia. *Blood, 6,* 213–227.

Scheinberg, P., Blackburn, I., Saslaw, M., Rich, M., & Baum, G. (1953). Cerebral circulation and metabolism in pulmonary emphysema and fibrosis with observations on the effects of mild exercise. *Journal of Clinical Investigation, 32,* 720–728.

Schmidt-Schonbein, H. (1977). Brain and Heart Infarct. Eds. Zulch, F., Kaufmann, M., Hossmann, K., and Hossmann, A. New York: Springer–Verlag.

______. (1981). Interaction of vasomotion and blood rheology in haemodynamics. In Clinical Aspects of Blood Viscosity and Cell Deformability. In Lowe, Barbenel, & Forbes (Eds.), *Clinical aspects of blood viscosity and cell deformability.* (pp. 49–66). New York: Springer–Verlag.

Shaw, D. B., & Simpson, T. (1961). Polycythaemia in emphysema. *Quarterly Journal of Medicine, 30,* 135–152.

Shimojyo, S., Scheinberg, P., Kogure, K., & Reinmuth, O. M. (1968). The effects of graded hypoxia upon transient cerebral blood flow and oxygen consumption. *Neurology* (Minneapolis), *18,* 127–133.

Skinhoj, E. (1968). CBF adaptation in man to chronic hypo- and hypercapnia and its relation to CSF pH. *Scandinavian Journal of Laboratory and Clinical Investigation,* (Suppl. 102), VIII:A.

Somer, T. (1975). Hyperviscosity syndrome in plasma cell dyscrasias. *Advances in Microcirculation, 6,* 1–55.

Thomas, D. J., Marshall, J., Ross Russell, R. W., Wetherley-Mein, G., Du Boulay, G. H., Pearson, T. C., Symon, L., & Zilkha, E. (1977a). Cerebral blood flow in polycythaemia. *Lancet, 2,* 161–164.

______. (1977b). Effect of haematocrit on cerebral blood flow in man. *Lancet, 2,* 941–943.

Thomas, D. J., Zilkha, E., Redmond, S., Du Boulay, G. H., Marshall, J., Ross Russell, R. W., & Symon, L. (1979). An intravenous 133 Xenon clearance technique for measuring cerebral blood flow. *Journal of Neurological Sciences, 40,* 53–63.

Tohgi, H., Yamanouchi, H., Murakami, M., & Kameyama, M. (1978). Importance of the haematocrit as a risk factor in cerebral infarction. *Stroke, 9,* 369–374.

Veall, N., & Mallett, B. L. (1965). The partition of trace amounts of Xenon between human blood and brain tissues at 37°C. *Physics in Medicine and Biology, 10,* 375–380.

Wade, J. P. H. (1981). Reactivity of the cerebrovascular bed to carbon dioxide in patients with primary high haematocrit before and after venesection. *Acta Neurologica Scandinavica, 63,* 306–314.

———. (1983). Transport of oxygen to the brain in patients with elevated haematocrit values before and after venesection. *Brain, 106,* 513–523.

Wade, J. P. H., Du Boulay, G. H., Marshall, J., Pearson, T. C., Ross Russell, R. W., Shirley, J. A., Symon, L., Wetherley–Mein, G., & Zilkha, E. (1980). Cerebral blood flow, haematocrit and viscosity in subjects with a high oxygen affinity haemoglobin variant. *Acta Neurologica Scandinavica, 61,* 210–215.

Wade, J. P. H., Pearson, T. C., Ross Russell, R. W., & Wetherley–Mein, G. (1981). Cerebral blood flow and blood viscosity in patients with polycythaemia secondary to hypoxic lung disease. *British Medical Journal, 283,* 689–692.

Weinreb, N. J., & Shih, C. F. (1975). Spurios polycythaemia. *Seminars in Hematology, 12,* 397–407.

Weisse, A. B., Moschos, C. B., Frank, M. J., Levinson, G. E., Cannilla, J. E., & Regan, T. J. (1975). Haemodynamic effects of staged haematocrit reduction in patients with stable cor pulmonale and severely elevated haematocrit levels. *American Journal of Medicine, 58,* 92–98.

Wetherley-Mein, G., & Pearson, T. C. (1982). The myeloproliferative disorders. In Hardisty & Weatherall (Eds.), *Blood and its disorders* (2nd ed.). Oxford: Blackwell Scientific Publications.

Whitmore, R. L. (1968). The flow behaviour of blood in the circulation. *Nature, 215,* 123–126.

13 Investigations of CBF in Various Medical Conditions

Stevo Knežević and Zdenko Mubrin
Department of Neurology, Clinical Hospital Center, and Pliva Research Institute, Zagreb, Yugoslavia

Cerebral blood-flow measurements have been performed in various fields of clinical medicine and some of these applications have already been described. In order to make this book as comprehensive as possible, this chapter will briefly review some of the less common uses of CBF measurements. It is accepted that CBF investigations provide reliable information which is closely related to cerebral metabolism (this is true at least for normal subjects, but it will be shown in this chapter that in various diseases the coupling of circulation and metabolism is severely disturbed). When used with the optimal number of detectors they can also supply information about regional cerebral metabolic activity with an acceptable spatial resolution. The modern methods can assess the functional integrity of the cortical structures of the brain and that makes them suitable for the investigations of encephalopathies in which the higher nervous functions are always disturbed.

Metabolic encephalopathies, as defined by Plum and Posner (1980) are the disorders of the brain function caused by direct or indirect interference with metabolism of wide areas of the brain. Most of them are caused by metabolic disorders and they are fully reversible if treated early and appropriately. Usually they begin as encephalopathies and may progress to stupor and coma. Plum et al. (1980) give an extensive list of the causes of these encephalopathies.

The first group of disorders are characterized by the deprivation of oxygen, substrate or metabolic cofactors. They include hypoxia, ischemia (interference with blood supply), hypoglycemia, and cofactor deficiency. Most of them have been discussed elsewhere in this book and they are not mentioned here.

The second group are the encephalopathies caused by diseases of some other organs. From this group we discuss the effects on CBF caused by liver and renal disease, diabetes, and thyroid disease. Of many other disorders that cause encephalopathies only the infections and effects of extracorporeal circulation during the open heart surgery on brain function are discussed here.

Not all encephalopathies present with the same clinical picture, but some features are common to all and are worth mentioning here. Their presence has allowed us to describe the whole heterogeneous group as suffering from encephalopathy. The most important first symptoms are the changes in mentation and awareness. The psychological manifestations often involve perception, memory, attention, alertness, orientation and affect. Methods for rCBF measurements have improved our knowledge of the pathogenesis of these symptoms and it has been shown that they are the result of both global and focal cerebral function abnormalities. A combination of diffuse and focal dysfunction probably underlies the cerebral symptoms of most patients with metabolic encephalopathy, and as they become more pronounced the patient's clinical state progresses to stupor and coma. When this happens, changes in respiration often accompany metabolic encephalopathies. Together with metablic changes caused by the underlying disease they lead to profound alterations in pH and blood gases. As the CBF is known to be critically dependent on these factors, they have to be taken into account when the results of CBF measurements are interpreted. These alterations are mentioned later in the discussion of various diseases.

HEPATIC ENCEPHALOPATHY

Hepatic encephalopathy occurs when the liver fails to detoxify substances which appear in the portal circulation. This happens when liver function fails or when the significant quantities of blood bypass the liver and reach the systemic circulation. The bypass may develop spontaneously or it may be surgically constructed as a treatment for portal hypertension. For this reason it has been suggested that the cerebral dysfunction syndrome is better called portal systemic encephalopathy (Conn & Liebertal, 1979).

Many possible toxic agents have been suggested as potential causes for hepatic encephalopathy. Ammonia was among the first and many authors still believe that even if some other agents are also responsible, and a multifactorial hypothesis has many advocates, raised arterial ammonia concentration is the sine qua non of the disorder. Morphological findings in the brain of these patients are few. The most important changes are seen in the astrocytes (Alzheimer type II) which are enlarged and increased in number. These changes are not specific for hepatic disease as they occur in response to hyperammonemia of any cause. Ammonia crosses the blood-brain barrier and enters the brain in proportion to its concentration in arterial blood. It is almost instantly converted into glutamine and presumably this happens in the astrocytes. This detoxifying mechanism becomes quickly exhausted if hyperammonemia is present and then even modest elevation of blood ammonia can cause toxic effects. It is believed that other substances can participate in the pathogenesis of hepatic encephalopathy and fatty acids, ketones, mercaptanes, several amino acids, false neurotransmitters and neurotransmitters (particularly GABA) have been studied (Conn & Liebertal, 1979; Eliasson, Prensky, & Hardin, 1978; Plum et al., 1980; Zieve, 1982).

Several studies have been published describing the changes of CBF and cerebral metabolism in hepatic disease and they will be reviewed here. In this presentation we shall proceed from mild to the more severe encephalopathy and liver disease.

Liver Disease

Rodriguez et al., (1983) have published recently the results of rCBF measurements in patients with subclinical hepatic encephalopathy. In all 10 patients the diagnosis of liver cirrhosis was established by liver biopsy. None of them had clinical signs of encephalopathy at the time of study but psychological tests showed minor cerebral impairment. The control group consisted of 32 normal volunteers who were matched for age. The measurements were done with the inhalation method, using ^{133}Xenon and 32 detectors to record the washout curves. The authors found a significant decrease in blood flow of the order of 20% in all detectors.

This study suggests that even patients without clinical signs of hepatic encephalopathy tend to have significantly lower CBF in both hemispheres and in all of the 32 regions studied. The authors admit that the pathophysiological background of this finding is not clear yet, but rCBF measurements appear to be a potential marker of subclinical hepatic encephalopathy and of the metabolic disturbances which are supposedly at the basis of this condition. It is possible that some toxic substances bypass the detoxification mechanisms of the liver and depress cerebral metabolism as reflected in the decline of psychological performance.

Fazekas, Ticktin, Ehrmantraut, and Alman (1956) found that the CBF was lower in patients with liver cirrhosis without encephalopathy than in normals. As the clinical state was deteriorating the CBF was found to be declining progressively and it was lowest in patients with coma.

Using a modification of the Kety and Schmidt's method, Posner and Plum (1960) studied 17 patients who were in different states of liver disease and encephalopathy. The values of CBF and cerebral oxygen uptake were normal for the patients who did not show signs of definite encephalopathy, but as hepatic encephalopathy developed and worsened CBF and cerebral oxygen uptake progressively decreased.

Maiolo, Bianchi Porro, Galli, Sessa, and Polli (1971) have studied in detail the progression of hepatic encephalopathy to a comatose state using the Kety-Schmidt technique. CBF was found to be within normal limits in patients with liver cirrhosis with or without encephalopathy, although it was slightly lower when encephalopathy was present. CMRO2 was significantly lower in patients with encephalopathy, compared with the values for cirrhotic patients without neuropsychiatric symptoms. The comatose patients were divided in four grades according to the level of neuropsychiatric involvement (grade I represents somnolence and grade IV coma). CBF was higher than normal in grade I and it was decreaseing progressively as the clinical state worsened, but it needs to be stressed that the standard deviations of their measurements were rather high (20%). CMRO2 showed similar trends. It was normal in grade I and decreased progressively with deepening coma.

TABLE 13.1
CBF in Liver Disease

Author	*Number of Patients*	*Method*	*Clinical State*	*CBF*
Fazekas et al. (1956)	51	Kety–Schmidt	Advanced cirrhosis. Patients without encephalopathy, with mild encephalopathy and comatose	As the brain involvement progressed, CBF declined
Posner et al. (1960)	47	Kety–Schmidt	Different states of liver disease and encephalopathy	As hepatic encephalopathy worsened, CBF progressively decreased
Maiolo et al. (1971)	8–48 in various groups	Kety–Schmidt	Various stages of encephalopathy and coma	CBF declined with the development of encephalopathy except for acute encephalopathy and acute coma when CBF was increased
Rodriguez et al. (1983)	10	Xe inhalation 32 detectors	Subclinical liver encephalopathy	CBF declined in all detectors in the order of 20%

When patients were divided according to the duration of their symptoms it was noted that CBF was very high in acute encephalopathy (up to 7 days of duration) and in acute coma (less than 24 hours from the beginning), and it was markedly depressed in chronic encephalopathy (at least 3 months of duration) and in chronic coma (more than 24 hours). CMRO2 results varied accordingly.

These results are different from the ones mentioned previously and they should be interpreted carefully because the variations in all measurements were very high in spite of the fact that the groups consisted of 8 to 48 subjects. The smallest variation was observed in the groups with chronic encephalopathy and coma.

Nevertheless the results seem to support the view that the onset of the comatose state was not the consequence of a primary depression of the brain energy metabolism, although such a metabolic impairment might occur later.

Portacaval Shunting

CBF investigations have also been performed in patients after the portacaval shunting. Polli, Bianchi Porro, and Maiolo (1969) reported interesting results using the Kety-Schmidt technique. In patients with liver cirrhosis who were mentally alert an increase in CBF was found, compared with the normal subjects (but the change was not statistically significant). When CBF was measured in 13 patients after the portacaval shunting (1–10 months after the operation) CBF increased by almost 80% and CMRO2 increased by 25% (but this again was not significant). None of the patients had ever had hepatic encephalopathy. These results are similar to the ones mentioned before for the patients in acute states of encephalopathy and coma, but as the disease persists for some time we have mentioned that CBF and CMRO2 tend to decrease. In this study, however, the patients were operated before the mental symptoms developed, and CBF was found to be increased even 1 or 2 years after surgery.

All the results of these studies seem to indicate that in chronic liver disease CBF and metabolism are depressed when psychological symptoms are present and as encephalopathy progresses they tend to decrease further. As the etiology is probably multifactorial and possibly different in every patient some of the various toxic substances may have different effects on brain metabolism. It seems possible that different pathogenesis lead to different disturbances in cerebral function. This might account for the inconsistencies found in measuring CBF and metabolism in various groups of patients. In acute portal-systemic encephalopathy the results are more consistent. They show that when the flow of toxic substances acutely increases the cerebral circulation and metabolism increase, possibly in order to improve the detoxification processes. When they fail and when the toxins and their metabolites accumulate the brain function becomes depressed and it is reflected in the measurements of CBF and metabolism.

Changes in Blood Gases

Hepatic encephalopathy is usually accompanied by hyperventilation and profound alterations in blood gases. The explanation for this hyperventilation is uncertain but it is very important in interpreting the CBF data and it is also necessary to consider anemia and hypoxemia, which are common in cirrhotic patients. Although the possible explanations for hyperventilation, hypocapnia, and alkalosis are very complex, it is clear that they enhance the toxicity of ammonia which more freely enters the tissues as the pH increases (Conn & Libertal, 1979). Respiratory alkalosis is difficult to treat but it has been suggested that it might be possible to correct or prevent it by breathing 5% CO_2. Posner and Plum (1960) studied the effect of CO_2 and acetazolamide and their results are very interesting.

They showed that the degree of alkalosis increased progressively as encephalopathy appeared and worsened. Five percent CO_2 or acetazolamide infusions produced no adverse effects on alert cirrhotics but the same treatment given to patients with hepatic encephalopathy caused both clinical deterioration and a severe decrease in cerebral oxygen uptake. The results suggest that toxicity of CO_2 and acetazolamide in hepatic encephalopathy directly results from increased cerebral tissue carbon dioxide tensions, and the authors postulate that respiratory alkalosis in advanced liver disease is compensatory, acting to prevent rather than to impair brain function.

Different results were published by James, Nashat, Sampson, Williams, and Garassini (1969), who claim that treatment with intravenous alkali (infusions of sodium bicarbonate) resulted in clinical improvement associated with an increase in cerebral oxygen consumption in patients with hepatic coma. These results were criticized by Conn & Liebertal (1979).

Similar experiments were also carried out later in normal models. In goats, Stanley, Salisbury, McHenry, and Cherniack (1975) found that CBF (measured with an electromagnetic flow meter) was consistently reduced during liver failure. The cerebral vessels were unable to dilate and the cerebral metabolism was reduced when the animals were challenged with CO_2. The authors suggest that the depression of CBF and metabolism is not due to hypocapnia. It is most likely that the effect is due to an accumulation of toxic metabolites caused by hepatic failure. The results also suggest that the depression of CO_2 responsiveness may be a result of a loss of the cerebrovascular smooth muscles reactivity to CO_2 or of the impairement of autonomic control mechanisms. It is also possible that the primary depression occurs in the brain stem as a result of its metabolic impairement.

Whatever the true mechanisms are, it seems reasonable that alkalosis should not be strictly corrected in the treatment of liver disease because the effects of alkalosis are probably beneficial. Though it must be emphasized that in some patients with very high levels of ammonia this might not always be true. It is also clinically important that the respiratory depressants and anesthetic agents should be administered to these patients with great care since they may not be able to compensate successfully for the hypercapnia which may appear, but this is a very well-known hazard that all clinicians are aware of.

Changes in Blood Pressure

Another interesting aspect of hepatic coma is the presence of arterial hypotension and increased intracranial pressure (Trewby, Hanid, Mackenzie, Mellon, & Williams, 1978). The clinical observation suggests that 88% of patients with fulminant hepatic failure have hypotension and 16% of the time they were in grade IV coma their systolic blood pressure was below 80 mmHG. Necropsy showed edema of the brain in 38% of the cases. It is expected that CBF and oxygen delivery to the brain are reduced in such states and that may result in further deterioration of the patients.

Trewby et al. (1978) investigated the effects of raised intracranial pressure and low systolic blood pressure on both CBF and cerebral metabolic rate for oxygen. The experiment was performed in pigs with induced hepatic failure and CBF was measured with the ^{133}Xenon method. They showed a marked derangement of cerebral autoregulation in response to both a low systolic blood pressure and a rise in intracranial pressure in the animals with liver failure. In the control animals the CBF did not fall with hypotension, but in the group of diseased hypotensive animals the CBF significantly decreased. The fall of CBF was also observed when the intracranial pressure increased and again the control animals did not show such a decrease in CBF. Furthermore in the animals with liver failure the oxygen extraction ratio did not increase as expected. The authors suggest that this effect could be explained with the opening of intracranial arteriovenous shunts or by the increased sensibility of cellular respiration to the buildup of metabolites that would accompany low CBF. The subsequent reduction in intracellular pH might be sufficient to lower CMRO2.

The clinical relevance of these findings is clear. Episodes of hypotension are to be prevented if secondary brain damage is to be avoided. The results that we have mentioned show how CBF investigations have proved to be valuable in the study of the pathogenesis of hepatic encephalopathy, in the understanding of the nature of the neuropsychiatric symptoms and in the evaluation of some possible treatments.

UREMIC AND DIALYSIS ENCEPHALOPATHY

Patients with end-stage renal disease and uremia, even without hypertension, sometimes have neurological symptoms of which encephalopathy, and even coma are the most important. Changes in CBF in these patients have received little attention. The work published by Heyman, Paterson, and Jones (1951) is still mentioned in current literature. In 16 patients with uremia they found either a normal CBF or an insignificant reduction, provided there was no hypertension or vascular change. When these complications developed, a moderate reduction in CBF was noted. In both groups of patients the cerebral oxygen consumption was significantly reduced, and the same results were found by Scheinberg (1954). It is interesting to note that the change did not correlate either with the mental state of the patients or with other biochemical tests performed.

Besides the uremic encephalopathies, dialysis dementia, and dialysis disequilibrium syndrome, there are also forms of encephalopathy which some of dialysed patients develop. Although a lot of other investigations have been done in these patients, CBF measurements have, as far as we are aware, not been performed. It seems that only one attempt has been made to measure rCBF before and after hemodialysis (Holzer, Marguc, Pogglitsch, Ott, & Katschnig, 1981). The results are difficult to interpret but the authors claim that before hemodialysis, patients show a distinct elevation of rCBF due to the severe anemia. After treatment the hematocrit was slightly increased and CBF returned to normal values. When all the results were corrected to a normal value of hemoglobin (160 g/l) predialysis CBF was found to be within the normal range. After the treatment it decreased to the low normal values. The authors also state that the fall of CBF was especially pronounced with increasing age of the patients and with the length of time on hemodialysis treatment.

It is difficult to judge the significance of these findings and until further studies are done the potential of CBF measurements in the explanation of the pathophysiology of these disturbances cannot be clearly established.

ENDOCRINOLOGIC ENCEPHALOPATHIES

Disturbances of the endocrine glands are known to have profound effects on brain metabolism and we shall mention here the studies of CBF performed on patients with diabetes mellitus and thyroid disease.

Diabetic Encephalopathy

Diabetes mellitus is characterized by abnormalities of carbohydrate, lipid and protein metabolism usually caused by the insulin deficiency. The complications of diabetes involving the brain, blood vessels, and many other organs were recognized many years ago and they were extensively studied. The term *diabetic encephalopathy* was introduced by De Jong in 1950. It was later supported by Reske Nielsen, Lundbaek, and Rafaelsen (1965) but others have also questioned its specificity (Warren & Le Compte, 1952). Bischoff and Zimmerman (1979) concluded that the lacunar state of the brain following multiple small infarcts in diabetics does not differ morphologically from a similar appearence in chronic hypertensive patients. However, the same authors propose that the characteristic finding in diabetics is that the lacunar state may develop in the absence of hypertension and it is probably due to unique pathophysiological conditions which seem to be established as a defective vasoreactivity.

It is well known that diabetes is one of the risk factors for the development of stroke and other cardiovascular diseases. That has been repeatedly shown and it was usually thought that the increased incidence of stroke is caused by the accelerated course of atherosclerosis (Cohen, 1968) and by the other associated risk ractors. The Framingham epidemiological study has revealed that when patients with diabetes have all the other risk factors corrected for they are still left with a two- to threefold net increase in the incidence of cardiovascular disease (Kannel & McGee, 1979). Similar results were later reported from the Whitehall study, in which the mortality from coronary heart disease and stroke in relation to glycaemia were studied (Fuller, Shipley, Rose, Jarrett, & Keen, 1983). A specific factor for this increased risk was not identified. As it is expected that this risk is connected with *circulatory regulation* it appears probable that CBF studies might provide a possible explanation for this specific disturbance.

Bentsen, Larsen, and Lassen (1975) investigated autoregulation of CBF in long-term diabetics, using the arteriovenous oxygen difference method. In 4 of the 16 patients studied they demonstrated a significant dependency of CBF on changes in mean blood pressures. The characteristic autoregulatory plateau seen in normals and even in hypertensive patients (where it is shifted, but still exists) was not present in 25% of the diabetics. The reason for the absence of the autoregulatory curve is not clear but the results indicate that diabetics may be unusually sensitive to variations in blood pressure, whether higher or lower than normal.

The other important factor in the regulation of CBF is CO_2. The effects of hypercapnia in diabetics were studied by Dandona, James, Newbury, Woolard, and Beckett (1978). They have used the ^{133}Xenon inhalation method to measure the global CBF in 28 control subjects and 59 diabetics. When the controls were challenged with the inhalation of 5% CO_2, 24 of the subjects showed a significant increase in CBF. After the same activation test, CBF increased in 23 patients, decreased in 26, and remained unchanged in 10 diabetics. It is important to mention that CBF decreased even in newly discovered diabetics in which characteristic signs of vascular and neuropathic changes were not yet developed. The authors concluded that this loss of reactivity is specifically linked to diabetes and that diminished cerebrovascular reserve may explain their increased risk for the development of cerebrovascular disease. Another interesting finding was that CBF declined similarly with age in both patients and controls. This suggests that diabetes does not affect the rate of decrease of CBF with age.

The results of this study have led us to investigate the changes of CBF in diabetics following another activation procedure (Knežević, 1985). We have chosen the motor activation of the right hand (by squeezing a rubber ball) to investigate the changes in the regional pattern of CBF. The CBF was measured with the ^{133}Xenon inhalation method using 32 detectors bilaterally. Following the activation procedure, the 16 control subjects increased their CBF in 5 regions in the left hemisphere and in 5 regions of the right hemisphere (in the motor areas of the brain contralaterally and ipsilaterally). The diabetic patients showed an unexpected finding in that the CBF increased significantly in almost all of the areas bilaterally (15 regions in the left and 14 in the right hemisphere). The exagerated and abnormally global response was seen in all groups of diabetics when they were divided according to age, duration of disease, and the therapy they were receiving. Our interpretation is that diabetics are able to increase their CBF when challenged by our activation procedure, but they are not able to restrict this response efficiently to the areas where metabolism is increased. Instead of being focal the increase in CBF was diffuse. The reason for this finding is not clear but it may be that either some biochemical abnormality is present in the regulation of rCBF, or the autonomic neuropathy leads to disturbances in regional regulation of CBF. It is also possible that the mean arterial blood pressure rises and CBF passively follows because the autoregulation is known to be abnormal as described earlier (blood pressure was not monitored in our study).

The variations of cerebral blood flow are known to be very small in any single individual and measured repeatedly after 6 hours to 6 weeks the coefficient of variation of CBF is in the order of 5%. But in insulin-dependent diabetics, Dandona, James, Woolard, Newbury, and Beckett (1979) showed that significant variations occurred in 10 of the 23 patients studied. The patients were studied 2–3 hours after insulin and breakfast and in 9 of them a significant fall in CBF was found and most of them had symptoms of impending faint without hypotension or hypoglycemia. It is interesting to note that this fall in CBF was not the result of hypoglycemia. In the other experiment reported in the same work they showed that CBF did not fall after and intravenous injection of a bolus of insulin despite the sharp fall in blood glucose concentration. These results suggest that the effects of insulin on CBF and the impaired regulation of CBF in diabetics is very complex and we shall need more information about the regulation of glucose metabolism in the brain in order to be able to understand these findings in all their complexity.

Diabetic coma is one of the most important complications of diabetes mellitus and it was one of the first clinical problems studied when methods for measuring CBF in humans were developed. In their classical work, Kety, Polis, Nadler, and Schmidt (1948) have investigated CBF in 14 patients in severe diabetic acidosis, 6 of whom were in deep coma. Their most important finding was that CBF was generally increased, arterial oxygen saturation was normal, and there was a 40%

reduction in cerebral utilization of oxygen. This is one of the few situations in which CBF is normal or even increased in deeply comatose studies.

Thyroid Disease

Several studies of CBF in thyroid disease were performed very soon after Kety and Schmidt had described the nitrous oxide technique. Scheinberg and Stead (1950), and Sokoloff, Wechsler, Balls, and Kety (1950) reported that CBF was not different in patients with hyperthyroidism when compared with normal subjects. Later, however, the same group (Sokoloff, Wechsler, Mangold, Balls, & Kety, (1953) attributed the increase to coincidental anemia. Scheinberg, Stead, Brannon, and Warren (1950) reported reduced CBF in myxedema. Sensenbach, Madison, Eisenberg, and Ochs (1954) have done the most complete investigation. They studied 22 males with hyperthyroidism and found that CBF was increased (42%), oxygen extraction was decreased (about 33%), and arterial O_2 content also fell (the significant fall in arterial O_2 content may be related to the alterations in pulmonary ventilation and gas exchange which occur in hyperkinetic states). In 11 male subjects with myxedema a decrease of CBF was found (22%) with increased oxygen extraction (19%). They also measured CBF after the treatment for both conditions and found it to be restored to normal. The conclusion that they offer was that the cerebral circulation shares in the overall hemodynamic alterations that occur as a consequence of an excess or deficiency of the thyroid hormones.

It is worth noting that the mean arterial blood pressure was 7% lower than normal in patients with hyperthyroidism, and 16% above normal in myxedema. Thus it does not seem so straightforward that CBF passively follows the cardiovascular changes in thyroid disease, and it appears probable that thyroxine has a direct effect on cerebral metabolism and circulation.

O'Brien and Harris (1968) have studied the CBF in myxedema using the ^{133}Xenon inhalation technique. They have also found that CBF decreased and in their review of the published studies on CBF and metabolism in thyroid disease they propose that the main effect on general and cerebral circulation is mediated by the changes in vascular resistance. They found that cerebrovascular resistance in myxedema is raised, the mean blood pressure does not comparably increase, and CBF consequently falls. The increased oxygen extraction compensates for the fall of CBF and they propose that this is one of the ways in which a form of autoregulation is expressed. In hyperthyroidism reversed events take place.

Using the modern terminology we can say that autoregulation of CBF to mean blood pressure changes is impaired, but without important changes in cerebral metabolism because the compensatory mechanisms seem to be adequate. The principal effect of the thyroid hormone in the brain is on the metabolism of proteins, which is negligible when compared with carbohydrate metabolism in the adult brain. That is probably the reason why compensatory mechanisms are sufficient in patients with thyroid disease in spite of the changes in CBF.

INFECTIONS

In the era before the introduction of sulfonamides and antibiotics the mortality from bacterial meningitis was so high that neurological complications in rare survivors were seldom studied. As the mortality in present times is in the order of 3–28% for various types of bacterial meningitis, clinicians have focused their attention on the nature and pathogenesis of various complications (Swartz, 1984).

In the context of this book our interest is in those complications which are more or less directly connected with changes in CBF and its regional distribution and regulation.

Shapiro and Eisenberg (1967) described a patient who was comatose due to St. Louis encephalitis. The CBF was normal (measured by a modification of the nitrous oxide technique), cerebral oxygen uptake was markedly reduced and the patient had a significant reduction of arterial CO_2 tension. They proposed that encephalitis with such a relative hyperemia should be included in the disorders which cause a luxury perfusion syndrome. The hyperventilation and consequent alkalosis were thought to represent a compensatory mechanism in the correction of acidosis and in preventing possibly damaging effects of further vasodilatation. But as hypocapnia was not able to exhibit its normal vasoconstriction effect, an alternative explanation for hypocapnia was proposed. Intense inflammation of the cerebral vessels may have altered their ability to respond to the hypocapnic stimulus, and the greater the vascular damage the more powerful the respiratory drive was. These findings were later confirmed in the report of the five patients with St. Louis encephalitis (Shapiro & Eisenberg, 1969).

Paulson, Brodersen, Lyders Hansen, and Sund Kristensen (1974) have used the intra-arterial Xenon method for the determination of CBF. Their study was done in 15 patients with acute bacterial meningitis and encephalitis. All patients were hyperventilating spontaneously and the average hemispheric blood flow was normal and CMRO2 slightly reduced in those with meningococal meningitis. Global CBF and CMRO2 were markedly reduced in pneumococal meningitis and encephalitis. (The studies were performed during general anesthesia and artificial ventilation was adjusted for the same level of pCO_2 as measured during spontaneous respiration prior to anesthesia.) Allowing the analysis of regional pattern this method has revealed focal rCBF abnormalities. They were infrequent in meningitis but frequent in encephalitis. In all patients these focuses were hyperemic and one patient also had ischemic focuses.

The functional tests were carried out and the activation with CO_2 and modifying blood pressure was performed. Globally and focally impaired autoregulation was found as well as impaired response to $PaCO_2$ changes. The increase in $PaCO_2$ was shown to induce focal loss of autoregulation. Impairement of autoregulation was much more common finding than impairment of the response to $PaCO_2$ changes. This has been described previously in patients with apoplexy and intracranial tumors and it was called *dissociated vasoparalysis*.

The results reported in this study differ from those mentioned before in the investigations of Shapiro and Eisenberg (1967, 1969). Global CBF was found to be decreased in several groups of patients and regional abnormalities of rCBF were also described. The reason is probably in the nature of the different forms of infections studied (viral vs. bacterial). Regional blood-flow patterns were not studied before as the techniques which were used allowed only the measurements of global circulation.

The work of Paulson et al. (1974) clearly shows that the brain is highly vulnerable in patients with acute meningitis and encephalitis. Especially, as autoregulation is lost, it is important to prevent rises in blood pressure, since it will be transmitted to the capillaries, thus increasing the risk of brain edema. It is also important to avoid hypercapnia because it induces acidosis and vasodilatation and may provoke loss of autoregulation. All the effects can potentiate brain edema with a rise in intracranial pressure.

EFFECTS OF EXTRACORPOREAL CIRCULATION

Although the techniques for extracorporeal circulation (ECC) are constantly being improved the evidence that brain damage often follows open heart surgery is accumulating. Stroke and encephalopathy are most frequent causes of morbidity and mortality. Major focal neurological sequelae of the operation occur probably in 2–5% of the patients (Sontaniemi, 1982). Although several investigations were done in order to define risk factors for the development of stroke in these patients, they have not been successful to the present time. For that reason the recognition of patients with increased risk is very difficult (Breuer et al., 1983).

Encephalopathy is a much more common complication and many patients have symptoms of diffuse brain damage following the oparation. Depending on the psychological and clinical criteria used, various proportions of patients were found to have postoperative encephalopathy. Tufo, Ostfeld, and Shekelle (1970) have found that 15% of patients had signs of cerebral damage at discharge from the hospital. They have also found that the symptoms were related to increasing age and depression of arterial pressure during the operation. In a recent prospective study Breuer et al. (1983) report 11.6% of patients with clinically detectable prolonged encephalopathy after open heart surgery. They have also found that a decrease in blood pressure was the only factor that statistically correlated with encephalopathy. Heller, Frank, Kornfeld, Malm, and Bowman (1974) described residual psychological abnormalities in as many as one-third of the patients examined 1 year after surgery.

McKay, Reves, Karp, Morawetz, and Lell (1983) published the results of rCBF measurements before, during, and after ECC. They used the ^{133}Xenon intra-arterial method for the measurement of rCBF. Their results showed that under anesthesia before ECC, rCBF was reduced but autoregulation was preserved. The reduction was attributed to the effect of anesthetic drugs and mild hypothermia. Blood pressure was within the limits of autoregulation and consequently CBF did not change. CBF was also associated with the cardiac output.

During all phases of ECC, rCBF was significantly reduced, and the reduction of 52% in rCBF is most likely related to the calculated 40% reduction in cerebral metabolic rate for O_2 at that time. It is interesting to note that during all stages of ECC there were poor associations of rCBF with $PaCO_2$, cardiac output and blood pressure. It appears that reactivity to CO_2 and autoregulation are lost during ECC. After the operation rCBF returned to the preoperation level and all the patients were neurologically intact.

Different results were obtained by Henriksen, Hjelms, and Lindeburgh (1983). They used the ^{133}Xenon intra-arterial method in 29 patients altogether. RCBF was measured five times in various periods during ECC in 24 patients. In 9 patients they observed a fall in CBF which is in accordance with the results of McKay et al. (1983) mentioned earlier. However, in 15 patients a marked increase of CBF was found during ECC. The decrease of CBF in 9 patients is not likely to be a result of mean arterial pressure being reduced below the autoregulation point. In all the patients CO_2 sensitivity was markedly reduced during ECC.

The highest values of CBF were found in the hypothermic phase of ECC (the mean increase was 67%) and this is clearly an unexpected finding. As metabolism must have been reduced at 29°C the increase in CBF probably reflects an uncoupling of flow and metabolism. The authors note that the observed hyperperfusion is not well understood and suggest that it may be the effect of luxury perfusion surrounding the areas of microvascular blockade (due to emboli, thrombocyte aggregation, or stagnant capillary flow). This hypothesis is similar to the likely explanation of luxury perfusion syndrome in patients with stroke as described by Lassen (1966). The authors do not mention the clinical condition of patients after surgery, and it would be interesting to know whether there were some clinical differences among the patients with various CBF findings. It is worth noting that the anesthetic procedure was also different in the two reports mentioned.

Henriksen (1984) has also used SPECT to measure regional cerebral blood flow in patients before and after open heart surgery. None of the 37 patients had major neurological deficits after the operation but the measurements of CBF showed a significant decrease in the first 10 days after the operation. The changes were uniform throughout the brain and no focal abnormalities of CBF were found. The reduction in CBF correlated positively with increasing age, duration of extracorporeal circulation and low mean arterial pressure during the operation. In the 11 patients investigated 1 year after surgery, CBF remained slightly reduced. The author believes that the marked changes in rCBF indicate the diffuse brain damage but lacking other supportive evidence (electrophysiological, psychometric, etc.) this has been questioned later (Wade & Ross Russell, 1984).

It seems clear that rCBF investigations may be helpful in further elucidation of brain damage which often occurs after the open heart surgery. Further improvements of the operating technique are to be expected and it seems that CBF investigations will be helpful in their development. Furlan and Breuer (1984) suggest that a reliable rCBF testing should be developed to assess autoregulatory capacity preoperatively and they expect that rCBF measurements might also allow a more rational approach to define optimal surgical and anesthesiological procedures.

REFERENCES

Bentsen, N., Larsen, B., & Lassen, N. A. (1975). Chronically impaired autoregulation of cerebral blood flow in long-term diabetics. *Stroke, 6,* 497–502.

Bischoff, A., & Zimmermann, A. (1979). Diabetic encephalopathy. Does it exist? *Acta Neurol. Belg., 79,* 469–474.

Breuer, A. C., Furlan, A. J., Hanson, M. R., Lederman, R. J., Loop, F. D., Cosgrove, D. M., Greenstreet, R. L., & Estafanuous, F. G. (1983). Central nervous system complications of coronary artery bypass graft surgery: Prospective analysis of 421 patients. *Stroke, 14,* 682–687.

Cohen, A. M. (1968). Myocardial infarction and carbohydrate metabolism. *Geriatrica, 23,* 158–160.

Conn, H. O., & Liebertal, M. M. (1979). *The hepatic coma syndromes and lactulose.* Baltimore: Williams & Wilkins.

Dandona, P., James, I. M., Newbury, P. A., Woolard, M. I., & Beckett, A. G. (1978). Cerebral blood flow in diabetes mellitus: Evidence of abnormal cerebrovascular reactivity. *Br. Med. J., ii,* 325–326.

Dandona, P., James, I. M., Woollard, M. L., Newbury, P., & Beckett, A. G. (1979). Instability of cerebral blood-flow in insulin-dependent diabetics. *Lancet, ii,* 1203–1205.

De Jong, R. N. (1950). The nervous system complications of diabetes mellitus with special reference to cardiovascular changes. *J. Nerv. Ment. Dis., 111,* 181–206.

Eliasson, S. G., Prensky, A. L., & Hardin, W. B. (1978). *Neurological pathophysiology* (2d ed.). New York: Oxford University Press.

Fazekas, J. F., Ticktin, H. E., Ehrmantraut, W. R., & Alman, R. W. (1956). Cerebral metabolism in hepatic insufficiency. *Amer. J. Med., 21,* 843–849.

Fuller, J. H., Shipley, M. J., Rose, G., Jarrett, R. J., & Keen, H. (1983). Mortality from coronary heart disease and stroke in relation to degree of glycaemia: The Whitehall study. *Br. Med. J., 287,* 867–870.

Furlan, A. J., & Breuer, A. C. (1984). Central nervous system complications of open heart surgery. *Current Concepts in Cerebrovascular Disease, 19,* 7–11.

Heller, S. S., Frank, K. A., Kornfeld, D. S., Malm, J. R., & Bowman, F. O., Jr. (1974). Psychological outcome following open-heart surgery. *Arch. Intern. Med. 134,* 908–914.

Henriksen, L. (1984). Evidence suggestive of diffuse brain damage following cardiac operations. *Lancet, i,* 816–820.

Henriksen, L., Hjelms, E., & Lindeburgh, T. (1983). Brain hyperperfusion during cardiac operations. *J. Thorac. Cardiovasc. Surg., 86,* 202–208.

Heyman, A., Patterson, J. L., & Jones, R. W. (1951). Cerebral circulation and metabolism in uremia. *Circulation, 3,* 558–563.

Holzer, H., Marguc, K., Pogglitsch, H., Ott, E., & Katschnig, H. (1981). The effects of haemodialysis on cerebral blood flow. *Proceedings of EDTA, 18,* 126–132.

James, I. M., Nashat, S., Sampson, D., Williams, H. S., & Garassini, M. (1969). Effect of induced metabolic alkalosis in hepatic encephalopathy. *Lancet, ii,* 1106–1108.

Kannel, W. B., & McGee, D. L. (1979). Diabetes and cardiovascular risk factors: The Framingham study. *Circulation, 59,* 8–13.

Kety, S. S., Polis, B. D., Nadler, C. S., & Schmidt, C. F. (1948). The blood flow and oxygen consumption of the human brain in diabetic acidosis and coma. *J. Clin. Invest., 27,* 500–510.

Knežević, S. (1985). Characteristics of cerebral circulation in patients with diabetes mellitus. Doctoral dissertation, University of Zagreb, Medical School, Yugoslavia.

Lassen, N. A. (1966). The luxury perfusion syndrome and its possible relation to acute metabolic acidosis localized within the brain. *Lancet ii,* 1113–1115.

Maiolo, A. T., Bianchi Porro, G., Galli, C., Sessa, M., & Polli, E. E. (1971). Brain energy metabolism in hepatic coma. *Exp. Biol. Med., 4,* 52–70.

McKay, R. D., Reves, J. G., Karp, R. B., Morawetz, R. B., & Lell, W. A. (1983). Effects of cardiopulmonary bypass on cerebral blood flow. *Anesth. Analg., 62,* 274–275.

O'Brien, M. D., & Harris, P. W. R. (1968). Cerebral-cortex perfusion-rates in myxedema. *Lancet, i,* 1170–1172.

Paulson, I. B., Brodersen, P., Lyders Hansen, E., & Sund Kristensen, H. (1974). Regional cerebral blood flow, cerebral metabolic rate of oxygen, and cerebrospinal fluid acid-base variables in patients with acute meningitis and with acute encephalitis. *Acta Med. Scand., 196,* 191–198.

Plum, F., & Posner, J. B. (1980). *The diagnosis of stupor and coma* (3d ed.). Philadelphia: F. A. Davis.

Polli, E., Bianchi Porro, G., & Maiolo, A. T. (1969). Cerebral metabolism after portacaval shunt. *Lancet, i,* 153.

Posner, J. B., & Plum, F. (1960). The toxic effects of carbon dioxide and acetazolamide in hepatic encephalopathy. *J. Clinic. Invest., 39,* 1246–1258.

Reske Nielsen, E., Lundbaek, K., & Rafaelsen, O. J. (1965). Pathological changes in the central and peripheral nervous system of young long-term diabetics. I. Diabetic encephalopathy. *Diabetologia, 1,* 233–241.

Rodriguez, G., Testa, R., Rosadini, G., Arvigo, F., Celle, G., Gris, A., Sannita, W. G., Sukkar, G., & Traverso, R. (1983). Reduction of regional cerebral blood flow in subclinical hepatic encephalopathy. *IRCS Med. Sci., 11,* 763.

Scheinberg, P. (1954). Effects of uremia on cerebral blood flow and metabolism. *Neurology, 4,* 101–105.

Scheinberg, P., & Stead, E. A., Jr. (1950). Cerebral metabolism in hyperthyroidism and myxedema. *Fed. Proc., 9,* 112.

Scheinberg, P., Stead, E. A., Brannon, E. S., & Warren, J. V. (1950). Correlative observations on cerebral metabolism and cardiac output in myxedema. *J. Clin. Invest., 29,* 1139–1146.

Sensenbach, W., Madison, L., Eisenberg, S., & Ochs, L. (1954). The cerebral circulation and metabolism in hyperthyroidism and myxedema. *J. Clin. Invest.,* 33, 1434–1440.

Shapiro, W., & Eisenberg, S. (1967). Cerebral blood flow and metabolism in the coma of St. Louis encephalitis. *JAMA, 202,* 145–147.

———. (1969). Pathophysiology of epidemic St. Louis encephalitis: III. Cerebral blood flow and metabolism. *Annals of Internal Medicine, 71,* 691–702.

Sokoloff, L., Wechsler, R. L., Balls, K., & Kety, S. S. (1950). The relation of cerebral O_2 consumption to the total body metabolism in hyperthyroidism. *J. Clin. Invest, 29,* 847.

Sokoloff, L., Wechsler, R. L., Mangold, R., Balls, K., & Kety, S. S. (1953). Cerebral blood flow and oxygen consumption in hyperthyroidism before and after treatment. *J. Clin. Invest., 32,* 202.

Sontaniemi, K. A. (1982). Neurological complications of open heart surgery. In A. Silverstein (Ed.). *Neurological complications of therapy* (pp. 293–315). New York: Futura.

Stanley, N. N., Salisbury, B. G., McHenry, L. C., Jr, & Cherniack, N. S. (1975). Effect of liver failure on the response of ventilation and cerebral circulation to carbon dioxide in man and in the goat. *Clinical Science and Molecular Medicine, 49,* 157–169.

Swartz, M. N. (1984). Bacterial meningitis. *N. Engl. J. Med., 311,* 912–914.

Trewby, P. N., Hanid, M. A., MacKenzie, R. L., Mellon, P. J., & Williams, R. (1978). Effects of cerebral oedema and arterial hypotension on cerebral blood flow in an animal model of hepatic failure. *Gut, 19,* 999–1005.

Tufo, H. M., Ostfeld, A. M., & Shekelle, R. (1970). Central nervous system dysfunction following open-heart surgery. *JAMA, 212,* 1333–1340.

Wade, J., & Ross Russell, R. W. (1984). Cerebral blood flow after cardiac surgery. *Lancet, i,* 1297.

Warren, S., & Le Compte, P. (1952). *The pathology of diabetes mellitus* (3d ed.). Philadelphia: Lea & Febiger.

Zieve, L. (1982). Hepatic encephalopathy. In L. Schiff & E. R. Schiff (Eds.). *Diseases of the liver* (pp. 433–459). Philadelphia: Lippincott.